SECOND EDITION

Introducing
Food
Science

SECOND EDITION

Introducing
Food
Science

Robert L. Shewfelt
Alicia Orta-Ramirez
Andrew D. Clarke

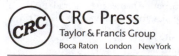

CRC Press
Taylor & Francis Group
Boca Raton   London   New York

CRC Press is an imprint of the
Taylor & Francis Group, an **informa** business

CRC Press
Taylor & Francis Group
6000 Broken Sound Parkway NW, Suite 300
Boca Raton, FL 33487-2742

© 2016 by Taylor & Francis Group, LLC
CRC Press is an imprint of Taylor & Francis Group, an Informa business

No claim to original U.S. Government works

Printed on acid-free paper
Version Date: 20150713

International Standard Book Number-13: 978-1-4822-0974-7 (Paperback)

Visit the Taylor & Francis Web site at
http://www.taylorandfrancis.com

and the CRC Press Web site at
http://www.crcpress.com

The second edition of this book is dedicated to

Betty and Sweetie who wait patiently each day while I write

before I can take advantage of being retired—Rob.

My students: past, present, and future—Alicia.

My wife Kristi and our children Alex, Maddie, and Liam—Andrew.

Contents

Section III   Functions of Food Scientists

Preface

This second edition has added two authors and three new contributors to specific chapters. We have also added a chapter on "Sustainability and Distribution" to acknowledge growing interest among the food science community in this topic. Much has happened in food science since the first edition was published. Processed foods have come under a more concerted attack from many sources, although most of these sources do not define what constitutes a processed food as opposed to a whole food. Consumers are confused by such a discussion and appear to make a distinction between processed and packaged foods that may not be merited. In this edition, we address such issues and provide our perspective as food scientists on processed, formulated, chilled, and prepared foods. We have updated the text of the first edition and almost half of the illustrations are new. A glossary has been added to this book and key terms are presented in bold when they first appear in the book.

Both editions were specifically designed to provide an overview of the field of food science for the major and non-major alike. The narrative proceeds from a nontechnical discussion of food issues that concern today's student to a more comprehensive technical overview of the basic principles as they relate to the study of food. Sandwiched in between are descriptions of the types of commercial products and processes with particular reference to nutritional consequences and primary functions of roles of food scientists. Each section builds on the previous section, providing a logical structure and cohesiveness. At the end of each chapter, we have included in the second edition a series of problems to help students test their ability to comprehend the material and to provide instructors a reservoir for assignments, class discussions, and test questions. All of these problems are stated in a format that can be linked to Bloom's taxonomy as it relates to IFT Core Competencies. At least one problem at the end of each chapter involves a calculation for instructors who bemoan the weakness in quantitative skills they see in their students.

Food science is unique among scientific disciplines in the heavy commercial orientation of the field. Food science serves as the technical arm of the food industry, where most food science graduates are employed. Although academicians acknowledge the importance of commercial aspects of the field, they are also dedicated to being a source of unbiased knowledge for the consumer and regulatory agencies. This book attempts to convey both commercial and scientific perspectives on the field in the interest of providing a true flavor of food science.

Food issues in the news comprise the first section of this book. From disease outbreaks to health benefits and detriments to international trade, foods and beverages provide a steady source of stories in every type of news medium. As consumers of foods and beverages daily, everyone has interests, concerns, opinions, and questions about what they eat. Unfortunately, most issues in the news pose nontechnical questions that defy technical answers. The purpose of this section is to enter the student's world and reframe food issues as presented from a journalistic viewpoint into a more scientific perspective. Stories are selected as illustrations for each chapter—Safety, Healthiness of Foods, and Foods We Eat. While widely held misconceptions are presented and corrected, the text avoids pat answers. Rather, emphasis is placed on separating what we know about such issues from what we don't know and how they can be reformulated into testable hypotheses. For greater depth on specific issues, the student is referred to specific passages later in the book.

The second section introduces students to commercial food products. Chapters 4 through 6—Processed Foods, Formulated Foods, and Chilled and Prepared Foods—provide the basic principles of food manufacture and food preservation with a strong emphasis on unit operations. Both traditional (canning, freezing, fermenting, and drying) and more modern (aseptic, irradiation, and high pressure) processes are presented. The importance of individual ingredients and how they are displayed on food labels are vehicles used to introduce formulated foods, a major component of the student diet. Sections on the moves of food companies to provide "clean labels" and "gluten-free foods" have been added to this edition. Foodservice operations, distribution systems, and packaging technology highlight the discussion on chilled and prepared foods. Material in these three chapters is sprinkled with flowcharts, diagrams, ingredient statements, and pictures to illustrate the major points. The importance of food preservation and sanitation in preventing food-associated outbreaks raised in Chapter 1 provides a major theme.

The profession of food science provides the basis for Section III. Career opportunities, necessary background, and professional perspective permeate these chapters. Chapter 7 on quality assurance introduces the topic of quality (nutritional, microbial, and sensory), its measurement, process control, Hazard Analysis and Critical Control Points (HACCP), shelf life, and commercial sanitation. Chapter 8 on product and process development describes the creative process and what is required to provide the wealth of options available to the modern consumer with sufficient quality and shelf life. Chapter 9 on sustainability and distribution brings attention to the demand for environmental responsibility and the industry response to that demand. Chapter 10 on government regulation and scientific research presents the importance of food regulations and a fundamental understanding of foods to ensure a healthy and safe food supply to include changes brought about by Food Safety Modernization Act (FSMA).

The book culminates with an introduction to the basic principles of the primary subdisciplines within food science. This section represents more in-depth technical detail needed to answer questions posed earlier in the book.

A chemical basis for safety, nutrition, preservation, ingredient functionality, and quality is provided in Chapter 11. The basic principles of nutrition and the contribution of foods to our health are presented in Chapter 12. An understanding of the factors that affect growth and inhibition of fermentative of spoilage, and pathogenic microorganisms is described in Chapter 13. Critical engineering concepts needed to understand the design and monitoring of food processes are described in Chapter 14 with a greater emphasis on the mathematical basis of the field than in the first edition. Fundamentals of sensory perception of foods and systematic means of measuring sensory attributes provide the basis of the final chapter. The section is designed to whet the student's appetite for a deeper taste of food science in more detailed books and courses.

While no single volume will satisfy needs for all introductory courses, this book offers a range of material that should be useful for many of those courses. Introductory courses for non-majors would focus on the first three sections and use the last section primarily as a reference source for scientific principles. In contrast, courses for food science majors would emphasize the final three sections and use the initial food issues section as a basis for outside readings and assignments. Courses that include both majors and non-majors would require more careful tailoring of course content to meet the specific needs of the students.

Acknowledgments

A book does not write itself. It is hard to recognize everyone who contributed to this effort.

First, we would like to thank Stephen Zollo who encouraged us to make major modifications and additions in this revision as well as Kari Budyk and everyone at CRC Press who helped us turn a multitude of electronic files into a finished book. We appreciate everyone who provided images that are used throughout the book. Also, we thank all of our students who have critiqued early versions of the chapters and have taught us as much about food and culture as we have taught them about food science.

Authors

Andrew D. Clarke is an associate professor of food science and the under-graduate advisor chairman in the food science program at the University of Missouri. He earned a BS and an MS degree in animal science from Texas Tech University in 1982 and 1984, respectively, before earning a PhD in animal science from the Colorado State University in 1987. He joined the University of Missouri program in 1987 to teach meat processing, conduct research on value-added products, and lead the Extension Program for meat processors in Missouri. He has taught seven different meat science courses and seven different food science courses covering topics from introductory levels up to a doctoral food preservation class. Currently, he emphasizes the undergraduate courses that cover the introduction to food science, the meat processing class, and the capstone course in food product development. He collaborates with colleagues in several states to offer Hazard Analysis Critical Control Points and Better Process Control School workshops for industry in Missouri. As a former director of graduate studies in food science (2003–2008), he continues to teach research methods to new graduate students in the Division of Food Systems and Bioengineering. Since 2008, he and colleague Ingolf Gruen have led six groups of students on study abroad trips to New Zealand and Germany that feature the meat, dairy, and wine industries of each country. He stays active in the American Meat Science Association (a director in 1995 and 1996) and the Institute of Food Technologists (chairman of St. Louis Section 2001–2002, chairman of Muscle Food Division 2005–2006) and once served as editor for *Food Science & Technology/LWT* (1997–2001).

Alícia Orta-Ramírez is the Louis Pasteur Lecturer in Food Microbiology and director of the undergraduate program in the Department of Food Science at Cornell University. She earned a DVM degree from the Universitat Autònoma de Barcelona, Spain, in 1989 and an MS and PhD in food science from Michigan State University, in 1994 and 1999, respectively. She joined the Cornell faculty in January 2007. Her responsibilities include teaching five undergraduate courses, coordinating advising and recruiting activities, and organizing workshops for science teachers. She has been an active member of the College of Agriculture and Life Sciences' Diversity and Inclusion Committee (including cochair in 2013–2014) and the Institute of Food Technologists' Education, Extension, and Outreach Committee (including chair in 2012–2013).

Robert L. Shewfelt is professor emeritus of food science and technology at the University of Georgia. He was a Josiah Meigs Distinguished Teaching Professor at the university when he retired at the end of May 2013. He conducted extensive research on postharvest physiology and handling of fruits and vegetables and was part of an interdisciplinary research team that introduced the systems approach to postharvest handling of fruits and vegetables. Professor Shewfelt taught more than 10 courses at the university including freshman seminars on chocolate science and coffee technology. He also taught a food processing lab as a virtual food company where each student had a position in the company that designed, manufactured, and tested the quality of four distinctly different processed food products. The marketing and information technology functions were outsourced to senior classes in the Terry College of Business on campus. He continues to write about food science in his retirement.

Contributors

Andrew D. Clarke
Food Science Department
University of Missouri
Columbia, Missouri

Angela E. Edge
Department of Food Science and Technology
University of Georgia
Athens, Georgia

Mark A. Harrison
Department of Food Science and Technology
University of Georgia
Athens, Georgia

Alicia Orta-Ramirez
Department of Food Science
Cornell University
Ithaca, New York

José I. Reyes-De-Corcuera
Department of Food Science and Technology
University of Georgia
Athens, Georgia

Robert L. Shewfelt
Department of Food Science and Technology
University of Georgia
Athens, Georgia

Section I

Food Issues in the News

1

Food Safety

It is 3 a.m. Nil's intimate companion for the last 90 minutes has been the porcelain throne. He has been intermittently spewing from both ends and feels horrible. The intense stomach cramps have just let up, but he is so nauseous he's afraid to venture out of the bathroom. His condition did not give him much warning. What had he done to deserve this? He had a decent meal downtown washed down by only two beers or so before turning in around midnight. His mind was a little foggy as he tried to think back to what else he had eaten. Maybe he should not have eaten that rare hamburger the day before yesterday. True, it looked a little sketchy, but man was it tasty! Besides, nothing he ate that long ago could be affecting him now. Oh no, it feels like something is coming back up again!

Alice grew up unnaturally thin and had persistent digestive issues. She couldn't figure out why she was in a constant mental fog as well. After many years of feeling helpless, she finally received confirmation via a blood test that she was part of the approximately 1% of people with celiac disease. Alice was forced to adopt a gluten-free diet as the only way to treat her condition. Although she feels much more energetic and healthier, sometimes it is difficult for her to go to events that have an abundance of pizza or eat out at local restaurants with friends. Frustrated with how limited she was, Alice decided to enter the field of Food Science where she could help develop new products for other celiacs and anyone else interested in following a gluten-free diet.

Alice and Nil represent millions of Americans who become sick because of the food they eat. Alice must avoid many foods that her friends consume in large quantities without fear. While Nil doesn't have the same dietary restrictions, he became ill because he ate some contaminated food, probably the rare hamburger. What is wrong with the American food supply? Why isn't the government doing anything to prevent this problem? Why do some foods go bad so quickly and others stay safe forever? What can we do to lower our risk? This chapter offers answers to these and other questions about the safety of the food supply. Some answers are simple. Others are clear but may be unexpected. Still others either require a deeper understanding of science than a simple answer can provide or are the basis of ongoing research at universities and governmental laboratories. Food Science is at the forefront of research and education programs on the safety of foods.

1.1 Food in the News

Newspapers, magazines, television, radio, and the Internet are filled with news stories about food-associated outbreaks. On the one hand, we hear that the American food supply is the safest ever. On the other hand, it seems like more people are getting sick every year. We hear about all these chemicals added to processed foods. Somebody must be hiding something. *Salmonella*, *Escherichia coli*, botulism, and *Listeria* have become household words. We know they make us sick, but it can be hard to establish how serious the risks are and how likely we are to get sick. Our response to the media bombardment varies from being afraid of everything we eat to ignoring any report on food.

Although we have access to detailed information on food-associated illness, not all of it is accurate or useful. It is often difficult to separate fact from fiction. Certain widely held beliefs about food poisoning are completely wrong. Other simple guidelines that could dramatically reduce food-associated illness are widely ignored. Consumers point fingers at the food industry and governmental agencies that point fingers back at the consumer. Blaming somebody else may make the pointer feel good, but it doesn't help solve food safety problems.

Bloggers and reporters are very good at raising awareness, but they are not as effective at providing solutions. It is easy to blame alarmists for this situation, but blame ignores simple problems in transmitting information. Primary limitations of communicating food issues are as follows:

- It is easier to grab attention and present a problem than it is to convey factual information and provide a solution.
- Up-close-and-personal stories are more likely to grab attention than more general ones.
- Obscure and unusual hazards tend to become amplified while more common and widespread ones tend to be diminished.
- Journalists are typically not trained in science while scientists are not usually good at communicating their stories in simple language.

Many food issues are complex and require an understanding of science. Journalists and bloggers looking for a killer topic become frustrated with scientists, who use big words, provide long answers to simple questions, and are reluctant to identify a simple cause and solution. Scientists become frustrated with a desire to oversimplify and the lack of appreciation for basic scientific principles on the part of a writer. Part of the problem is that many of the questions consumers ask are not answerable by science, while many of the answers science can provide do not fit into a sound bite a journalist can

Cranberries	Elton John
Miranda Lambert	Steven Tyler
William Shattner	Selena Gomez
Daniel Radcliffe	Lady Gaga
Katy Perry	Mandy Moore

http://foodpoisoningbulletin.com/2012/food-poisoning-of-the-rich-and-famous/
http://www.learn2serve.com/blog/3-celebrities-who-got-food-poisoning-in-2012/
http://voices.yahoo.com/food-poisoning-nightmares-stars-11089484.html

INSERT 1.1
These celebrities have something in common. They were all victims of food poisoning. For more details, see the websites listed at the bottom of the insert.

communicate. See Insert 1.1 for some celebrities who have been in the news in the past few years.

The remainder of the chapter will introduce us to

- How food makes us sick
- Some common misconceptions about the safety of our foods
- Some of the causes for the apparent rise in food-associated illnesses in the United States in recent years
- How food scientists work to decrease our chances of getting sick from the food we eat
- Some simple rules we can follow to reduce our risks associated with foods

This chapter provides a food science perspective on the subject. More scientific details will follow in Chapters 4, 7, 12, and 13.

1.2 Unsafe Foods

Simply put, an unsafe food is one that makes us sick when we eat it. There are at least five ways a food can make us sick, including the presence of

- Harmful microbes (including viruses and parasites)
- Harmful additives (such as preservatives)
- Environmental contaminants (such as pesticides)
- Natural toxins
- Compounds (such as allergens) that induce sensitivities in susceptible individuals

Food scientists are much more concerned about illness caused by microbes than other sources, as it is estimated that more than 95% of food-associated illnesses are caused by microbes. In addition, food scientists believe that natural toxins present a greater risk to consumers than either pesticides or preservatives.

There is a general belief that foods are inherently safe in their natural state and that they become unsafe when exposed to technology. Food scientists believe that many natural foods like those derived from animals are inherently unsafe and that a scientific understanding of what causes safety problems leads to development of technology that provides safer foods. A goal of this book is to provide a better understanding of our foods and what we can do to keep foods safe.

1.3 Microbial Hazards

It comes as a surprise to most consumers to learn that fresh foods are more likely to contain harmful microbes than processed products (Insert 1.2 ranks the relative safety of several foods). The primary sources of harmful microbes in foods can be traced back to feces (human or animal waste). When food microbiologists start to look for a microbe of interest, they frequently collect soil or feces samples to isolate their microbe of choice. The reason we wash raw foods is to remove soil and feces from their surface. Unfortunately, even if we remove all visible evidence of the soil or feces, the associated microbes may cling to the surface of the food. Fresh fruits, vegetables, and grains may become contaminated from the soil; from insect, rodent, or bird droppings; or from organic fertilizers.

1. Alfalfa sprouts
2. Undercooked chicken
3. Raw cookie dough
4. Rare hamburger
5. Salad from a food bar
6. Unpasteurized orange juice
7. Chocolate éclair
8. Pasteurized milk
9. Refrigerated yogurt
10. Canned tuna fish

INSERT 1.2
Listed above are 10 different foods ranked in order from most likely to cause food-associated illness (1) to least likely (10) according to Dr. Michael P. Doyle, Director of the Center for Food Safety at the University of Georgia.

As disgusting as it may seem, when we eat meat, we are eating the muscle tissue of formerly live animals. Theoretically, the inside of the muscle is sterile and does not pose a threat to human health. Unfortunately, all these animals produce feces as well as muscle. During livestock production and during the harvesting (slaughter) process, the surface of meat is likely to become contaminated with feces. Some advocates for safer foods believe that it is careless handling of animal carcasses in fresh meat and poultry packing plants that causes contamination with visible feces, but this belief is not accurate. It is doubtful that we could provide sterile steaks, pork chops, or chicken thighs (or even less contaminated ones than commercial packing operations) if we harvested our own steers, hogs, or chickens and then dressed and cut up the meat. See Insert 1.3 for some common microbes responsible for food-associated illness.

Pathogen	Cases			Hospitalizations		Deaths	
	No.	Incidence*	Objective†	No.	(%)	No.	(%)
Bacteria							
Campylobacter	6621	13.82	8.5	1010	(15)	12	(0.2)
Listeria	123	0.26	0.2	112	(91)	24	(19.5)
Salmonella	7277	15.19	11.4	2003	(28)	27	(0.4)
Shigella	2309	4.82	N/A§	450	(19)	3	(0.1)
STEC O157	552	1.15	0.6	210	(38)	2	(0.4)
STEC non-O157	561	1.17	N/A	76	(14)	2	(0.4)
Vibrio	242	0.51	0.2	55	(23)	2	(0.8)
Yersinia	171	0.36	0.3	55	(32)	4	(2.3)
Parasites							
Cryptosporidium	1186	2.48	N/A	227	(19)	4	(0.3)
Cyclospora	14	0.03	N/A	2	(14)	0	(0.0)
Total	**19,056**			**4200**		**80**	

Abbreviations: N/A = not available; STEC = Shiga toxin–producing *Escherichia coli.*

Note: Data for 2013 are preliminary.

* Per 100,000 population.

† Healthy People 2020 objective targets for incidence of *Campylobacter, Listeria, Salmonella,* STEC O157, *Vibrio,* and *Yersinia* infections per 100,000 population.

§ No national health objective exists for these pathogens.

INSERT 1.3
Number of cases of culture-confirmed bacterial and laboratory-confirmed parasitic infection, hospitalizations, and deaths, by pathogen—Foodborne Diseases Active Surveillance Network, United States, 2013. (From Crim, S.M. et al., MMWR, 63:328–32, 2014.)

Food products are processed primarily to kill microbes or at least slow their growth in or on foods. Proper handling and storage of perishable products such as fresh produce and raw meats slows the growth of microbes. The most effective weapons used to control food-associated illnesses are proper sanitation and storage during handling and distribution from the farm to the consumer. Proper sanitation involves doing everything to reduce contamination at each step along the way. Proper storage involves maintaining conditions that lower the chance of a food becoming unsafe, usually by quick cooling and keeping it in a cold chain. Packaging of foods helps prevent microbes from touching the food, but even packaged foods can become dangerous if mishandled.

1.4 Spoiled: When Good Food Goes Bad

Another misconception most consumers have about food is the idea that it is easy to tell if a food is safe by looking at it, smelling it, or taking a small bite. If it looks, smells, or tastes nasty, then it must be dangerous, right? Not necessarily! When we say a food has gone bad, we are probably talking about spoilage (see Insert 1.4). Spoiled food is no longer pleasant to eat. While it is never a good idea to eat spoiled food, a spoiled food is not necessarily an unsafe food. Even more important, an unsafe food is not necessarily spoiled. If all unsafe foods were spoiled, there would be much less food poisoning than we have currently. If we remember the example of Nil at the beginning

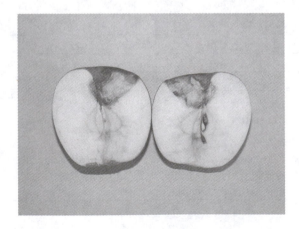

INSERT 1.4
Spoiled apple as found at http://ars.usda.gov/images/docs/15133_15327/Image12.jpg.

of the chapter, he did not report anything tasting strange leading to his illness.

What spoiled and unsafe foods have in common is that microbes probably caused the problem. The difference is that the types of microbes that cause spoilage are not usually the same ones that make foods unsafe. By now, it should be clear that spoilage is not a good indicator of a safety risk because many of the microbes that make food unsafe do not change the color, taste, or smell of the food. However, the handling and storage conditions that lead to growth of spoilage microbes tend to be similar to those that lead to the growth of microbes that make the food unsafe.

1.5 Food Poisoning

Before discussing food poisoning, we need to know what it is and what it is not. Food poisoning is a sickness caused by consuming a contaminated food. There are many possible causes, but the most likely cause is microbial. When we talk about food poisoning, we are not talking about the stomach turning we might get when we smell spoiled food. We are talking about symptoms that send us to bed or the bathroom for about 24 hours or to something that can lead to a coma or death. Most cases result in severe gastric distress with accompanying diarrhea or vomiting or both. What people refer to as a stomach virus is usually the result of food poisoning.

Microbial food poisoning occurs as an **infection** or **intoxication**. An infection happens when a microbe is present in a food or beverage, we eat the contaminated item, and the microbe grows in us like a typical infectious disease. An intoxication is one in which the microbe grows in the food or beverage and produces a toxin. After the toxin has been produced, the item might be heated to the point the microbe is killed, but the toxin is still present. We then consume it, and the toxin makes us sick.

There are many things about food poisoning that most people do not know. For example, the last meal consumed is not usually the meal responsible for the outbreak. When people get sick and suspect food poisoning, they tend to blame the last thing that they ate. One type of food poisoning, a staph intoxication, can happen within 1–6 hours after the offending food was eaten. Most other food poisoning outbreaks take at least 12 hours after the offending food is eaten to cause distress, like those encountered by Nil. Some outbreaks take as much as a week to develop. At that point, it can be hard to figure out the cause. Symptoms and incubation times of common food-associated illnesses are shown in Insert 1.5.

Microbe or toxin	Symptoms	Incubation times
Campylobacter jejuni	Nausea, vomiting, stomach cramps, intense diarrhea	2–5 days
Clostridium botulinum	Blurred vision, breathing and swallowing difficulties, dry mouth, respiratory failure	12–36 hours
Escherichia coli O157:H7	Vomiting, watery turning to bloody diarrhea, kidney failure	1–8 days
Listeria monocytogenes	Slight fever, stomach cramps, diarrhea, abortion, meningitis, etc.	1 day to many weeks
Salmonella enterididis	Chills, fever, nausea, vomiting, stomach cramps, diarrhea	24–36 hours
Staphylococcal enterotoxin	Sweating, chills, nausea, vomiting, stomach cramps, diarrhea	1–6 hours

INSERT 1.5
Symptoms and incubation times of some common food-associated illnesses.

1.6 Tracking Down the Culprits

Scientists who try to track down the cause of an outbreak are called epidemiologists. An **outbreak** is defined by the Centers for Disease Control and Prevention as an occurrence of two or more cases of a similar illness resulting from the ingestion of a common food. **Epidemiologists** go to the scene of an outbreak and compile a list of those who became sick to get a clue to the responsible organism. They also list foods and beverages consumed by those who became sick and those who did not get sick to help narrow down the number of suspected foods.

Food handling and preparation practices are studied to identify possible causes while potential offending foods are collected and tested. Samples from the patient and the food are compared to see if there are microbe matches. In addition, the distribution patterns of the offending foods back to their sources are studied to find the main point of contamination. Most outbreaks are caused by a combination of several food handling errors, permitting contamination and growth of one of a small number of harmful microbes. The longer the time lapse between food consumption and illness, the more difficult it is to find the cause.

1.7 Expiration Dates

Many packaged foods, particularly the more perishable ones, come with an expiration date. The expiration date represents the food scientist's best guess on how long a food will last before it spoils. A food scientist calculates the expiration date by first determining the product's shelf life (how long it will last under typical storage). The expiration date is usually set before the end of shelf life, but it is not as simple as being acceptable to eat the day before the expiration date and unacceptable the day after the date. Too many things can affect spoilage of food products. The food scientist does not want to cut the day too close as consumers get very upset when they find something has spoiled before the date on the package. On the other hand, if the date is set long before it actually spoils, then consumers are unlikely to buy it, and perfectly good food will get thrown out before it has spoiled. Premature tossing of good food leads to increased costs for the food company, prices for the consumer, and food waste.

1.8 Food Preservation

Food preservation involves reducing the chances that food will spoil or become unsafe. One way to preserve food is to kill microbes by heating the food or beverage. Canned foods are essentially sterile. Canning refers to the process and not necessarily the package. Many products in plastic or glass jars have also been canned and are thus considered to be commercially sterile. Other methods of heating that lower the number of microbes include cooking (in either a microwave or regular oven) and pasteurization. Pasteurization kills harmful microbes but not spoilage microbes.

Another way of preserving foods involves slowing or preventing the growth of microbes. A refrigerator slows the growth of microbes in highly perishable foods. Freezing and drying are much more effective in slowing microbial growth than refrigeration, but it is important to realize that microbes are still present. Once we thaw a frozen food or add water to a dried food they are just as likely to spoil or become unsafe as any other unprotected food. Even canned food can become contaminated after it has been opened. Another method of food preservation actually encourages the growth of microbes. In fermented products (yogurt, alcoholic beverages, most pickles, some sausages, and sauerkraut), beneficial microbes are added to produce that particular product, and they grow so fast that spoilage and harmful microbes don't have a chance to grow.

Processed foods are handled, prepared, treated, and packaged under carefully controlled conditions. These processes must be approved by the appropriate governmental agency. A safeguard used in approving such processes is that a processed food should be designed to spoil before it becomes unsafe to make it less likely that someone will eat the unsafe food and become sick. An important part of any food is its package. The primary purposes of any package are to contain the food and to protect it from contamination by microbes. Once a food has been removed from the container, it can become contaminated quickly by kitchen utensils, the air, or touching contaminated food or water. Improper storage can cause harmful microbes to grow, leading to spoilage or unsafe foods.

1.9 Preservatives

The word *preservative* is considered a dirty word by many consumers. Many look for the words "no preservatives" on food labels. Actually, preservatives are food ingredients that slow spoilage and help prevent food-associated illnesses. They achieve this effect by preventing or slowing the growth of microbes. The two most common preservatives are sugar and salt. Preservatives are food additives that extend shelf life and lower costs, which can lead to less waste, more profit for the food company, and lower prices for the consumer. Food additives must not be added to conceal diseased, decayed, or other defective products. These additives must serve a useful purpose and must be effective for the intended use.

One reason consumers object to preservatives and other food additives is that they are chemicals, many with hard-to-pronounce names. Everything in our foods and in our bodies is a chemical including water, sugar, salt, vitamins, minerals, and proteins. Food scientists are not concerned about the actual presence of chemicals in our food, but they are concerned about reducing the ones that are harmful and increasing the ones that are beneficial. Awareness among consumers regarding suspicious ingredients approved for use is sometimes raised by bloggers and watchdog organizations that lead to reactions that may alter how companies formulate their products.

In one recent case, lean finely textured beef (LFTB) was described as being "pink slime" in news reports although it has been strictly regulated and produced in a wholesome manner for almost two decades. The product is made by exposing meat to small amounts of food grade ammonium hydroxide to control harmful bacteria that may be present in the beef. Misunderstanding spreads because consumers equated the process to adding household ammonia to the meat and the furor was compounded because LFTB is usually not identified separately as an ingredient on food labels. The government and industry view was that the product is safer than untreated beef after *E. coli* gained prominence, and because LFTB is 100% beef, it is not singled out on a label.

Another example of consumer pressure that did result in a major company removing a specific food additive was the "yoga mat chemical" incident. Azodicarbonamide (ADA) is an approved food additive used to bleach flour and make dough stronger and more rubbery. ADA was widely criticized when it was identified as an industrial chemical that is also used in the manufacture of yoga mats and similar nonfood products. In reaction to the negative publicity, some foodservice operations required that their suppliers reformulate products to drop the ADA component. Food scientists believe that consumers are unduly concerned about the safety of preservatives and other additives. Food additives are required by law to undergo rigorous safety testing and be effective for their intended use, but this concept has not been communicated well to the general public.

1.10 Safety of the American Food Supply

If we know so much about food poisoning, then why do we have so much of it? In fact, it seems like food is getting more dangerous, not safer. The American food supply has undergone revolutionary changes in the last 30 years. Several possible reasons for this situation have been advanced, but the truth is we really don't know. Some of the possible reasons for more food-associated illness today than 30–40 years ago include the following:

- New and newly recognized harmful microbes have come into our food supply.
- Greater consumption of imported foods such as fruits, vegetables, and seafood.
- Consumption of more raw and undercooked foods.
- Factory farms lead to concentration of microbes in raw foods.
- Less knowledge by food preparers on proper food handling techniques.
- Increased use of antibiotics in animals leading to greater resistance of microbes to antibiotics.
- Our food supply has fewer microbes; thus, we are less likely to build up resistance to them when we are young.
- More people are exposed to other diseases (such as AIDS) that compromise the body's ability to resist harmful microbes.
- Increased reporting by consumers affected.
- Higher coverage in news reports.

Changing circumstances have led to food poisoning outbreaks that were unheard of just a few years back, but in many instances, it is very difficult to identify a specific cause. Advanced knowledge has led to more effective control of microbes in food processing plants and restaurants. However, greater centralization has led to more people becoming sick when a mistake does occur.

Many food scientists do not believe that there has been a great increase in cases of food poisoning. They believe that we are just becoming more aware of the dangers that lurk in our foods. Epidemiologists have become more effective in identifying the cause of food-associated illnesses that might have been blamed on some other cause. The long times between eating the food and the start of the illness are not as big a problem in identifying the cause as they once were. Physicians have also become better at diagnosing food-associated illnesses.

Research in food microbiology has led to the discovery of microbes that we did not know were harmful. These microbes may have been causing illnesses for years, but we did not know it. One very important contributing factor to detection of modern-day food-associated disease outbreaks that would previously have gone undetected is a national/international network (PulseNet) that collects molecular subtyping results of human isolates of food-associated pathogens. Finally, sophisticated news-gathering organizations have the ability to tell us about small outbreaks in faraway places that previously would only be known in the local town or city where they occurred.

1.11 Safety in the Home

If we are going to decrease the number of cases of food poisoning, then everyone who interacts with the food in any way from the farm to the table must take responsibility for the safety of his or her food. Food scientists believe that one of the least controlled steps from farm to table is in the home or wherever consumers handle and prepare the food after they buy it. This belief goes back to the idea that foods are inherently unsafe in their natural state and that a scientific understanding of what causes safety problems leads to development of technology that provides safer foods. Food companies that produce the packaged foods we buy and restaurants that prepare the meals we eat have access to this knowledge, but many consumers do not.

When food inspectors went into homes using the same forms they use in restaurants, they found that more than 99% failed! See what the inspectors were looking for in Insert 1.6. There are some simple rules we can follow in our apartments, dorm rooms, or homes that can reduce our chances of getting sick from the food we eat. Our efforts should start in the supermarket. We want to make sure that no juices from raw meats (which will eventually be cooked) drip on fresh fruits and vegetables that we plan to eat raw. If we worry about raw meat contaminating other foods, we can always buy precooked meats as long as we are willing to pay extra for them. Damaged packages can lead to contamination of a packaged food, either deliberate or accidental. Foods that should be refrigerated but are not cold provide evidence that the product has been mishandled by the supermarket.

Critical violation examples:

☐ Cross-contamination of foods that will not be cooked,

☐ Failure to wash hands,

☐ Failure to keep hot foods hot,

☐ Failure to properly cool leftovers,

☐ Use of swollen or rusty cans,

☐ Preparation of foods by someone who is sick.

Major violation examples:

☐ Evidence of roaches, other insects or mice,

☐ Eating or drinking by person preparing food,

☐ Failure to have separate towels for drying hands and for wiping counters,

☐ Failure to properly store leftovers,

☐ Failure to use thermometers to monitor cooking of meats,

☐ Use of foods beyond the stated expiration date,

☐ Refrigerated storage temperatures too high.

INSERT 1.6
How many homes could pass inspection from the health department? If the food preparation area was investigated by the local health department, it would fail a home with one critical or four major violations. (Adapted from Daniels, R.W., *Food Technol.*, 52(2), 54, 1998.)

After we buy our food and take it to our vehicle, we want to make sure that we don't become guilty of food abuse. Perishable foods (anything normally stored in a refrigerator or freezer) begin to spoil rapidly in a hot environment. It is a good idea to make the supermarket the last stop on the way home. Highly perishable foods such as raw meats should never be left out of refrigerated conditions for more than 1 hour. The longer perishable foods are left at room temperature, the more quickly they will spoil and the more likely they are to become a safety hazard. When we get home, it is important to put away the perishables as quickly as possible. Again, we need to make sure juices from raw meats do not come in contact with any food that will not be fully cooked.

The most frequent factors in food poisoning outbreaks are improper storage temperatures, poor personal hygiene, too low cooking temperatures, cross-contamination, and food from unsafe sources. Personal hygiene means we should wash our hands thoroughly before handling any foods and make sure that all surfaces that will touch the food are clean. Frequent hand washing during meal preparation is a good idea, particularly after touching raw meat or uncooked eggs. The towel we use for hands and counters should never be used to dry dishes. Tasting while fixing a meal is not a good idea, either, particularly if a heated food has not been cooked enough to kill the harmful microbes. Care should be taken not to use the same cutting boards or surfaces for raw meats and salad materials unless they have been thoroughly cleaned. Adequate cooking is needed to kill harmful microbes in raw foods.

When the meal is over, food should be put away but not in the container in which it was prepared. Cooking followed by contamination and improper storage can accelerate growth of harmful microbes. Proper refrigeration slows growth of harmful microbes in leftovers. Two simple rules for handling food are (1) to keep hot food hot and cold food cold and (2) when in doubt, throw it out. Despite concerns about increasing incidents of food poisoning, the recommendations described above have not changed much in the last 50 years.

1.12 Pesticides and Other Contaminants

It would be nice to live in a world where we did not need pesticides, but pests represent the greatest threat to availability of food worldwide. Many poor people in countries with adequate food supplies are unable to obtain sufficient food, partly because insects, rodents, and plant diseases get to the food first. Insects devour crops before or after harvest in the fields and damage food in storage. Rodents can spread disease and consume food meant for humans. Plant diseases lower yield in the field and spoil harvested crops. Stress to plants in the field from flooding, drought, low temperature, or high temperatures also lower yields and increases susceptibility to pests. Pesticides are used to help prevent crop loss caused by insects, rodents, and diseases. Contaminated food and water cause illness and death.

Pesticides are applied to crops to kill pests. They are carefully monitored to ensure the safety of the food supply. Pesticides are very toxic chemicals when applied to the plant. Pesticides are designed to break down into harmless chemicals before they reach the consumer. Federal and state governmental agencies carefully monitor residue levels of pesticides in raw and processed products. Many techniques such as Integrated Pest Management (IPM) are practiced to reduce pesticides on food crops and their residues in our foods. When pests are particularly numerous, IPM can result in increased pesticide use, but it usually results in much less pesticides than more conventional practices. Steps in food processing tend to decrease pesticide levels in foods but do not eliminate them. While pesticides poison and kill agricultural workers who don't take proper precautions when applying them, there have been few cases of consumers becoming ill as a result of pesticides in the foods they ate.

Organic food production attempts to reduce the use of fossil fuels and synthetic chemicals. Animal manure and composted plant materials serve as fertilizers for organic crops while synthetic nitrogen products are used in modern agriculture that produces most of the food we eat. Organic fertilizers that come in contact with food present a hazard, and contaminated irrigation wastes are a primary source of harmful microbes. Proper composting of animal waste should kill all harmful microbes. Some of the most serious *E. coli* outbreaks have occurred by contamination of a water supply by animal manure. Most crop production in the United States relies on pesticides, while organic production emphasizes biological and cultural alternatives. Organically grown products are desired by many consumers, but these products usually cost more, have a shorter shelf life, and may not look as nice as those grown with pesticides.

1.13 Natural Toxins

Despite the widespread belief that natural is better than artificial, food scientists see little scientific evidence to support this claim. The idea that natural is good and artificial is bad is at best oversimplistic and at worst dangerous. That concept does not stop food companies and makers of dietary supplements from taking advantage of our admiration of all things natural. Some of the deadliest chemicals are natural, like the botulinal or paralytic shellfish toxins. Some foods that are normally safe become poisonous under special conditions. Documented cases of deaths from poisonous shellfish and green potatoes provide examples. A series of lawsuits challenging foods labeled as *natural* is beginning to make an impact on this designation leading to the use of more ambiguous marketing terms like *naked*, *pure*, and *simple*.

Whole foods generally provide a complementary package of nutrients with minimal toxic consequences and maximum bioavailability. Safety risks increase when natural compounds are separated (extracted) from a plant or animal source and concentrated. Chemical solvents may be needed to separate the natural compound from the plant, animal, or insect (cochineal is an approved natural red food coloring extracted from beetles). Many of these solvents are toxic and remain in the final product at trace levels. Natural extracts are usually less pure than chemical synthetics, and some of the impurities are toxic. We should not be worried about the safety hazard of these compounds when present at the low levels in nature. When natural chemicals are used as ingredients, they must be concentrated. During concentration and purification of these ingredients, the natural toxins can also be concentrated and purified. Toxins that pose no risk when at low levels in whole foods can be dangerous at the higher levels in natural ingredients.

Finally, there is no such thing as natural cooking just as there is no natural food processing or natural synthesis of artificial compounds. Cooking is a form of food preservation whether it happens in the home, in a restaurant, or at a food manufacturing plant. *Homo sapiens* is the only species that has developed the sophistication to modify its environment to overcome natural barriers for good or for ill. Food scientists think that it makes more sense to judge a chemical by understanding its properties than by whether it is natural or artificial.

1.14 Allergies and Food Sensitivities

Individual sensitivities to foods are controversial. Skin or blood tests can determine true allergies to specific foods. More general reactions to foods may occur, but these sensitivities are more difficult to diagnose. Many physicians and scientists who study allergens are skeptical about food sensitivities (called atopic responses), suggesting that such sensitivities reside only in the mind of the victim. Suffering victims are likely to seek help outside the medical or scientific community when told they are making up their illness.

True food allergens induce an abnormal immune response in susceptible individuals. Eggs, fish (including shellfish), grains (corn, wheat, and rice), legumes (soybeans and peanuts), milk, and various tree nuts are common sources of food allergens. Other foods such as celery, strawberries, and yeasts are also reported as allergenic. We link an allergy to a complete food, but usually only a few proteins in a food product are responsible for the allergic reaction. Symptoms of allergic reactions are triggered when specific protein molecules in the food are linked on the surface of special cells in the intestine. These cells then send out signals to other cells leading to an allergic reaction. Many of these reactions result in gastroenteritis leading to stomach aches, diarrhea, and other intestinal difficulties. Similar reactions can also occur in the food processing workplace through inhaling of the allergen from the air. Some allergies, particularly an allergy to peanut proteins, can be very serious, leading to anaphylactic shock and death in less than an hour after exposure.

Although not a true allergic reaction, celiac disease is an autoimmune disorder in which microvilli in the intestinal tract react with gliadin, a component of gluten found in wheat and other grains. The damage done to the intestine by this disease not only results in cramping, diarrhea, and general intestinal discomfort, it interferes with absorption of nutrients leading to anemia and other nutrient deficiency diseases. At present, the only cure is a gluten-free diet as Alice learned when she was told she was a celiac. Some individuals have been diagnosed with asymptomatic sensitivity to gliadin/gluten, but the extent of this condition remains controversial. A number of gluten-free products are available on the market now for anyone who desires to eliminate or reduce gluten in their diet as shown in Insert 1.7.

Some consumers have atopic reactions to foods or additives that are not true allergens. Sulfites can induce severe reactions including abdominal pain, diarrhea, cramping, nausea, difficulty in swallowing, headache, chest pain, faintness, and loss of consciousness in a few very susceptible consumers. Consumption of large amounts of monosodium glutamate on an empty stomach has been referred to as Chinese restaurant syndrome leading to headaches, burning neck, chest tightness, nausea, and profuse sweating.

Despite widespread publicity, the Feingold hypothesis, which claims an association between artificial colors, other additives, and sugar to hyperactivity in

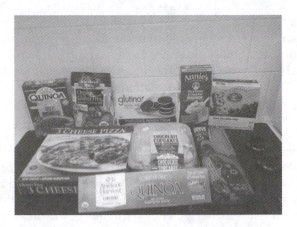

INSERT 1.7
An array of gluten-free products for celiacs and others who wish to avoid gluten. (Photo courtesy of Robert Shewfelt.)

children, has not been proven in controlled tests. These atopic responses are much more difficult to study than true allergies, which produce true antibodies that can be measured in the blood. That is why many scientists and physicians are skeptical about them.

One clearly documented sensitivity is lactose intolerance. Many Africans, Asians, American Indians, and their descendants lose the ability to break down lactose.

Consuming a diet that eliminates any food or beverage that might cause a reaction is the surest way of preventing allergic reactions. Skin tests narrow down the number of possible true allergens but do not always work for atopic responses. All foods implicated by the skin tests are eliminated from the diet, with a single food added back each week. If no reaction occurs, another food is tested. In addition, shots are given to lessen the chances of reactions. A combination of shots and dietary restrictions works for many individuals, while others must quit eating the suspected food. Atopic responses are usually tested by placing a small amount of the suspected food in the mouth and then waiting for symptoms to develop. This type of test is less likely to provide results than those looking for true allergic reactions.

1.15 Governmental Regulation

Many governmental agencies are responsible for monitoring the safety and quality of our food supply. The terms **safety** and **quality** are frequently used synonymously and interchangeably. In reality, these two things are very different to food scientists. Safety is focused on the aspect of keeping the food we eat free from hazards that would cause us to become ill if we were to consume it. Quality is the area where companies emphasize certain attributes such as flavor, appearance, and other consumer-driven factors. Different laws and subsequent regulations are set forth to govern each of these areas.

The Food and Drug Administration determines which food additives are allowed in foods and matches the ingredient statement on the label with the ingredients in the product. The United States Department of Agriculture (USDA) regulates all meat plants that distribute meat across state lines. USDA inspectors look at every carcass of fresh meat harvested in the country to ensure that diseased animals are not distributed to the American public. The Environmental Protection Agency regulates pesticides in foods.

Restaurants are inspected by the local or state health department. These inspections involve conditions in a restaurant that could result directly in a health hazard or those that are indications of poor sanitation practices. Restaurants can be shut down until adequate corrections are made if serious infractions are found. Poor sanitation practices result in lower health rating scores. Most restaurants are required to post their most recent inspection results.

Governmental agencies are not perfect, but they provide a strong basis for a safe food supply. Agencies like those mentioned above can provide guidelines, inspect processing plants or restaurants, and investigate companies that are violating the law or regulations. They do not have the budgets to constantly inspect every food operation every day, week, month, or even year. They can't place agents in every public or commercial restroom to make sure we all wash our hands. They can't be in every field, backyard, or kitchen to make sure proper procedures are being followed. Every company and every consumer needs to assume the responsibility of improving the safety of our food.

1.16 Remember This!

This chapter is filled with much information, and it is not easy to remember it all, but we should try to remember the key points listed below:

- Many governmental agencies are responsible for monitoring the safety and quality of our food supply.
- Although not a true allergic reaction, celiac disease is an auto-immune disorder in which microvilli in the intestinal tract react with gliadin, a component of gluten found in wheat and other grains.

- Pests represent the greatest threat to availability of food, worldwide.
- Preservatives are food ingredients that slow spoilage and help prevent food-associated illnesses.
- A processed food should be designed to spoil before it becomes unsafe to make it less likely that someone will eat the unsafe food and become sick.
- The last meal consumed is not usually the meal responsible for an outbreak of food poisoning.
- An expiration date represents the food scientist's best guess about how long a food will last before it spoils.
- The most effective weapons in control of food-associated illnesses are proper sanitation and storage during handling and distribution from the farm to the consumer.
- Spoilage is not a good indicator of a safety risk.
- Fresh foods are more likely to contain harmful microbes than processed products.

1.17 Looking Ahead

This chapter was designed to introduce us to issues in food safety and entice us into reading further. Chapter 2 will introduce health issues associated with food, while Chapter 3 will explore reasons why we choose the foods we eat. For more information on food preservation, flip to Chapter 4. For more on quality testing procedures to reduce the chances of spoilage and safety hazards, check out Chapter 7. Greater detail on the effects of food preservation on the environment can be found in Chapter 9, whereas governmental regulations are discussed in Chapter 10. We will find more on preservatives, natural toxins, and chemical reactions that occur in foods in Chapter 11. Chapter 13 discusses in much greater detail the types of microbes in foods and how the food and its environment affect their growth.

Testing Comprehension

1. Select a story reported in the news or over the Internet in the last 2 months that is about food. Is this story credible? Why or why not? Find another story on the same subject that presents an alternate

view. Analyze the alternative view for its credibility. What can we do to help analyze whether a news story is credible?

2. Compare and contrast the characteristics of spoiled and unsafe foods. Is there any difference between a spoiled food and an unsafe one? Explain. Is the discussion in the chapter on spoiled and unsafe foods likely to change personal eating habits? Why or why not?

3. Find a packaged product that has an expiration date on it. Is it currently past that expiration date? Should it be consumed on or after the expiration date? Why or why not? What reasons would cause the product to expire? What would the dangers be to consuming it after its expiration date? Are there any problems associated with just throwing it away after its expiration date? Why or why not?

4. Outline the benefits and limitations of food preservation. Identify at least five methods of food preservation. Is food preserved in the home safer or less safe than food preserved in a food manufacturing plant? Why?

5. Alice wakes up on a Saturday morning at 10 with stomach cramps. Her roommate finds that she has a fever and shortly thereafter learns she has diarrhea. They go to a nearby health clinic for diagnosis and treatment. The medical staff indicates that she has food poisoning. Identify the probable cause of her illness. When was it likely that she consumed the food responsible for it? Why is her roommate not sick?

6. Diagram how a specific food could become contaminated. Identify the actions that could be taken to prevent this contamination and who should take these actions to prevent it.

7. Devise a strategy for a fast-food chain to avoid a potential boycott organized by activists who claim that the chain is poisoning its customers. A blog posted on the Internet claimed that methanol, a highly toxic component of antifreeze and biodiesel fuel, is produced in diet drinks sweetened with aspartame when the molecule breaks down to lose its sweetness. A comment in response to the blog indicates that methanol at similar concentrations is also a component of fresh, sliced tomatoes. A food scientist, interviewed on both NPR and Fox News, confirms that the blog and the comment are correct with regard to the presence of methanol in diet drinks losing their sweetness and in fresh-cut tomatoes.

8. Describe a personal experience or incident reported in the news about someone with food poisoning, an allergic reaction, or other sensitivity to a food or ingredient. How was the cause of the incident properly identified and diagnosed? How was it treated? How could a similar problem be prevented in the future?

9. Calculate the average percentage yield of meat from beef cattle if 2.6 million head are harvested each year to produce 2.0 billion pounds of beef with the average weight per head of 1306 pounds. What are the intended and unintended consequences of the removal of LFTB from ground beef?

References

Crim, S. M., M. Iwamoto and J. Y. Huang, 2014. Incidence and trends of infection with pathogens transmitted commonly through food—Foodborne Diseases Active Surveillance Network, 10 U.S. Sites, 2006–2013. MMWR 63,328.
Daniels, R. W., 1998. Home food safety. *Food Technol.*, 52(2):54.

Further Reading

Ali, N., 2014. *Understanding Celiac Disease: An Introduction for Patients and Caregivers,* Lanham, MD: The Rowman & Littlefield Publishing Group.
Colville, J. and D. Berryhill, 2007. *Handbook of Zoonoses: Identification and Prevention,* St. Louis, MO: Mosby.
Doyle, M. P. and R. L. Buchanan, 2012. *Food Microbiology: Fundamentals and Frontiers,* 4th ed., Washington, DC: ASM Press.
Madsen, C., R. Crevel, C. Mills and S. Taylor, 2013. *Risk Management for Food Allergy,* San Diego, CA: Academic Press.
Montville, T. J., K. R. Matthews and K. E. Kniel, 2012. *Food Microbiology, an Introduction,* 3rd ed., Washington, DC: ASM Press.
Morris, J. G. and M. Potter, 2013. *Foodborne Infections and Intoxications,* 4th ed., San Diego, CA: Academic Press.
Ray, B. and A. Bhunia, 2013. *Fundamental Food Microbiology,* 5th ed., Boca Raton, FL: CRC Press.
Wheeler, W. B. 2007. *Pesticides in Agriculture and the Environment,* New York: Marcel Dekker.

2

Healthiness of Foods

Garrett is into working out. He is the backup first baseman on his university baseball team, and he needs to bulk up to get more power in his swing. He works the weight machines every day, but he realizes that exercise is only part of a healthy lifestyle and that nutrition is the other part. He learns that most foods are unhealthy for one reason or another and that the best way to bulk up is to get rid of carbohydrates and get his energy from protein. He likes fresh, whole foods, particularly meat and dairy products.

Jennifer is giving up meat. She is becoming disgusted with the American fast-food culture that features fatty burgers, greasy fries, and sugar-laden drinks. She knows these foods are unhealthy. At first, she just eliminated red meats from her diet. A little later, after hearing about the gross things that happen to chickens on the farm, she now only eats fish. Then, in talking with some of her newfound friends who were also shunning meats, she is thinking about eliminating all dairy products—eggs and anything else that comes from animals. When she stopped hanging out with Garrett because he insisted on keeping his carnivorous habits, she became even more serious. One of the things she likes the best is that this diet is so simple. All she would need to do is to eat anything that is not from animals. She was surprised at the diversity of products available. There are lots of grains, fruits, and vegetables, and they are actually very tasty. At first she was hungry all the time, but after a while the hunger pangs went away.

Malik decided to weigh himself on the scale so thoughtfully provided by the cafeteria. He knew he had been gaining weight (or all his jeans were shrinking), but he wasn't sure how much. He looked down and couldn't believe it. He was only halfway through his freshman year, and he had already gained 13 pounds of the dreaded Freshman-Fifteen! It was time for some serious weight loss. What could he do? He'd read that carbohydrates were the problem and decided to try the latest diet, which replaces all those "nasty" carbohydrates with protein. It was time to start eating healthy and get away from all that pizza and other junk food served up by the cafeteria.

Garrett, Jennifer, and Malik think that their diets are reasonably healthy, but they all have misconceptions. This chapter will explore what healthiness means. We'll introduce the basic nutrients and describe what we need to consider in designing a healthy diet.

2.1 Looking Back

The previous chapter focused on issues concerning the safety of foods. The following key points in that chapter help prepare us for understanding processed foods:

- Preservatives are food ingredients that slow spoilage and help prevent food-associated illnesses.
- A processed food should be designed to spoil before it becomes unsafe to make it less likely that someone will eat the unsafe food and become sick.
- An expiration date represents the food scientist's best guess about how long a food will last before it spoils.
- Spoilage is not an indicator of a safety risk.
- Fresh foods are more likely to contain harmful microbes than processed products.

2.2 Healthy Foods and Unhealthy Foods

Many of us are interested in eating healthier, but sometimes it is difficult to know what is healthy and what is not healthy. Foods like carrots, apples, lettuce, sprouts, whole wheat bread, and yogurt have a healthy image whereas colas, beer, chocolate bars, pizza, hamburgers, fries, and most appetizers in our favorite restaurants don't. It seems that healthy foods are often unappetizing or tasteless, but unhealthy foods are temptingly flavorful. Is it possible to eat healthy foods and enjoy them too?

When we talk about eating healthy, we are talking about nutrition. Good nutrition involves getting the proper nutrients without consuming too many calories. Obviously, any food that has a good balance of nutrients but can cause food poisoning is not very healthy. Thus, a food must be safe as well as nutritious to be healthy. Food scientists and nutritionists tend to discuss healthy and unhealthy diets rather than healthy and unhealthy foods. Healthy diets require a balance of nutrients and yet allow for a few foods that might not qualify as healthy foods. Unhealthy diets generally do not provide adequate amounts of some nutrients while other nutrients may be present in excess.

2.3 Energy from Foods

In a time when it seems that everyone is either overweight, on a low-calorie diet, or both, it is easy to forget the main reason for eating—to get energy. We get energy from food in the form of calories. There are three main sources of calories—carbohydrates, proteins, and fats. Carbohydrates and proteins provide approximately 4 calories of energy per gram (114 calories per ounce). Fats provide approximately 9 calories per gram (255 calories per ounce), more than twice as much as carbohydrates or proteins. That's why we are more likely to lose weight if we cut back on fat instead of proteins or carbohydrates. However, we need a balance in the sources of our calories.

Although most of us could stand to cut back on the fat we consume, we do need some fat in our diet. Overall, though, we need to keep in mind that a small amount of fat in our diet (usually no more than 30% of the total calories) is not only healthy but necessary. Despite its deficiencies, fat contributes to satiety; that is, it slows down digestive processes and prolongs stomach-emptying time. Meals with a modest amount of fat will need more time to digest, resulting in longer between periods of hunger. Fats are also the vehicle of absorption for vitamins A, D, E, and K (fat-soluble vitamins) as well as other healthy compounds like lycopene. Certain fats have been associated with improved health. Among these fats are omega-3 fatty acids, conjugated linoleic acid, and flaxseed, hemp, and fish oils.

We also need protein to perform other functions in addition to providing calories. However, when protein becomes the major source of energy, we may not produce enough glucose in the blood to maintain proper brain functioning. A special class of proteins called enzymes speeds up chemical reactions in the body. These enzymes need special substances (cofactors) to help them perform properly. The enzymes and other molecular components in our bodies are constantly under construction.

The other main nutritional reason for eating food is to get vitamins and minerals. Vitamins and minerals are needed to support bodily processes. Essential vitamins and minerals serve as enzyme cofactors or components of these cofactors.

A third nutritional component is **dietary fiber**. Fresh fruits and vegetables are high in dietary fiber as are products containing whole grains. Dietary fiber is chemically a carbohydrate that comes from the cell walls of plants; much of it is indigestible by the body so it contributes fewer calories than other carbohydrates like sugars and starch. Dietary fiber adds bulk to the diet to help keep bowel movements regular. It also helps remove toxins from the intestines and may help in the prevention of many of the diseases associated with overnutrition. Too much dietary fiber, however, can bind vitamins and minerals, thus making a malnourished condition worse.

Basic nutrition is more simple and straightforward than it is portrayed in the media and in popular books. On the other hand, human physiology and metabolism (what happens to those nutrients inside our bodies) is more complex than the oversimplified explanations in the same media and books. It is also a good idea to include an exercise plan as part of an overall diet plan.

2.4 Food and Disease

One thing many of us are concerned about is how the food we eat will affect our health. Although food-borne diseases can be a concern, when we talk about healthy foods, we are talking about foods that will help us avoid the diseases of civilization (cancer, diabetes, heart disease, and obesity). Hunger, malnutrition, and infection are the major killers in less industrialized societies. More industrialized countries tend to have higher standards of sanitation and better healthcare. As a result, the citizens tend to live longer and are

Country	Life expectancy 2006	Life expectancy 2014	Infant mortality 2009
Angola	37.6	55.3	180.2
South Africa	42.5	49.6	44.4
Nigeria	47.4	52.6	94.3
Kenya	55.3	63.5	54.7
Bangladesh	62.8	70.6	59.0
Russia	65.9	70.2	10.5
India	68.6	67.8	30.1
Iran	70.6	70.9	35.7
China	72.9	75.2	20.2
Mexico	75.6	75.4	18.4
United States	78.0	79.6	6.2
United Kingdom	78.7	80.4	4.8
France	79.9	81.7	3.3
Canada	80.3	81.7	5.0
Australia	80.6	82.1	4.7
Japan	81.4	84.7	2.8

INSERT 2.1
Life expectancy (at birth in years) in 2006 and 2014 and infant mortality rate (infant deaths per 1000 births) in 2009 for selected countries. (Adapted from http://www.infoplease.com as derived from US Census Bureau, International Database.)

more likely to become obese and develop cancer, diabetes, or heart disease. During the last 100 years, there have been major increases in life expectancy (see Insert 2.1 for changes in the last decade in selected countries), and quality of life in our aging years is being seen as a more important goal as the aging population grows.

Most of the health problems associated with food are caused by either not getting enough food or getting too much. First, our bodies must get enough energy to supply our needs. The unit of energy is the calorie (more appropriately, the **kilocalorie**). Energy provided by food comes from the macronutrients (carbohydrates, fats, and proteins), not caffeine or other stimulants. Acute malnutrition resulting in growth failure is attributed to inadequate calories, protein, or both. Overnutrition leads to the development of obesity and associated diseases.

Most people get enough protein and calories, but they still can be malnourished. Not getting enough of specific vitamins or minerals can result in a deficiency disease. For example, not getting enough vitamin C can result in scurvy, which is characterized by bleeding gums, blotchy bruises, and failure of wounds to heal. Lack of vitamin A can prevent cells from developing properly and lead to night blindness. Anemia can result from not enough iron or a lack of vitamin B_{12}. Osteoporosis is the result of a calcium insufficiency. Such deficiency diseases are worldwide problems. Deficiency diseases can be devastating, but the cause, preventive measures, and treatments are clear.

Cancer is the most dreaded disease of civilized societies. It has been estimated that approximately 20% of the deaths in the United States are attributed to cancer. Cancer is not a single disease; rather, it is a term that groups many similar diseases characterized by abnormal cellular growth and malignancy. The good news is that many cancers are attributed to environmental causes and are presumed to be preventable. The bad news is that the causes, treatment, and prevention of cancer are not as simple as for deficiency diseases. Cancer is not a deficiency disease of a vitamin or mineral. It is not usually caused by the ingestion of a single carcinogen or prevented by a single food, nutrient, or drug. Although diet plays a role in either increasing or decreasing the risks associated with a type of cancer, rarely is it the specific cause.

Heart disease is the leading killer in the world. It must be understood that in the classification of causes of death, no one dies of old age. If Garrett lives until the age of 93 when his heart stops beating and nothing else is seriously wrong with him, he will be classified as dying of heart disease. Generally speaking, overconsumption of food, particularly fatty foods, increases the chances of developing heart disease. Smoking and excessive consumption of alcohol are also risk factors for heart disease. Similar factors increase the risk of developing diabetes. Diabetes is a disease with several levels of treatment: diet, medication, and insulin injection. Although a diabetic must be very careful with dietary intake, it is not clear that overconsumption of sugar in a prediabetic state is the cause of the onset of the disease. As with cancer, the cause, treatment, and prevention of heart disease and diabetes are not as clear as for malnutrition.

A word here about cause and effect might be appropriate. An article from the Internet proclaims, "Tea Consumption Doubles the Chance of Conception." The article points out that tea drinkers (presumably women) are twice as likely to become pregnant as people who do not drink tea. Now, most of us are sophisticated enough to know that it takes more than drinking tea for a woman to conceive. Is there something in the tea that makes a woman more fertile? Is tea really an aphrodisiac? The lack of a cause-and-effect relationship in this example is clear, but in many things, we see in the media that it is more difficult to separate the cause from the effect.

2.5 Weight Loss without Pain

Whether it is fighting the "Freshman Fifteen" or trying to maintain one's appearance for the next social outing, there is a great deal of pressure for weight control and keeping "in shape" on any college campus. Although most of us realize controlling our weight is about diet and exercise, we still hope that there is an easier way to lose weight. Many advertisements for supplements, foods, or weight-loss programs offer remedies without pain. Unfortunately, there is no simple way to lose weight. Fad diets, fat burners, and other miracle weight-loss regimes make empty promises. Counting calories is still the most effective way of monitoring food intake, and knowledge of food composition, keeping a sensible exercise plan, and showing willpower are the three most successful elements of a good weight-loss program.

Maintaining a healthy body weight is important in remaining fit and in feeling good about ourselves. We can determine if we have a healthy body weight by locating our body mass index in Insert 2.2. As an athlete, Garrett works out frequently (more than two vigorous sessions of 30 minutes or longer a week) in addition to the time spent in baseball practice and appears to be overweight by the chart, but he realizes that the chart does not allow for extra muscle mass. Jennifer, however, is not heavy enough. She is probably not eating enough food and could be malnourished. Being underweight may be as much of a health risk as being overweight. Another serious health problem is weight cycling: the repeated loss and regain of body weight.

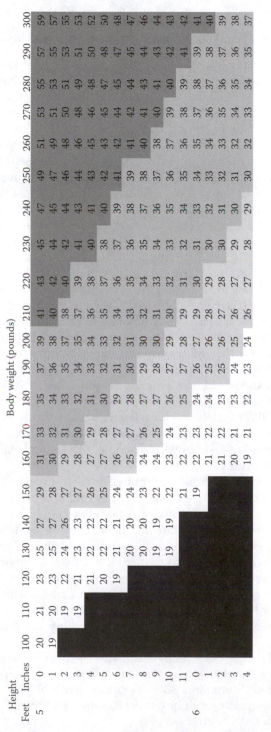

INSERT 2.2
Body mass index chart. (From Body Mass Index and Health, Nutrition Insights, vol. 13, No. 2, USDA 2001. www.cnpp.usda.gov/FENR/FENR/FENRv13n2/fenrv13n2p52.pdf.)

2.6 Popular Diets, Food Fads, and Their Consequences

The concept of a diverse and balanced diet appears to be giving way to diets tailored to meet unique nutritional needs. Of course, there may be a few individuals with special dietary needs, but, in general, our nutritional requirements tend to be very similar. An overexaggeration of different dietary requirements leads to food fads and can result in malnutrition.

The Appalachian Trail Diet (Insert 2.3) is effective, but it is not popular because there are many competing diets that promise quick weight loss with much less exertion. Malik adopted one of the most popular diets by cutting down on carbohydrates and increasing proteins. The idea is that consumption of carbohydrates stimulates insulin production, which leads the body to convert the carbohydrates to stored fat. The diet assumes that consumption of proteins stimulates glucagon production, which leads the body to use proteins and fats for energy. Although this theory sounds good, it ignores the energy needs of the body and the calorie levels of food. Most food scientists, nutritionists, and dieticians are skeptical about the effectiveness of low-carbohydrate/high-protein diets and are concerned that these diets can cause long-term damage to strict followers. Unfortunately, these diets are very popular with many physicians, who tend to have limited training in nutrition but serve at the front lines of dietary guidance.

In many parts of the world, the average person takes in 70% or more of their calories from carbohydrates, whereas the average American tends to take in less than 50% of daily calories from carbohydrates. Nevertheless, Americans are more likely to be overweight than people from other countries. If low-carbohydrate diets can trick people into losing weight, why are they considered harmful?

When we don't consume enough carbohydrates and consume too much protein, our bodies begin to use the protein as fuel and not as material to make new proteins. Too much protein in our diet also leads to excretion of excessive urea in urine, which can lead to severe kidney damage. High-protein diets can also lead to a loss of calcium, and they also frequently contain high levels of fat. In addition, the body cannot store protein; thus, it converts the excess protein to fat and then stores it. Furthermore, low-carbohydrate diets result in an imbalanced state called **ketosis**. In ketosis, the body cannot maintain enough blood sugar to meet the needs of the brain, with extended periods of ketosis possibly resulting in brain damage.

Eating a balanced diet does help us make the most of what we have. Claims that food or supplements can make us smarter or help us concentrate are exaggerated. Stimulants such as caffeine can help us stay awake and increase our attention level; however, too much caffeine can make us irritable and lead to anxiety attacks.

Toll of the trail

How do eight weeks of hiking affect the human body? Prior to setting out on the Appalachian Trail, reporter Scott Huler, 35, dropped by the Raleigh Athletic Club to have some vital statistics recorded. Then, within a week after completing his 410-mile stint, Huler, who is 6'3", was re-examined. Some key findings:

Stat	Before (3/20)	After (5/10)
Chest	36½"	34½"
Arm (flexed)	12¾"	12"
Waist	34½"	30"
Hips	37¾"	36¼"
Thigh (flexed)	22¼"	21⅛"
Calf	15"	14½"
Weight	172 lbs.	162 lbs.
Blood pressure (resting)	106/76	110/72
Heart rate (resting) (in beats per minute)	62	66
Body-fat analysis	8.6%	6.2%
Bench press (max.)	160 lbs.	175 lbs.
Leg extension (max.)	135 lbs.	155 lbs.

Trail diet

An average day of food consumption for a hiker looks something like this:

Food	Calories	Calories from fat	Protein (grams)	Carbohydrates (grams)	Fat (grams)
BREAKFAST					
Oatmeal	160	16	4	33	2
Tangerine	65	0	1	16	0
Pop-Tart	210	70	3	34	7
LUNCH					
Cheese	300	210	21	3	24
Bread	140	5	6	31	0.5
Peanut butter	380	260	16	14	32
Jelly	50	0	0	0	0
Dried-meat stick	280	110	7	0	12
SNACKS					
Snickers bars (2)	560	240	8	72	28
Gorp*	1,240	320	30	174	49
DINNER					
Freeze-dried Lipton dinner	500	60	20	80	8
Total	**3,885**	**1,291**	**116**	**457**	**162.5**

* Includes raisins, peanuts, M&Ms and granola

The U.S. Department of Health and Human Services recommends a normal daily diet of about 2,000 calories.

A person Huler's size, carrying his backpack, walking 3 mph, would burn about 354 calories per hour. By comparison, he might expect to burn 432 calories per hour doing calisthenics or 630 calories per hour swimming.

INSERT 2.3
Appalachian trail diet. (From Huler, S., "Appalachian Adventures," *Charlotte News and Observer*, 1995. With permission.)

Academy of Nutrition and Dietetics, http://www.eatright.org

Center for Nutrition Policy and Promotion, http://www.cnpp.usda.gov

FITDAY, http://www.fitday.com

Food Insight, http://www.foodinsight.com

Nutrition.gov, http://www.nutrition.gov

Sports, Cardiovascular and Wellness Nutrition, http://www.scandpg.org/sports-nutrition/

USDA, ChooseMyPlate.gov, http://www.ChooseMyPlate.gov

Weight Watchers, http://www.weightwatchers.com

INSERT 2.4
Some websites to consult to get more information on nutritional quality of foods and developing reasonable diet plans.

Lack of enough calories interferes with our ability to stay alert and attentive. On the other hand, too many calories can lead to sleepiness and laziness. Inadequate consumption of vitamins and minerals can also affect our ability to concentrate. There is some evidence that certain foods (or their components) can affect our mood, but the linkage has not been clearly established. There are few if any magical foods, but a balanced diet contributes to health and well-being, whereas a poor diet can lead to laziness, inattentiveness, and a bad attitude.

The sad part about many food fads is that people who intend to eat healthy do not know the nutritional benefits or detriments of a particular food, supplement, ingredient, or component in the context of an overall diet. Thus, by trying to improve their health, they may actually be harming it. There is much good information about health in the news media, but there is also much misinformation. For some useful websites on nutrition, see Insert 2.4.

2.7 Fake Fats

If low-carbohydrate/high-protein diets don't work, then should we lower fat consumption? Since an ounce of fat contains twice the calories as an ounce of protein or carbohydrate, we can cut back our calorie consumption twice as fast if we cut out fats. There are many ways we can reduce calories in our diet. One way is to just do without them. Another way to avoid fats is to eat foods typically low in fats. The main problem with low-fat diets, however, is that most people get easily discouraged and give up because they miss the flavor that fat provides and end up cheating on their diet.

The technological solutions designed by food scientists are low-fat versions of typically fatty foods, which would allow Malik to enjoy his favorite foods without consuming large amounts of fat. It is not as simple as just removing the fat, however. For example, removing all the fat and sugar in a large cup of frozen yogurt results in a very small cup of yogurt that is not nearly as appetizing and flavorful. Still, there are several ways to lower the fat content in foods. One way is to replace the fat with carbohydrates, proteins, or a combination of both. Unfortunately, this approach does not always result in caloric reduction. Another way of lowering the fat is by replacing it with something that adds bulk to the product but does not provide calories. However, there is a price to pay for consuming too much of these delicious treats—bloating and digestive distress.

Reducing fat consumption can also be achieved by using the so-called *fake fats* like Olestra®. These fake fats have all the taste sensations of true fats in the mouth, but the body is not able to absorb them; thus, they have no calories. Olestra is in many products, but probably the product that most people are familiar with is fat-free potato chips. Unfortunately, Olestra interferes with the body's ability to use vitamins A and D properly. This problem is remedied by replacing these vitamins. Another problem with Olestra is that its lubricating properties in the mouth are duplicated in the lower intestines, resulting in some rather loose stools. This problem is not usually a major one for people who refrain from eating large amounts at a single sitting.

Although fat reduction can be an important part of a disciplined weight-loss plan, there are some typical mistakes dieters make with foods. First, the more they lower fats in their diet, the harder they find it to stick with the diet because fats contribute to the enjoyment of foods. Generally, a reduced-fat food is more likely to satisfy than one that is fat-free. Regardless of how fats are reduced in the diet, weight loss will not occur unless there is a reduction in calories. That is, if we cut half the fat, yet eat twice as much, we will not lose weight.

2.8 Dietary Supplements, Nutraceuticals, and Functional Foods

Dietary supplements are substances that are taken to supply a need or reinforce one's diet. Until recently, the term was used to describe pills that were consumed to make up for an essential nutrient that was not supplied by the diet. In the past, parents provided their children with vitamins and minerals in a single pill a day (sometimes in the form of a favorite cartoon character) to make sure they were not deficient in any essential nutrients. Now, we can supplement the nutritional quality of our diet with protein powders, medicinal herbs, supernutritious chocolate bars, and many other foods that make nutritional claims.

Most dieticians prefer that we obtain our vitamins and minerals from whole foods. Sometimes, however, supplements of specific nutrients are needed in special circumstances. For example, women of childbearing age typically need additional iron and folic acid, vegetarians need more iron and vitamin B$_{12}$, and lactose-intolerant individuals need additional calcium. Dietary supplements have now gone beyond the supplying of essential nutrients. We are now consuming garlic for infections and prevention of atherosclerosis, cranberries to maintain a healthy urinary tract, echinacea for the treatment of sore throats and colds, and St. John's wort for depression. We are beginning to think that we can treat our symptoms at home for most diseases without the need of a physician.

Nutraceuticals are foods specifically designed to act as drugs. Nutraceuticals are the food industry's answer to the health-food market. Many of these ingredients are added to improve mood. Although there appears to be a relationship between foods and mood, the linkage has not been clearly established. With the potential profitability of nutraceuticals, food companies have rushed in to gain their share of the market. One problem that food scientists face in designing nutraceuticals is producing a truly healthy product that also has good sensory quality because many of the ingredients used to formulate a product have a nasty flavor. Food scientists need to find ways to build in flavor without losing the nutritional value or health benefits of the product.

Functional foods are marketed to perform a specific function. Two of the hottest trends in food products today are nutrition and convenience. Vitamin- and mineral-filled chocolate bars and drinks provide quick, easy nutrition with the extra fat and sugar providing a pleasant way to get all the nutrients one needs. Likewise, sugared and fortified breakfast cereals perform a similar function. Sports drinks supply vitamins and minerals, as well as electrolytes to replenish the ones lost in sweat during a workout. Calcium-fortified orange juice provides an alternative to dairy products for consumers who dislike or have sensitivities to milk. With the discovery of additional benefits of certain components, some traditional foods are now being promoted as functional foods. For example, ketchup is high in lycopene, which is a powerful antioxidant, and mustard is now being touted as being healthful because of the presence of antimicrobial compounds and antioxidants.

With all this information available, how is the consumer supposed to cope with it when even professionals have trouble sorting through it all? There are some guidelines we should consider next time we buy a supplement, nutraceutical, or functional food:

- It is a fallacy that if a little is good, a lot is better (it might even be toxic—just like drugs, leading to an overdose).
- Many of these substances have not been thoroughly studied, and when studied have generally been tested in isolation and not in the presence of the wide variety of substances that make up a typical diet.

- A substance may be present but not at a high enough level to be effective (much more may be needed to cure depression, acne, or warts than is available in that herbal tea).
- An effectively high dose may be doing other damage (some of these supplements cause serious interactions with prescription drugs).
- There may be other components present that could have adverse effects when consumed at too high a level.

As the medical and nutritional sciences advance, we will find substances and combinations of substances that are truly beneficial to health. Presently, however, there are more products available that consumers trust and are willing to buy than there are products with proven health benefits.

It remains to be seen if the growth of dietary supplements and functional foods is a fad, a fundamental change, or a springboard for new products that will be permanently incorporated into our diets. It is hard to believe that the original Kellogg's and Post breakfast cereals that are so much a part of our culture today were part of the health-food craze that affected Americans of the late 1800s.

2.9 Enhancing Athletic Performance

There is one group of consumers who is particularly interested in nutrition and in dietary supplements—athletes. They are looking for performance enhancement through dietary supplements. The most important nutritional need of an athlete is additional calories. Insufficient calories to replace the ones burned off during exertion and exercise will result in weight loss, and excessive weight loss results in loss of strength. The increased calories of an athlete's diet require increased levels of vitamins, but there is little information to support megadosing with vitamins. Women athletes generally can benefit from extra calcium and iron. It appears that athletes have a greater need for dietary iron than nonathletes.

Increased protein consumption may lead to increases in muscle nitrogen balance in active athletes. Protein supplements are available as whole proteins or amino acids in the form of pills, powders, and potions. Protein powders are likely to contain nonfat dried milk, soy products, and other non-animal sources. Consumption of large amounts of animal proteins, like a big juicy steak, is likely to add excess fat and cholesterol to the diet. The building blocks of proteins are amino acids. Our digestive system breaks down the proteins we consume into amino acids. The consequences of consuming large doses of amino acids have not been widely studied, although some, like tryptophan, can have toxic impurities that can lead to illness or death. Consumption of individual amino acids is not recommended, as they may lead to metabolic imbalances. Branched-chain amino acids are particularly popular, as they are thought to be more likely to serve as energy sources and to enhance serotonin production. Serotonin may enhance performance and raise the threshold for pain, but the short-term gain could have undesirable long-term consequences.

Optimal diets for athletes in training are 60%–70% calories from carbohydrates, 25%–30% calories from fat, and 10%–15% calories from protein—not the low-carbohydrate, high-protein diets many are trying. Whether we are participating in intercollegiate athletics or just working out on our own, our diet should meet both our long-term and short-term health needs. There are many good books on sports nutrition that are based on solid nutrition science. One is listed in the Further Reading section of this chapter. There are many not-so-good books, articles, and individuals who have strange ideas about sports, training, exercise, and nutrition. We shouldn't let them experiment on us with their untested ideas, as we could be suffering the consequences many years after we are finished with competitive sports.

2.10 Six Glasses a Day

Water is the major component of most foods. Next to oxygen, it is the most important nutrient for our body. We can only live a few minutes in the absence of oxygen and a few days without water. It is recommended that we drink one and one-half quarts (approximately six glasses) of water per day. The idea that we can only get water from the bottle or the tap is misguided, though; we can obtain sufficient water from foods and beverages; however, we must not think we are getting sufficient water when we drink caffeinated or alcoholic beverages.

Caffeine and alcohol are diuretic, which means they increase the frequency of urination. Thus, some of the water goes down the toilet rather than meeting our daily needs. That is why our trips down the hall or stops at the rest areas are more frequent when we drink too much coffee, cola, sweet tea, beer, or similar refreshments. Another problem with consuming too many sugared or alcoholic beverages is that we may be adding excess calories and thus adding to a potential weight problem. In dry climates, we need to consume more water because we lose more of it through the pores in the skin than in moist climates. Although water collects on our skin as beads of sweat in humid climates, it evaporates immediately into the dry air in dry climates. Electrolyte (sodium and potassium) balance is essential in maintaining proper water balance in our tissues. An extreme case is where individuals have consumed too much water (water intoxication or **overhydration**), which can lead to death owing to low levels of sodium in the blood.

2.11 Fasting

People of many religious faiths practice fasting as a way to purify the mind and the body. Fasts usually involve the elimination, for a period, of all solid foods. Juice fasts permit the consumption of nutritious beverages, but strict fasts do not even permit the consumption of water. Ramadan is a month of strict fasting from sunup to sundown practiced by Muslims. Every Jewish person over 13 is expected to fast for 24 hours at Yom Kippur. Drinking of water is permitted. Fasting is an integral part of the Hindu religion. It was an important part of the early Christian church, but fasting is not as widely practiced by Christians today.

Even for a short time, fasting is an effective expression of self-sacrifice. Spiritualists who fast recommend starting with small fasts before progressing to extended ones. Fasting, combined with meditation, tends to help us focus on the things that are really important in life, but it can have nutritional consequences. Fasting is self-starvation and can result in severe nutritional deficiencies. When we consume more energy than we burn, we store excess calories as glycogen (animal and human reserve of glucose) and fat. During a fast, the body breaks down glycogen first, followed by fat. As stated previously, the brain needs glucose to function properly. When blood glucose is low, it sends signals out to break down fat and protein. In an extended fast, proteins are broken down, producing ketone bodies leading to ketosis. During a total fast, up to a half-pound of fat can be burned at the potential cost of loss of brain function as the ketone bodies are not an adequate substitute for glucose.

2.12 Eating Disorders

Eating disorders develop when peer pressure clashes with biological needs. The most common eating disorder is anorexia. It involves a self-induced fast to lose weight. Advanced stages of anorexia can interfere with normal sleep, induce depression, and lead to malnutrition. In the second stage of anorexia, anorexics become desensitized to hunger pangs and develop an aversion for most foods, eating just enough to survive but not enough to thrive. The body shuts down vital processes to conserve energy. The final stage of anorexia results in wasting, withering, and death, similar to starvation associated with famines.

A related disorder, bulimia, results in anorexia through self-induced vomiting or excessive use of laxatives, enemas, or diuretics. Since the food is not in the body long enough for most of the nutrients to be absorbed, weight loss and other symptoms of anorexia result.

Binge eating is a frequent response to stress (exams, grades, dysfunctional personal relationships, and peer pressure), resulting in weight gain. Binge-and-starve diets result in nutritional imbalances and interfere with the body's normal metabolic processes. People with this disorder are particularly susceptible to zinc deficiencies.

Studies have shown that women, particularly those of college age, tend to be more susceptible to eating disorders than men owing to hormonal secretions and greater social pressure to be thin. It is very important to catch an eating disorder before it gets out of hand. Treatment is painful and serious digestive problems, such as spastic colon, can persist after a normal diet has been resumed. Most college campus health centers have

Signs and symptoms of anorexia nervosa
- Weight loss leading to a body weight of 85 percent of what's considered acceptable
- Intense fear of being "fat" or gaining weight
- Frequent weighing
- Develops ritualistic eating habits, such as cutting food into tiny pieces, eating alone, and dragging out meals
- Loss of menstrual period
- Excessive exercise
- Increased sensitivity to cold
- Refuses to admit eating patterns are abnormal
- Withdraws socially

Signs and symptoms of bulimia
- Preoccupation with food, weight, and appearance
- Eats large volumes of food and then "gets rid" of it by vomiting, fasting, exercising, or taking laxatives
- Experiences mood swings and depression
- Dental problems
- Stomach and digestive problems—such as bloating, constipation, diarrhea
- Scratched or scarred knuckles from scraping against teeth to induce vomiting
- Irritation of the esophagus and throat
- Realization that eating pattern is abnormal
- Irregular menstrual periods

How to help a friend with an eating disorder
- Choose a time and place to talk away from distractions and other interruptions.
- Don't be judgmental.
- Be a good listener, but don't promise to keep serious information confidential.
- Don't assume the role of a therapist or nutritionist.
- Don't oversimplify the problem by saying, "All you have to do is eat."
- Don't engage in a battle, but don't ignore the problem.

INSERT 2.5
Signs and symptoms of anorexia and bulimia and how to help. (Excerpted in part from Litt, A.S., *The College Student's Guide to Eating Well on Campus*, Revised and Expanded Edition, Tulip Hill Press, Bethesda, MD, 2005, Chapter 6. With permission.)

programs that will provide counseling. For more insight into eating disorders, see Insert 2.5.

2.13 Natural, Organic, and Whole Foods

Many consumers are concerned about the foods produced by modern food
technology. They long to return to simpler, more "pure" foods. These consumers reject many of the commercially packaged foods, believing that natural, organic, or whole foods provide more nutritious and safe alternatives.
However, food scientists do not believe such alternatives are necessarily
more nutritious or safe. Although natural, organic, and whole foods are similar, they also have distinct differences. Sometimes, it is difficult to distinguish the difference between these foods. To confuse matters further, some
consumers use different definitions to identify certain foods. Classifying the
foods in Insert 2.6 is not as simple as it first seems.

Natural foods can be found in nature, unlike colas, potato chips, snack
cakes, breakfast beverages, nutritional bars, and frozen entrees. What "natural" means, however, is not always clear and, in fact, there are no standards
or regulations regarding the production of "natural" products, especially if
they do not contain meats or eggs. Few would argue that fresh garden vegetables, meat from animals hunted in the wild, or mushrooms and herbs
gathered in the woods would qualify as natural foods. Most, but not all, consumers would consider fresh vegetables grown in greenhouses, beef steaks
from a supermarket, or dried spices also to be natural. Items such as canned
corn, breads, pastas, and juices are more difficult to classify.

Are natural products more nutritious or safer than "unnatural" ones? Food
scientists believe that we need more information to make that determination.
A freshly picked ear of corn is more nutritious if it is cooked properly shortly
after harvest than if it is canned. Overcooking the ear of corn, however, can
be just as damaging to the nutrients as the canning process. If we quickly
blanch and freeze the ear of corn, it will retain its nutrients much better than
if it is stored for several days in the refrigerator. Most food scientists would
take their chances with a fresh beef steak from the supermarket that has
been inspected by the United States Department of Agriculture (USDA) over
a fresh venison steak from a weekend hunter who has slaughtered and cut
up the deer in a neighborhood deer cooler.

According to the USDA, "Organic is a labeling term that indicates that the
food or other agricultural product has been produced through approved
methods. These methods integrate cultural, biological, and mechanical
practices that foster cycling of resources, promote ecological balance, and
conserve biodiversity. Synthetic fertilizers, sewage sludge, irradiation, and
genetic engineering may not be used." Organic food production attempts

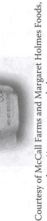

Courtesy of The Beef Checkoff

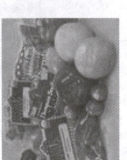

Courtesy of Melissa's Organics, Melissa's World Variety Produce, http://www.melissas.com

Silk and Silk Live! are registered trademarks of WhiteWave Foods Company; use of photo is authorized

Courtesy of McCall Farms and Margaret Holmes Foods, http://www.margaretholmes.com

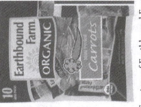

Courtesy of Earthbound Farm, http://www.ebfarm.com

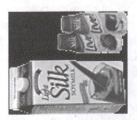

Courtesy of Moringa Nutritional Foods, Inc., http://www.morinu.com

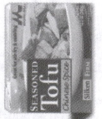

INSERT 2.6

Which of the following products are natural, organic, processed, or whole foods? Natural: fruit, steak, and carrots; organic: fruit and carrots; processed: soymilk, tofu, and peanuts; whole: fruit, corn, carrots, and peanuts; whole: fruit, corn, carrots, and steak. Based on the information provided and the definitions of the terms.

to minimize inputs of fossil fuels and synthetic chemicals. Animal manure and composted plant materials serve as fertilizers for organic crops. Organic products have a marketing advantage, but they tend to cost more and have a shorter shelf life than their conventional counterparts.

As described above, a freshly harvested plant part is likely to be more nutritious than one that has been shipped and stored for a longer period. However, there is little, if any, scientific evidence to support the claim that organic foods are more nutritious and safer than conventional products. For example, the use of animal manure as a fertilizer certainly does not make a crop safer, particularly a root crop like potatoes or carrots.

The term *organic* is also used to describe meat products that come from animals that have not been treated with antibiotics or synthetic growth hormones and have consumed feeds that were not treated with pesticides. There are legitimate concerns about the overuse of antibiotics because it has been shown that antibiotic overuse can produce drug-resistant strains of bacteria, which threaten human health. Meats that claim to be "hormone-free" are misleading because hormones are natural components of any plant or animal. Thus, the only truly "hormone-free" foods are distinctly "unnatural."

Whole foods are those foods that are readily identifiable by their original components. Milk, fresh or processed fruits and vegetables, as well as whole or ground meats would be considered whole foods. Generally speaking, whole foods have more nutrients with less sugar and fat than many snack foods. There are exceptions, such as ripe bananas, which have very high levels of sugar; avocados (or guacamole); and butter, which are very high in fat. Also, fortified breakfast cereals could hardly be considered whole foods, but they contain an extensive list of vitamins and minerals. Food scientists consider synthetic nutrients to be just as effective as natural ones. Once again, a name such as "whole food" does not guarantee better nutrition. We need more information about the product before we can determine how nutritious or how safe it is.

2.14 Reading the Label

Nutrition labels can help us with the nutritional quality of our diets. Fresh fruits, vegetables, and meats do not have nutrition labels, but there are many resources we can refer to for these values. The Nutrition Facts part of the label indicates the serving size, how many servings per container, calories per serving, and the fat calories per serving in the left column. Then there is a chart that provides the amount per serving of the macronutrients (total fat, total carbohydrate, and protein). Fat is further broken down into saturated fat, polyunsaturated fat, monounsaturated fat, and *trans* fats. Although a controversial issue in nutrition, it is recommended that we limit our intake of *trans* fats. At best, they count as saturated fatty acids; at worst, they could be toxic.

Product A

Nutrition Facts

Serving Size (21g)
Servings Per Container

Amount Per Serving

Calories 70	Calories from Fat 0

	% Daily Value*
Total Fat 0g	0%
Saturated Fat g	
Trans Fat g	
Cholesterol 0mg	0%
Sodium 170mg	7%
Total Carbohydrate 15g	5%
Dietary Fiber 1g	4%
Sugars 2g	
Protein 4g	

Vitamin A 10%	•	Vitamin C 15%
	•	Iron 30%

*Percent Daily Values are based on a 2,000 calorie diet. Your daily values may be higher or lower depending on your calorie needs:

		Calories	2,000	2,500
Total Fat	Less Than		65g	80g
Saturated Fat	Less Than		20g	25g
Cholesterol	Less Than		300mg	300 mg
Sodium	Less Than		2,400mg	2,400mg
Total Carbohydrate			300g	375g
Dietary Fiber			25g	30g

Calories per gram:
Fat 9 • Carbohydrate 4 • Protein 4

Product B

Nutrition Facts

Serving Size (236g)
Servings Per Container

Amount Per Serving

Calories 130	Calories from Fat 45

	% Daily Value*
Total Fat 5g	8%
Saturated Fat 3g	15%
Trans Fat g	
Cholesterol 20mg	7%
Sodium 130mg	5%
Total Carbohydrate 13g	4%
Dietary Fiber g	
Sugars 12g	
Protein 8g	

Vitamin A 15%	•	Vitamin C 4%
Calcium 30%		

*Percent Daily Values are based on a 2,000 calorie diet. Your daily values may be higher or lower depending on your calorie needs:

		Calories	2,000	2,500
Total Fat	Less Than		65g	80g
Saturated Fat	Less Than		20g	25g
Cholesterol	Less Than		300mg	300 mg
Sodium	Less Than		2,400mg	2,400mg
Total Carbohydrate			300g	375g
Dietary Fiber			25g	30g

Calories per gram:
Fat 9 • Carbohydrate 4 • Protein 4

Product C

Nutrition Facts

Serving Size (213g)
Servings Per Container

Amount Per Serving

Calories 210	Calories from Fat 50

	% Daily Value*
Total Fat 6g	9%
Saturated Fat 2g	10%
Trans Fat g	
Cholesterol 20mg	7%
Sodium 840mg	35%
Total Carbohydrate 31g	10%
Dietary Fiber 2g	8%
Sugars 14g	
Protein 9g	

Vitamin A 6%	•	Vitamin C 6%
Calcium 6%	•	Iron 8%

*Percent Daily Values are based on a 2,000 calorie diet. Your daily values may be higher or lower depending on your calorie needs:

		Calories	2,000	2,500
Total Fat	Less Than		65g	80g
Saturated Fat	Less Than		20g	25g
Cholesterol	Less Than		300mg	300 mg
Sodium	Less Than		2,400mg	2,400mg
Total Carbohydrate			300g	375g
Dietary Fiber			25g	30g

Calories per gram:
Fat 9 • Carbohydrate 4 • Protein 4

Product D

Nutrition Facts

Serving Size (121g)
Servings Per Container

Amount Per Serving

Calories 20	Calories from Fat

	% Daily Value*
Total Fat g	
Saturated Fat g	
Trans Fat g	
Cholesterol mg	
Sodium 390mg	16%
Total Carbohydrate 4g	1%
Dietary Fiber 2g	8%
Sugars 2g	
Protein 1g	

Vitamin A 6%	•	Vitamin C 4%
Calcium 2%	•	Iron 4%

*Percent Daily Values are based on a 2,000 calorie diet. Your daily values may be higher or lower depending on your calorie needs:

		Calories	2,000	2,500
Total Fat	Less Than		65g	80g
Saturated Fat	Less Than		20g	25g
Cholesterol	Less Than		300mg	300 mg
Sodium	Less Than		2,400mg	2,400mg
Total Carbohydrate			300g	375g
Dietary Fiber			25g	30g

Calories per gram:
Fat 9 • Carbohydrate 4 • Protein 4

Product E

Nutrition Facts

Serving Size (302g)
Servings Per Container

Amount Per Serving

Calories 200	Calories from Fat 90

	% Daily Value*
Total Fat 10g	15%
Saturated Fat 2g	10%
Trans Fat g	
Cholesterol 40mg	13%
Sodium 110mg	5%
Total Carbohydrate 7g	2%
Dietary Fiber 3g	12%
Sugars g	
Protein 21g	

•

*Percent Daily Values are based on a 2,000 calorie diet. Your daily values may be higher or lower depending on your calorie needs:

		Calories	2,000	2,500
Total Fat	Less Than		65g	80g
Saturated Fat	Less Than		20g	25g
Cholesterol	Less Than		300mg	300 mg
Sodium	Less Than		2,400mg	2,400mg
Total Carbohydrate			300g	375g
Dietary Fiber			25g	30g

Calories per gram:
Fat 9 • Carbohydrate 4 • Protein 4

Product F

Nutrition Facts

Serving Size (35g)
Servings Per Container

Amount Per Serving

Calories 210	Calories from Fat 190

	% Daily Value*
Total Fat 21g	32%
Saturated Fat 3g	15%
Trans Fat 0g	
Cholesterol 0mg	0%
Sodium 160mg	7%
Total Carbohydrate 4g	1%
Dietary Fiber 0g	0%
Sugars 4g	
Protein 0g	

Vitamin A 0%	•	Vitamin C 0%

*Percent Daily Values are based on a 2,000 calorie diet. Your daily values may be higher or lower depending on your calorie needs:

		Calories	2,000	2,500
Total Fat	Less Than		65g	80g
Saturated Fat	Less Than		20g	25g
Cholesterol	Less Than		300mg	300 mg
Sodium	Less Than		2,400mg	2,400mg
Total Carbohydrate			300g	375g
Dietary Fiber			25g	30g

Calories per gram:
Fat 9 • Carbohydrate 4 • Protein 4

INSERT 2.7
Nutritional labels for products A through F as described in more detail in Insert 2.8.

The two categories listed under carbohydrates are dietary fiber and sugars. The amount per serving of sodium must also be listed. In addition, the percent daily value is included for all the nutrients except sugar and sodium. The percent daily values for vitamin A, vitamin C, calcium, and iron are also given as well as for the micronutrients that contribute significantly to our diet from this product.

It is important to keep in mind that all values are stated in terms of the amount per serving. A bag of chocolate chip cookies may contain 75 cookies, but the serving size may be only 5 cookies. The label indicates that the product provides 4% of the daily value of iron, 11% of the daily value of fat, and 150 calories. Five cookies can be a nice snack, but, if we eat the whole bag, we will get 60% of our iron, 165% of our fat, and 2250 calories! We probably should look elsewhere to get our iron.

Look at the Nutrition Facts statements of the six items in Insert 2.7. From them, Malik designed a simple meal plan for a day. He had a big bowl of breakfast cereal containing three servings and a single serving of 2% milk. He drank some water but was hungry by midmorning. He resisted the temptation to hit the vending machine. Lunch was rushed between classes, so he heated the lasagna entree for 90 seconds in the microwave and chased it with the entire can of green beans, which is two servings. He, of course, had another two glasses of water with the lasagna and green beans. In the afternoon, he ignored his hunger pangs and looked forward to his evening meal.

For supper, he went to his favorite fast-food restaurant to consume a healthy grilled chicken salad topped with basil vinaigrette dressing along with more water. They gave him two packs (one serving each) of the salad dressing, but he only used one.

There are other significant items on a food label. One is the ingredient statement as shown in Insert 2.8. The ingredients are listed by quantity— from the most to the least. The milk and canned beans are very simple processed products, whereas the cereal, lasagna, and salad dressing are complex

Item A—Breakfast cereal

Rice, wheat gluten, sugar, defatted wheat germ, salt, high fructose corn syrup, dried whey, malt flavoring, calcium caseinate, ascorbic acid (vitamin C), reduced iron, niacinamide, zinc oxide, pyridoxine hydrochloride (vitamin B_6), riboflavin (vitamin B_2), thiamin hydrochloride (vitamin B_1), vitamin A palmitate, folic acid, and vitamin D. Quality protected with BHT

Item B—2% milk

Reduced fat milk, vitamin A palmitate and vitamin D_3 added

Item C—Lasagna with meat sauce

Tomatoes (water, tomato paste), lasagna macaroni product (semolina, water, egg whites, glyceryl monstearate), cooked beef, sugar, corn oil flavoring, salt, parmesan cheese (pasteurized cultured milk, salt, enzymes), citric acid, spices, autolyzed yeast, hydrolyzed corn, soy, and wheat protein, olive oil, mushroom flavor (maltodextrin and mushroom juice powder)

Item D—Canned green beans

Green beans, water, salt (for flavor)

Item E—Grilled chicken salad

Lettuce, chicken tenders, tomatoes, carrots, celery, diced onions

Item F—Basil vinaigrette dressing

Soybean oil, balsamic vinegar (preserved with sulfites), olive oil, basil, water, high fructose corn syrup, sugar, salt, dehydrated garlic, spice, xanthan gum, iron, niacinamide, zinc oxide, pyridoxine hydrochloride (vitamin B_6), riboflavin (vitamin B_2), thiamin hydrochloide (vitamin B_1), vitamin A palmitate, folic acid, and vitamin D. Quality protected with BHT

INSERT 2.8
Ingredient statements for items in Insert 2.7.

formulated foods with many ingredients. Note that some ingredients like the lasagna product have ingredients of their own, which are listed in parentheses. Parentheses are also used to help explain the common names of some strange-sounding chemicals like the vitamins listed in the cereal and dressing. Each label must also include the company address of the distributor. This address is not necessarily where the product was manufactured.

2.15 Designing a Healthy Diet

In developing a healthy diet, we want to get enough protein, vitamins, and minerals without getting too much fat, sugar, and sodium or too many calories. Reliance on any one food is not a good idea, and it is best to eat a wide variety of foods in moderation.

MyPlate (www.ChooseMyPlate.gov) is a useful tool to help us balance our diets and make healthier food choices (see Insert 2.9). MyPlate is designed to simulate a single dining setting with plate, fork, and cup. The plate is divided into four sections with grains and vegetable servings slightly larger than fruits and protein, thus indicating the proportionality of the servings. The cup suggests milk as the beverage of choice. MyPlate replaced MyPyramid in 2011 and represents a slight departure and simplification from previous guidelines. For example, while six groups were specified in MyPyramid (fruits, vegetables, grains, dairy, meat and beans, as well as oils), MyPlate is less restricted and allows inclusion of vegetarian diets and the website provides information on how to eat healthy on a budget and supplementary material including recipes, menus, and daily food plans.

Overall, MyPlate (as well as previous programs) was developed to follow the *Dietary Guidelines for Americans*, a Federal initiative started on 1980. The Guidelines "encourage Americans to focus on eating a healthful diet—one

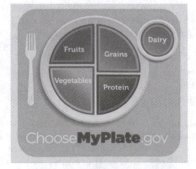

INSERT 2.9
MyPlate from http://ChooseMyPlate.gov (USDA 2014d).

that focuses on foods and beverages that help achieve and maintain a healthy weight, promote health, and prevent disease." These guidelines are revised every 5 years and a new version is expected to be released in 2015.

With obesity in an epidemic rise, it is never too early to adopt healthy food choices and, in an effort to help the United States to raise a healthier generation of children, federal efforts have expanded to encourage healthy eating at schools. In 2012, the USDA Food and Nutrition Service launched the *Nutrition Standards in the National School Lunch and School Breakfast Programs*, which was aimed to require "most schools to increase the avail-ability of fruits, vegetables, whole grains, and fat-free and low-fat fluid milk in school meals; reduce the levels of sodium, saturated fat and trans fat in meals; and meet the nutrition needs of school children within their calorie requirements." The standards address the most current nutrition guidelines and take into consideration the American school's situation.

In summary, keeping in mind key words like *variety* and *moderation*, we are very fortunate to have access to a plentiful and safe food chain as well as information on which and how much of those foods to consume for a healthy life. It is then up to us to make healthy food choices!

2.16 Remember This!

- It is never too early to adopt healthy eating habits!
- The Nutrition Facts part of the label indicates the serving size, how many servings per container, calories per serving, and the fat calo-ries per serving.
- Organic food production minimizes the input of fossil fuels and synthetic chemicals.
- Eating disorders occur when peer pressure clashes with biological needs.
- Fasting is self-starvation and can result in severe nutritional deficiencies.
- Nutraceuticals are foods specifically designed to act as drugs.
- There are few, if any, magical foods, but a balanced diet contributes to health and well-being, whereas a poor diet can lead to laziness, inattentiveness, and a bad attitude.
- There is no simple way to lose weight.
- Although food-borne diseases can be a concern, generally, though, when we talk about healthy foods, we are talking about foods that will help us avoid the diseases of civilization (cancer, diabetes, heart disease, and obesity).

• Good nutrition requires an adequate consumption of nutrients without consuming too many calories.

2.17 Looking Ahead

In the next chapter, we'll find how people decide what foods to eat. In Chapters 4 through 6, we will learn how the foods we find on supermarket shelves are processed or formulated. In Chapters 7 through 9, we will learn how food scientists ensure the quality and safety of foods, how they develop new products, and how the government regulates them. More detailed information on nutrition will be presented in Chapter 12.

Testing Comprehension

1. Analyze the perspectives on diet and nutrition of Garrett, Jennifer, and Malik. Identify the strengths and weaknesses of their ideas. What potential health consequences could result from their approach?

2. List the differences between a healthy and an unhealthy food and between a healthy and an unhealthy diet. The authors suggest that we should focus our attention on the healthiness of the diet and not of individual foods. Describe and critique their rationale.

3. Provide three examples each of a natural food, an organic food, a processed food, and a whole food. Rank in order these four categories of foods from healthiest to unhealthiest. Explain the reasons for this order. Would the authors of the book and the instructor of the class agree with this order? Why or why not?

4. Outline a personal nutritional strategy to maintain good health. What are the major barriers to implementing this strategy? How can these barriers be overcome?

5. Develop a 1-day meal plan for Jennifer that consists of whole foods and provides her with 1500–2000 calories, at least 100% of her Daily Value for calcium, iron, vitamin A, and vitamin C and no more than 100% of her Daily Value for fat and sodium. Analyze her plan for healthiness, cost, safety, and desirability.

6. Calculate the number of calories Malik consumed on the basis of the information provided in Insert 2.7 and the associated discussion in the text. Calculate the percentage of his calories that came from carbohydrate, fat, and protein as well as the %DV (Daily Value) for sodium,

protein, vitamins C and D, iron, calcium sodium, and dietary fiber. Assess the healthiness of his diet on the basis of these calculations.

7. List and describe the benefits and limitations of dietary supplements. Why do most dieticians recommend that we get our nutrients from foods and not supplements? What makes it so difficult to rely only on foods to get enough nutrients?

8. List and describe the nutritional consequences of fasting and the eating disorders described in the chapter. What obligation do we have when we see a friend or family member who is engaged in unhealthy eating practices?

9. Between the time this book was written and the time it is read, the Nutrition Facts statements will probably have had a makeover. Compare and contrast the labels shown in this chapter with those now available. Which of these styles is more useful? Why? Redesign the current label to make it more useful.

10. Select a sport. Provide a step-by-step guideline for a diet of an athlete of that sport to achieve an optimal weight. Note that, in certain team sports, weight may vary because of a specific position. What determines the length of time needed to achieve an optimal weight? What are the dangers of achieving this weight in too short or too long a period?

References

Litt, A. S., 2005. *The College Student's Guide to Eating Well on Campus*, rev. and expanded ed., Bethesda, MD: Tulip Hill Press.

USDA, 2014a. Center for Nutrition Policy and Promotion. Available at http://www .cnpp.usda.gov/DietaryGuidelines.

USDA, 2014b. Food and Nutrition Service. 2014. Nutrition Standards for School Meals. Available at http://www.fns.usda.gov/school-meals/nutrition-standards -school-meals.

USDA, 2014c. National Organic Program. Available at http://www.ams.usda.gov /AMSv1.0/.

USDA, 2014d. MyPlate. Available at http://www.choosemyplate.gov/.

Further Reading

Gardner, Z. and M. McGuffin, 2013. *American Herbal Products Association's Botanical Safety Handbook*, 2nd ed., Boca Raton, FL: CRC Press.

Ohr, L. M., 2014. Fats for fitness. *Food Technol.*, 68(9):65–70.

Roday, S., 2012. *Food Science and Nutrition*, Oxford: Oxford University Press.

Somer, E., 2012. *Eat Your Way to Happiness*, Toronto, ON, Canada: Harlequin.

UNICEF, 2014. Clinical Forms of Acute Malnutrition. Available at http://www.unicef
.org/nutrition/.

Whitney, E. N. and S. R. Rolfes, 2012. *Understanding Nutrition*, 13th ed., Boston:
Cengage Learning.

Wolinsky, I. and J. A. Driskell, 2012. *Sports Nutrition: Energy Metabolism and Exercise*,
Boca Raton, FL: CRC Press.

3

Foods We Eat

Ignacio likes to try and prepare new foods. He always goes to new restaurants and tries the latest thing. Nothing is too exotic for him. When he watches television, he is more likely to watch the ads than the actual programs. When he tastes something he really enjoys, he won't shut up until everyone he knows tried it. He's also very vocal about the foods he doesn't enjoy.

Selina is taking advantage of an opportunity of a lifetime. She is an exchange student in Ghana. When she first arrived, she was a very picky eater because most of the food was so strange to her. She longed for the foods she had grown up with and took every opportunity to eat fast food, but the burgers in the fast-food chains in Ghana were just not the same as in the chains at home. For the first time in her life, she was slimming down. As she adjusted and made new friends, she decided she was missing an important part of the cultural experience. She discovered millet, a crunchy yellow grain, and *nshima*, a mashed corn dish with an interesting flavor. It was delicious. She's having a great time now and is beginning to dread going home when the term is over. She's also regained the pounds she lost during the first couple of months.

Kyle avoids all preservatives and *processed* foods. He will read all the labels of the foods he is considering purchasing when shopping. He doesn't want all those "nasty chemicals" in his body. When he can, he shops at the natural foods market, where he can buy lots of dietary supplements to improve his health. The problem is that he ends up with more expensive products that take a lot of time to prepare, and although he wants to eat healthy, he also wants to do other things with his life. He often eats at a vegetarian restaurant down the street where the food is good, but it eats into his budget, and by the time he walks there and back, it takes almost as much time as it would have if he had just prepared it himself. Maybe he could move in with someone who shares his views on food and loves to cook!

When choosing the foods we eat, like Ignacio, Selina, and Kyle, we find that our food choices are influenced by many factors—our culture, our budget, and our time, among others. Moreover, sometimes our views about healthy eating are distorted, leading to inappropriate food choices.

3.1 Looking Back

- The Nutrition Facts part of the label indicates the serving size, how many servings per container, calories per serving, and the fat calories per serving.
- Eating disorders occur when peer pressure clashes with biological needs.
- Fasting is self-starvation and can result in severe nutritional deficiencies.
- There are few, if any, magical foods, but a balanced diet contributes to health and well-being, whereas a poor diet can lead to laziness, inattentiveness, and a bad attitude.
- There is no simple way to lose weight.
- Good nutrition requires an adequate consumption of nutrients without consuming too many calories.
- Preservatives are food ingredients that slow spoilage and help prevent food-associated illnesses.
- The last meal consumed is not usually the meal responsible for an outbreak of food poisoning.
- Spoilage is not a good indicator of a safety risk.
- Fresh foods are more likely to contain harmful microbes than processed products.

3.2 Food Choices

Eating can be one of the most enjoyable times of the day, but it can also get in the way of more important things. Although the foods we eat can affect our health and happiness, we do not always choose the foods based on logic or even much conscious thought. In his research on food behavior, Dr. Brian Wansink of Cornell University estimates that we make as many as 200 decisions a day about what we will eat, most of which are reactions and not thought through.

According to the International Food Information Council Foundation's 2014 Food & Health Survey, the main factors affecting food and beverage choices in the United States are taste (90%), price (73%), and healthfulness (71%), with convenience (51%) and sustainability (38%) following far behind. Also according to the survey, at least 60% of Americans put some thought on planning their meals—dinner being the most planned meal of the day. Although a vast majority of Americans are trying to lose weight, less than

30% understand that calories contribute to weight gain equally regardless of the source (i.e., proteins, fat, or carbohydrates). On the other hand, only 40% of consumers give food and beverage safety "a lot" of thought, with women and college graduates being the most likely groups among them.

It may be of interest to point out that Europeans take a slightly different approach when choosing their food. According to the Pan-European Survey of Consumer Attitudes to Food, Nutrition, and Health, the main drivers are quality/freshness (74%), price (43%), taste (38%), "trying to eat healthy" (32%), and "what my family wants to eat" (29%).

Regardless of where we come from, this chapter will look at why we choose the foods we do and how these choices affect the healthiness of our diet. Today may actually be a good time to take a good look at our eating habits and become aware of the different factors that affect our own dietary choices.

3.3 Sensory Characteristics

As seen above, taste is the number one factor that determines our food choices. In other words, no matter how nutritious, safe, and high quality a product is, if it does not taste good, we will not be very likely to choose it. It is not just the taste but the combination of all the sensory characteristics (i.e., flavor, appearance, and texture) that influence our choice of food. Sensory quality affects what we are willing to put into our mouths, how much we enjoy it, whether we will spit it out or consume more, and even how much benefit we will derive from it. Digestion of food begins in the mouth. Better-tasting food will actually be more likely to be digested than food that does not taste as good.

The first sensory characteristic is color or appearance. Before we put anything in our mouths, we tend to look at it to see if it is acceptable. Certain foods are expected to display certain colors. We like our spinach green, but not our meats. Consumers prefer red tomatoes, although orange tomatoes are higher in vitamin A. Other factors that affect acceptability are blemishes, splotches, bruises, bugs or obvious bug holes, rotten parts, and so on. Color of fruit-flavored beverages can affect the perception of sweetness. A darker red drink is perceived to be sweeter than the one with normal color. On the other hand, the appearance of a product may look so good that it increases our expectations beyond what the flavor can deliver. If a product is not as good as it looks, we then become disappointed when we eat it.

Flavor is the combination of the senses of taste and smell. When we say something tastes good, we are usually referring to flavor and not taste. Taste is perceived by the taste buds on the tongue. The aroma (smell) is perceived through our nostrils before we put in the food in our mouth and also during chewing. Additionally, chemical sensations like heat (spicy) or astringency (the puckering feeling after drinking cranberry juice for example) will contribute to the overall perception of foods in our mouth.

The texture of a food relates to how it feels to our sense of touch—either to the hand or in the mouth. At first glance, texture does not seem to be so important, but it is one that leads to the rejection of many foods. Most of us do not like lumpy mashed potatoes, slimy boiled okra, grainy ice cream, or mealy apples. Either a food feels right or it doesn't, and if it does not feel right, we are likely to reject it.

3.4 Price

Price is also an important determinant of food choice and is usually related to income and social status. Most students are on tight budgets and can't afford to spend much on food. Students looking for bargains often buy canned and dry food because fresh meat, fruits, vegetables, and frozen foods tend to be more expensive. Some students are better at budgeting time and money than others. Many students may eat well at the beginning of the month, but they are reduced to feasting on ramen noodles toward the end. For students and others that must carefully budget their money, it pays to develop a strategy to balance nutritional concerns with preferences and economics. Items are less expensive when purchased in bulk, but it is no bargain if the leftovers are allowed to spoil because of improper handling or because they are not consumed within a reasonable time.

3.5 Health

As we learned in Chapter 2, the fundamental role of foods is to provide our bodies with energy in the form of calories and nutrients like protein, vitamins, minerals, and dietary fiber that are important in maintaining good health. A nutritious diet to most people is one that avoids "bad" foods like white breads, salted snacks, foods with added sugars, burgers, and fries and embraces "good" foods like multigrain breads, fruits, and vegetables. Most foods have a nutritional image, and energy bars, yogurt, and fruit drinks have better reputations than others like hamburgers, eggs, and canned vegetables. Nutritional information is provided for a serving of several items in Insert 3.1. It is not that easy to distinguish "good" foods from "bad" ones just by looking at the label.

Using just "good" and "bad" foods to decide on our diet narrows our selection to a point where it can result in nutrient imbalances. It can be

Product G

Nutrition Facts
Serving Size (226g)
Servings Per Container – 1

Amount Per Serving

Calories 200 — Calories from Fat 70

	% Daily Value*
Total Fat 8g	12%
Saturated Fat 2g	10%
Trans Fat 0g	
Cholesterol 40mg	13%
Sodium 660mg	28%
Total Carbohydrate 14g	5%
Dietary Fiber 3g	12%
Sugars 5g	
Protein 18g	

Vitamin A 90% • Vitamin C 25%
Calcium 20% • Iron 8%

*Percent Daily Values are based on a 2,000 calorie diet. Your daily values may be higher or lower depending on your calorie needs:

		Calories	2,000	2,500
Total Fat	Less than		65g	80g
Saturated Fat	Less than		20g	25g
Cholesterol	Less than		300mg	300mg
Sodium	Less than		2,400mg	2,400mg
Total Carbohydrate			300g	375g
Dietary Fiber			25g	30g

Calories per gram:
Fat 9 • Carbohydrate 4 • Protein 4

Product H

Nutrition Facts
Serving Size (50g)
Servings Per Container – 1

Amount Per Serving

Calories 210 — Calories from Fat 60

	% Daily Value*
Total Fat 7g	11%
Saturated Fat 4g	20%
Trans Fat 0g	
Cholesterol 0mg	0%
Sodium 320mg	13%
Total Carbohydrate 24g	8%
Dietary Fiber 1g	4%
Sugars 14g	
Protein 14g	

Vitamin A 50% • Vitamin C 200%
Calcium 6% • Iron 0%

*Percent Daily Values are based on a 2,000 calorie diet. Your daily values may be higher or lower depending on your calorie needs:

		Calories	2,000	2,500
Total Fat	Less than		65g	80g
Saturated Fat	Less than		20g	25g
Cholesterol	Less than		300mg	300mg
Sodium	Less than		2,400mg	2,400mg
Total Carbohydrate			300g	375g
Dietary Fiber			25g	30g

Calories per gram:
Fat 9 • Carbohydrate 4 • Protein 4

Product I

Nutrition Facts
Serving Size (40g)
Servings Per Container – 17

Amount Per Serving

Calories 100 — Calories from Fat 0

	% Daily Value*
Total Fat 0g	0%
Saturated Fat 0g	0%
Trans Fat 0g	
Cholesterol 0mg	0%
Sodium 5mg	0%
Total Carbohydrate 24g	8%
Dietary Fiber 3g	12%
Sugars 12g	
Protein 1g	

Vitamin A 10% • Vitamin C 0%
Calcium 2% • Iron 2%

*Percent Daily Values are based on a 2,000 calorie diet. Your daily values may be higher or lower depending on your calorie needs:

		Calories	2,000	2,500
Total Fat	Less than		65g	80g
Saturated Fat	Less than		20g	25g
Cholesterol	Less than		300mg	300mg
Sodium	Less than		2,400mg	2,400mg
Total Carbohydrate			300g	375g
Dietary Fiber			25g	30g

Calories per gram:
Fat 9 • Carbohydrate 4 • Protein 4

Product J

Nutrition Facts
Serving Size (49g)
Servings Per Container – 9

Amount Per Serving

Calories 170 — Calories from Fat 10

	% Daily Value*
Total Fat 1g	2%
Saturated Fat 0g	0%
Trans Fat 0g	
Cholesterol 0mg	0%
Sodium 0mg	0%
Total Carbohydrate 40g	13%
Dietary Fiber 6g	24%
Sugars 0g	
Protein 6g	

Vitamin A 0% • Vitamin C 0%
Calcium 2% • Iron 6%

*Percent Daily Values are based on a 2,000 calorie diet. Your daily values may be higher or lower depending on your calorie needs:

		Calories	2,000	2,500
Total Fat	Less than		65g	80g
Saturated Fat	Less than		20g	25g
Cholesterol	Less than		300mg	300mg
Sodium	Less than		2,400mg	2,400mg
Total Carbohydrate			300g	375g
Dietary Fiber			25g	30g

Calories per gram:
Fat 9 • Carbohydrate 4 • Protein 4

Product K

Nutrition Facts
Serving Size (130g)
Servings Per Container – 3.5

Amount Per Serving

Calories 130 — Calories from Fat 50

	% Daily Value*
Total Fat 6g	9%
Saturated Fat 1g	5%
Trans Fat 0g	
Cholesterol 0mg	0%
Sodium 300mg	13%
Total Carbohydrate 21g	7%
Dietary Fiber 8g	32%
Sugars 1g	
Protein 8g	

Vitamin A 15% • Vitamin C 0%
Calcium 8% • Iron 15%

*Percent Daily Values are based on a 2,000 calorie diet. Your daily values may be higher or lower depending on your calorie needs:

		Calories	2,000	2,500
Total Fat	Less than		65g	80g
Saturated Fat	Less than		20g	25g
Cholesterol	Less than		300mg	300mg
Sodium	Less than		2,400mg	2,400mg
Total Carbohydrate			300g	375g
Dietary Fiber			25g	30g

Calories per gram:
Fat 9 • Carbohydrate 4 • Protein 4

Product L

Nutrition Facts
Serving Size (56g)
Servings Per Container – 8

Amount Per Serving

Calories 180 — Calories from Fat 140

	% Daily Value*
Total Fat 16g	25%
Saturated Fat 0g	0%
Trans Fat 0g	
Cholesterol 35mg	12%
Sodium 600mg	25%
Total Carbohydrate 2g	1%
Dietary Fiber 0g	0%
Sugars 0g	
Protein 6g	

Vitamin A 0% • Vitamin C 0%
Calcium 2% • Iron 2%

*Percent Daily Values are based on a 2,000 calorie diet. Your daily values may be higher or lower depending on your calorie needs:

		Calories	2,000	2,500
Total Fat	Less than		65g	80g
Saturated Fat	Less than		20g	25g
Cholesterol	Less than		300mg	300mg
Sodium	Less than		2,400mg	2,400mg
Total Carbohydrate			300g	375g
Dietary Fiber			25g	30g

Calories per gram:
Fat 9 • Carbohydrate 4 • Protein 4

INSERT 3.1

Nutrition Facts for 11 products. Minor nutrients in products H, J, M, and O are not shown. Products include the following: G, Lean Cuisine Baked Chicken Florentine; H, Zone Perfect Strawberry Yogurt All Natural Nutrition Bar; I, Sunsweet Gold Label Dried Plums; J, Post Healthy Classics The Original Shredded Wheat Spoon Size; K, Kuner's of Colorado Southwestern Black Beans with Cumin & Chili Spices; L, Bryan Juicy Jumbos Franks.

(Continued)

Product M

Nutrition Facts
Serving Size (27g)
Servings Per Container – 1

Amount Per Serving

Calories 100	Calories from Fat 10
	% Daily Value*
Total Fat 1g	2%
Saturated Fat 1g	5%
Trans Fat 0g	
Cholesterol 0mg	0%
Sodium 125mg	5%
Total Carbohydrate 24g	8%
Dietary Fiber 1g	4%
Sugars 13g	
Protein 1g	

Vitamin A 8%	•	Vitamin C 10%
Calcium 0%	•	Iron 20%

*Percent Daily Values are based on a 2,000 calorie diet. Your daily values may be higher or lower depending on your calorie needs:

	Calories	2,000	2,500
Total Fat	Less than	65g	80g
Saturated Fat	Less than	20g	25g
Cholesterol	Less than	300mg	300mg
Sodium	Less than	2,400mg	2,400mg
Total Carbohydrate		300g	375g
Dietary Fiber		25g	30g

Calories per gram:
Fat 9 • Carbohydrate 4 • Protein 4

Product N

Nutrition Facts
Serving Size (227g)
Servings Per Container – 1

Amount Per Serving

Calories 240	Calories from Fat 20
	% Daily Value*
Total Fat 2g	3%
Saturated Fat 1.5g	8%
Trans Fat 0g	
Cholesterol 20mg	7%
Sodium 110mg	5%
Total Carbohydrate 49g	16%
Dietary Fiber 0g	0%
Sugars 40g	
Protein 7g	

Vitamin A 0%	•	Vitamin C 0%
Calcium 20%	•	Iron 0%

*Percent Daily Values are based on a 2,000 calorie diet. Your daily values may be higher or lower depending on your calorie needs:

	Calories	2,000	2,500
Total Fat	Less than	65g	80g
Saturated Fat	Less than	20g	25g
Cholesterol	Less than	300mg	300mg
Sodium	Less than	2,400mg	2,400mg
Total Carbohydrate		300g	375g
Dietary Fiber		25g	30g

Calories per gram:
Fat 9 • Carbohydrate 4 • Protein 4

Product O

Nutrition Facts
Serving Size (62g)
Servings Per Container – 14

Amount Per Serving

Calories 100	Calories from Fat 25
	% Daily Value*
Total Fat 3g	5%
Saturated Fat 3g	15%
Trans Fat 0g	
Cholesterol 10mg	3%
Sodium 50mg	2%
Total Carbohydrate 14g	5%
Dietary Fiber 4g	16%
Sugars 4g	
Protein 3g	

Vitamin A 8%	•	Vitamin C 0%
Calcium 8%	•	Iron 0%

*Percent Daily Values are based on a 2,000 calorie diet. Your daily values may be higher or lower depending on your calorie needs:

	Calories	2,000	2,500
Total Fat	Less than	65g	80g
Saturated Fat	Less than	20g	25g
Cholesterol	Less than	300mg	300mg
Sodium	Less than	2,400mg	2,400mg
Total Carbohydrate		300g	375g
Dietary Fiber		25g	30g

Calories per gram:
Fat 9 • Carbohydrate 4 • Protein 4

Product P

Nutrition Facts
Serving Size (52g)
Servings Per Container – 6

Amount Per Serving

Calories 200	Calories from Fat 110
	% Daily Value*
Total Fat 12g	18%
Saturated Fat 0.5g	3%
Trans Fat 0g	
Cholesterol 5mg	2%
Sodium 95mg	4%
Total Carbohydrate 22g	7%
Dietary Fiber 1g	4%
Sugars 10g	
Protein 2g	

Vitamin A 0%	•	Vitamin C 2%
Calcium 6%	•	Iron 4%

*Percent Daily Values are based on a 2,000 calorie diet. Your daily values may be higher or lower depending on your calorie needs:

	Calories	2,000	2,500
Total Fat	Less than	65g	80g
Saturated Fat	Less than	20g	25g
Cholesterol	Less than	300mg	300mg
Sodium	Less than	2,400mg	2,400mg
Total Carbohydrate		300g	375g
Dietary Fiber		25g	30g

Calories per gram:
Fat 9 • Carbohydrate 4 • Protein 4

Product Q

Nutrition Facts
Serving Size (35g)
Servings Per Container – 6

Amount Per Serving

Calories 130	Calories from Fat 45
	% Daily Value*
Total Fat 5g	8%
Saturated Fat 0g	0%
Trans Fat 0g	
Cholesterol 0mg	0%
Sodium 65mg	3%
Total Carbohydrate 20g	7%
Dietary Fiber 4g	16%
Sugars 5g	
Protein 5g	

Vitamin A 0%	•	Vitamin C 0%
Calcium 0%	•	Iron 4%

*Percent Daily Values are based on a 2,000 calorie diet. Your daily values may be higher or lower depending on your calorie needs:

	Calories	2,000	2,500
Total Fat	Less than	65g	80g
Saturated Fat	Less than	20g	25g
Cholesterol	Less than	300mg	300mg
Sodium	Less than	2,400mg	2,400mg
Total Carbohydrate		300g	375g
Dietary Fiber		25g	30g

Calories per gram:
Fat 9 • Carbohydrate 4 • Protein 4

INSERT 3.1 (CONTINUED)
Nutrition Facts for 11 products. Minor nutrients in products H, J, M, and O are not shown. Products include the following: M, Kellogg's Froot Loops; N, Breyers Fruit on the Bottom Mixed Berry Lowfat Yogurt; O, Edy's No Sugar Added Vanilla Flavored Light Ice Cream; P, Krispy Kreme Doughnuts Original Glazed Doughnuts; Q, Kashi Peanut Butter Chewy Granola Bars.

overwhelming when we hear contradictory statements about certain food components. Fad diets promote the ingestion of certain groups of foods over others (i.e., high protein, low carbohydrate). Some diet recommendations claim that increasing vitamin and mineral intake is the secret to good health. However, the healthiest diet is one in which adequate calories are balanced with proper levels of protein, vitamins, and minerals. We all know that too little of any particular nutrient is unhealthy, but too much of a nutrient, particularly vitamins A and D and certain minerals, can also be unhealthy.

3.6 Safety

As discussed in Chapter 1, foods can make us ill. Foods that exhibit an unfamiliar odor, color, or texture can be suspicious although spoiled foods are not necessarily unsafe and unspoiled foods are not necessarily safe. Cooking helps ensure that our meats are safe, and rinsing and washing fresh fruits and vegetables help make them safer. Other storage and sanitation practices are used during the handling of food to decrease the chances of our becoming ill from contaminated food. More than 80% of Americans believe that brand-name foods or those from chain restaurants are safe although almost 40% have changed their food habits after the brand or chain is linked to a case of food poisoning.

Not all of our efforts to avoid unsafe foods are successful, however, as there are still too many people who get sick and die each year by consuming contaminated foods. Myths like those mentioned in Chapter 1 lead to many of these food-borne illnesses. Some of the myths include the following:

- Rare burgers and raw eggs are safe to eat.
- Preservatives make foods unsafe.
- Natural foods are safer than processed foods.
- Mishandled foods that look and smell all right are safe.
- Cooked foods are sterile and don't need to be refrigerated.
- Drinking alcohol protects shellfish eaters from contamination.

Commercial establishments are held responsible for complying with regulatory guidelines for the proper handling and storage of foods. Consumers must share part of the burden by following simple practices like

- Washing our hands after using the bathroom, changing diapers, or playing with our pets before preparing food
- Keeping cold foods cold and hot foods hot
- Avoiding cross-contamination of raw and cooked items in the kitchen

3.7 Weight Loss

As discussed in Chapter 2, many of us are unhappy with our weight. It is estimated that more than 30% of the American population is obese and a similar percentage is overweight. Selecting a healthy diet is the first step. Next, we need to find the foods that fit into that diet. Dieters use many methods to lose unwanted pounds: fasting; skipping meals; avoiding fat, sugar, and carbohydrates; increasing proteins; taking appetite suppressants or dietary supplements; counting calories; and exercise.

Skipping meals, particularly breakfast, can be self-defeating because breakfast skippers tend to eat "small" snacks throughout the day, which ultimately add up to a greater number of calories. A better strategy, skipping foods with high fat and sugar content, is a way to reduce calories. There are numerous products on the market that are low in fat and sugar; however, most of these items are also low in fiber. Diets low in fiber and fat contribute to hunger pangs because the stomach becomes empty more quickly. In addition, diets with less than 15%–20% calories from fat are difficult to maintain because they tend to be unappetizing. Increasing fiber content with some fat, preferably from plant sources, will help keep one satisfied without adding too many calories.

It is very common for dietary supplements to promise that the pounds will drop off without cutting back on calories or working out. Unfortunately, the phrase "no pain, no gain" is probably closer to the truth. Appetite suppressants do decrease our desire for food, but they are expensive and may also have unwanted side effects.

The best way of monitoring diets is by counting calories. Those of us who are trying to lose weight look for foods that are nutrient dense and restrict high-calorie foods and beverages (particularly alcohol, which provides lots of calories and few other nutrients). To see how food choices affect calorie consumption, see Inserts 3.2 and 3.3.

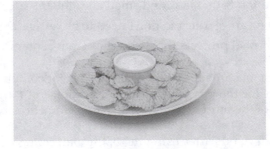

INSERT 3.2
A snack of chips and dip containing 175 calories. (From Rolls, B., *The Volumetrics Eating Plan*, New York: Harper-Collins, New York, 2005. Photo courtesy of Michael A. Black. With permission.)

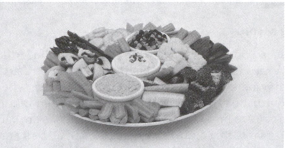

INSERT 3.3
A veggie platter also containing 175 calories. Which option is healthier, this one or the chips in Insert 3.2? (From Rolls, B., *The Volumetrics Eating Plan*, New York: Harper-Collins, New York, 2005. Photo courtesy of Michael A. Black. With permission.)

Foods that help reduce weight are those that are tasty, filling, and low in calories. Fruits, vegetables, and whole grains are high in fiber and water but low in calories. When combined with a protein source and some fat, they can fill up our stomachs and slow the emptying time to delay hunger. The most effective weight-loss diet is one that is low in calories, satisfying, and adaptable. It should also be high in nutrients. Guidelines for designing a diet to maintain a healthy lifestyle were provided at the end of Chapter 2. A sensible exercise program, combined with a sound diet, is still the most effective and healthiest way to lose weight.

3.8 Weight Gain

Believe it or not, some people are underweight and would be healthier with some weight gain. Many athletes are interested in bulking up. Since the best way to lose weight is to decrease calorie consumption, the best way to gain it is to increase calorie consumption. It is ironic that those who wish to bulk up tend to turn to proteins, the same source of calories for those who wish to lose weight. One reason for the emphasis on proteins is that muscle is primarily protein. It is the combination of impact exercise (e.g., weight lifting) and excess consumption of carbohydrates, however, that is more effective in building muscle. As in dieting to reduce weight, it is recommended that the dieter set realistic weight goals when dieting to bulk up. A realistic goal for healthy weight gain is 20% of body mass for a young male and 10%–15% for a young female per year. Such increases in weight should be coupled with resistance (weight) training to ensure that the gain is lean body mass and not fat.

3.9 Social Factors

Friends and social occasions affect what we eat and thus influence our long-term health. A recommendation of a new food from a trusted friend or family member may be the best introduction to that food, whereas a negative comment may turn us off to a certain product. When in a crowd, we may feel social pressure to break our normal diet. If friends are eating fast food or dining at restaurants that feature high-calorie appetizers and main courses, it is hard to eat healthy. Likewise, when everyone around us is eating sensible meals and watching what we choose, it is harder to splurge.

Parties tend to have food and beverages that are high in calories and low in vitamins and minerals. Sporting events tend to increase the need to have tailgate and postgame parties and lots of calorie-laden food. Late night snacking can also have devastating consequences on the waistline. Foods help people mix and mingle by creating a comfort zone. When we are enjoying the company of others, we are less likely to monitor just how much we are eating and drinking. In many social situations like weddings, funerals, and professional receptions, food serves as an icebreaker, but we are restricted by the food choices offered at the venue. Although most social occasions now offer lower-calorie alternatives (e.g., celery and carrot sticks without the dip), which can be consumed slowly, these items are not usually the most popular ones.

3.10 Religious Influences

Food traditions are associated with many religions: eating fish on Fridays by Catholics, abstinence from pork and other products by Jews and Muslims, avoidance of all meats except seafood by Buddhists, vegetarianism embraced by Hindus, and the potluck suppers of many faiths. Many religious groups abstain from alcoholic beverages, whereas others incorporate them into their ceremonies. Bread and olive oil are considered sacred foods for some groups. Feasts and holidays associated with religions introduce specific foods and traditions. Christians in North America consume turkey and cranberry sauce at Thanksgiving; Jews, unleavened bread during Passover; and Hindus, sweets and puddings in celebration of Divali. In addition, fasting is associated with many religious groups such as the Jews, Muslims, Buddhists, and Hindus. A comparison of some dietary habits of different religions is shown in Insert 3.4.

Kosher laws govern the foods that Jews are permitted to consume. Kosher laws specify types of animals that are permissible and forbidden for food, prohibit the consumption of blood, and forbid the consumption of dairy and

Occasion	Religion	Significance	Associated foods
Ash Wednesday	Christian	Beginning of Lent	Abstinence from certain foods for six weeks until Easter
Christmas	Christian	Celebration of birth of Christ	Varies widely; usually centered around meat like turkey
Divali	Hindu	Darkest night of the year	Many delicacies including *roti*; flatbread with curry
Easter	Christian	Celebration of resurrection	Varies widely; usually centered around meat like ham
Eid al-Fitr	Muslim	Breaking of Ramadan fast	Large feast
Passover	Jewish	Celebration of freedom	*Seder*: chicken soup, matzo balls, unleavened bread
Pravarana	Buddhist	End of the rainy season	Buns and sweets
Ramadan	Muslim	Month of fasting	No food or water between sunrise and sunset
Rosh Hashanah	Jewish	Beginning of the New Year	Apples dipped in honey, sweets, nothing sour or bitter
Sabbath	Jewish	Day of rest and day of prayer	Cooked meals prepared evening before
Yom Kippur	Jewish	Day of atonement	No food or water from sunset to sunset

INSERT 3.4

Religious occasions associated with feasting or fasting. (Adapted from Kittler, P.G. and Sucher, K.P., *Cultural Foods*, Belmont, CA: Wadsworth/Thomson Learning, 2000.)

meat products at the same meal. Among the animal restrictions for kosher foods are wild birds, shark, dogfish, hog, lobster, shrimp, crab, and insects. Strict guidelines must be followed during the slaughter of animals, and these processes must be approved by a rabbi to be considered kosher. Salt of a specific grain size (small enough to cover the entire surface but large enough to prevent dissolving within 30 minutes after application), known as kosher salt, is applied to the meat to draw out any remaining blood in the meat. Orthodox Jews serve meat on a separate set of dishes than those they use to serve dairy items. Pareve foods are those that can be consumed with either meat or dairy products. In addition, there are special rules governing the foods that can be consumed during Passover. Kosher practices are far-reaching and prescribed for the way food is prepared and served.

Halal laws govern those foods that Muslims are permitted to consume. Halal refers to permitted foods, and **haram** refers to those that are forbidden. Kosher and halal practices have many similarities with some noticeable differences. For example, locusts, shrimp, and lobster are halal. Pork, cats, dogs, birds of prey, carrion, blood, intoxicants, and inappropriate drugs are haram. There is no requirement to separate meat and dairy products in Islam. Slaughter of animals for meat must be done in a humane fashion by a sane Muslim who invokes the name of Allah during slaughter. The blood must be drained from the animal before any cutting, but soaking and salting, which are required for kosher products, are not required for halal. Hunting is permitted if it is for meat but not if it is solely for sport.

3.11 Ethnicity

Food is an integral part of our cultural heritage. Many factors contribute to a specific cuisine. Staples are foods that form the basis of a cuisine such as meat and potatoes in the Midwestern United States, beans and corn in many parts of Latin America, and rice in many other parts of the world. Specialty foods round out a cuisine, giving it its flair and desirability to people of other cultures and certain flavors and dishes become associated with it. Frequently, these flavors are acquired tastes that are not acceptable to outsiders. When ethnic cuisine becomes popular (Mexican, Chinese, and Italian in the United States, or hamburgers and fried chicken outside the United States), it tends to be an adaptation and interpretation of the authentic diet. Foods popular in the northeastern United States reflect the immigration of Europeans. Tea, beer, and whiskey come from the United Kingdom; many cheese, sauces, and spices come from France; pizza and pasta come from Italy. Southern cooking has its roots in "soul food" from Africa. An emphasis on pork products, fried foods, and boiled leafy green vegetables are products of the slave culture.

Cajun cuisine, a specialty in Louisiana, features such foods as pralines, beignets, and gumbo.

The staples of the central plains are a mix of Native America, central Europe, and Scandinavia. Popcorn, nuts, and many of our vegetables were contributed by plains Indians; sausages and potatoes came from Germany; milk and preserved fish are common foods from Scandinavia. Latinos have had considerable influence on American cuisine, particularly in the southwest. Tacos, tortillas, burritos, and enchiladas are products of Mexico; starchy vegetables such as cassava and chili-based sauces and jerked meats come from the Caribbean islands; coffee, chocolate, and tropical fruits are part of Central and South American culture. The West Coast has seen the influence of Asian cultures. Soy sauce, fried rice, and stir-fry vegetables are just a few of the contributions to the American diet from China; ramen noodles and sushi come from Japan; noodle soups, coconuts, curries, and fermented fish have been introduced from other Asian cultures. Although there are still regional differences, most of these cultures have diffused throughout the American diet. See Insert 3.5 for more information on ethnic foods in America.

3.12 Family Traditions

Early exposure to foods has a profound effect on our preferences. Foods that we did not like but were forced to eat when we were young are ones we frequently reject later. Likewise, foods that we enjoyed as a child are those that provide special comfort as we age. Family traditions establish many of our attitudes toward foods and provide a basis upon which we judge new foods. Family traditions around holidays may differ from the traditions of ethnic groups. Most of us accept unquestioningly that the foods we ate at home when we were young are the ones we are supposed to eat although we are becoming more adventurous at experiencing new flavors.

3.13 Advertising

Advertising may play a bigger role in our food choices than many of us are willing to admit. Advertising like that shown in Insert 3.6 can be particularly effective at introducing new food products. If we are not aware that a product exists, we are not going to buy it. Obviously, advertising can be a source of both information and misinformation when it comes to food choices. Different media, and television, particularly, have a great influence on sensitive groups like children and teenagers. It has been estimated that

Food	Ethnicity	Description
Arroz con pollo	Cuban	Chicken with rice with seasonings like peppers and saffron
Brunswick stew	Southern	Made from squirrel meat and onions
Burrito	Mexican	Shredded meat, cheese and/or beans in a flour tortilla
Cracklin' bread	African American	Yellow cornmeal bread with added pork cracklings (crisp fat or skin)
Gumbo	Cajun	Stew with many vegetables particularly okra and tomatoes
Gyro	Greek	Minced lamb in pita bread
Jerky	Native American	Salted, dried meat, originally primarily buffalo
Kasha	Central European	Roasted buckwheat groats (whole or ground)
Kimchi	Korean	Spicy-hot fermented cabbage or turnips
Oatmeal	British/Scottish	Also known as porridge
Pasta	Italian	Wide variety of noodles served with a variety of sauces
Peanut butter	Southern	Blend of ground peanuts, oil, and salt
Pierogi	Polish	Boiled, stuffed dumpling with onions and cabbage
Pita bread	Middle Eastern	Flat, leavened bread with an internal pocket
Sushi	Japanese	With rice, frequently associated with raw fish (*sashimi*)
Taco	Mexican	Shredded meat, cheese and/or beans in a folded corn tortilla
Tofu	Asian	Curds from soybean milk

INSERT 3.5
Ethnic foods in the United States. (Adapted from *Cultural Foods: Traditions and Trends* and *Food Lover's Companion*).

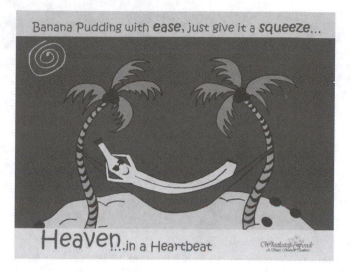

Banana Pudding with **ease**, just give it a *squeeze*...

Heaven!..in a Heartbeat

INSERT 3.6
Food advertisement for banana pudding designed by Laura McKinley, Lauren Hill, Chris Zachary, and Ben Sherrill as part of a class assignment.

the average American kid spends more hours watching TV than in school, which accounts for significant exposure to food advertising and affects the food purchase requests from children to parents. Fortunately, some of the most influential food corporations have initiated the advertising of healthy products and encouraging healthier lifestyles. Overall, there is a move toward more regulations and decreasing unhealthy food marketing.

3.14 Time and Trends

As society changes, so does the food. Diets today are quite different from those of 20 or 30 years ago. Many factors have affected what we eat today. Technology has transformed our food supply (see Insert 3.7). The food industry now produces more formulated foods that are more convenient for meals prepared in minutes rather than hours. The foods can be eaten on the run and don't require a sit-down, home-style dinner. We tend to be more health conscious, yet we are heavier than our counterparts of yesteryear. Part of the reason we carry extra weight is because we have more sedentary lives than our predecessors.

We also eat more meals away from home than we once did. Going to a restaurant used to be a once-a-week or even a once-a-month treat. Fast-food restaurants that featured only hamburgers, fries, or chicken now have a wide range of menu options with larger sizes. Ethnic restaurants have taken over

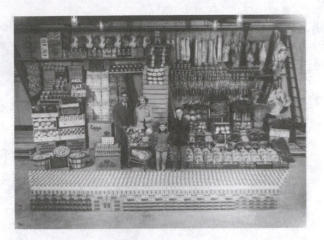

INSERT 3.7
Photo of food for a family of four in the United States in the 1950s. Notice the absence of processed and formulated foods. Picture is of Steve Czeklinski, a DuPont worker, and his family. (Reprinted by permission of Hagley Museum and Library. Photo courtesy of Alex Henderson.)

the dining scene, offering more exotic options that appeal to more adventurous eaters. The variety for such products as yogurt, fresh salads, prepared dishes, sushi, and energy bars are too numerous to list—products that were not even available to our parents.

3.15 Personal Philosophy

Our diets are affected by our personal beliefs. Some of us are sensitive to nature and can't bring ourselves to eat meat, but most of us have no such qualms. Others like Kyle eat "organic" foods or those with less packaging because of concerns about pollution and the environment. Our food choices are influenced by our politics, our friends, the media, and many other sources. Many of these influences may be rational, but others are not. Regardless, our beliefs have an effect on what we choose to eat and those choices affect our nutritional status.

3.16 Convenience

Throughout history, a large part of people's lives was taken up with finding food, preparing it, and consuming it. Many of us today have ready access to food 24/7, and yet we are still looking for ways to make our foods more convenient. In the age of multitasking, we see no problem in eating while on social media, driving down the road, or waiting in line. Technology has provided us with many options not available to previous generations or other parts of the world.

Convenience comes in packages that have the food portioned into single servings to avoid measuring out what we need. We have packages that have everything we need for a meal for eating directly or for ready preparation. Many packages are developed for use in the microwave, and the package serves as a disposable eating container. Other foods are designed to be eaten with our fingers. These innovations were designed primarily to free us from the drudgery of the kitchen and the confinement of the sit-down meal. For many of us, meals have become just another task to accomplish and scratch off our lists rather than just for pure enjoyment of food.

Fast-food restaurants provide convenience by delivering a fully prepared meal quickly. These operations minimize the time between order and delivery of a meal. Thus, the main factor that distinguishes fast food from other restaurants is the speed of service. Nutritional concerns are less important at fast-food restaurants than other foodservice outlets. The types of foods popular at fast-food outlets tend to be high in fat, high in salt, and low in fiber, although salads are now provided as an option in many chains. Yet, some consumers are rejecting the fast-food world and convenience foods. The slow-foods movement started in Italy in 1982 and is finding enthusiasts elsewhere. This movement avoids shortcuts in shopping, preparing, and enjoying food. It emphasizes quality—the quality of the ingredients and the food. It stresses the social aspects of enjoying a good meal together with family and friends. For many of us, however, preparing meals are not a high priority in our lives, and we prefer to spend that time on more interesting activities.

3.17 Pathogenic Eating

As mentioned before, mealtime serves as a source of pleasure and offers an opportunity for socializing. Unfortunately, some people develop bad food habits that seriously affect their health. Food scientists and nutritionists stress moderation in food consumption and eating a wide variety of foods. Athletes are also at risk, with some estimates indicating 60% have unhealthy diets. Football linemen may consume massive amounts of food to achieve their weight goals, while wrestlers and gymnasts may sweat off pounds to lose weight. Supplements are sought as the magic answer to gain or lose weight and enhance performance or endurance, but rapid changes in weight place undue strain on our bodies.

Pathogenic eating can extend to being overconcerned about healthiness leading to unhealthy habits. *Orthorexia nervosa*, an obsession with healthful eating, leads to the elimination of "bad" foods, greatly reducing the amount of "good" foods available. Foods may be classified as "bad" because of social concerns, real or perceived safety issues, desire to get closer to nature, and food sensitivities. Likewise, foods may be classified as "good" to eat right for our type, macrobiotics or body purification, and spiritual gratification. Each of these concerns can be legitimate in the right context. We live in a complex world and must be careful with what we put into our bodies, but when concerns and strict adherence to a rigid set of rules become more important than our overall health, they become an obsession.

3.18 Psychological Factors

Psychological factors like stress and mood can also greatly affect our food choices. Stress seems to have become a common player in our daily lives and affects the way we eat in addition to having other health-related consequences. Different people respond differently to stress, and while some may tend to eat more, others tend to eat less. Mood also has a significant impact on food choices (i.e., cravings), but it is worth noticing that food can indeed affect our mood as well.

3.19 Meal Patterns around the World

Meal patterns vary widely across cultures as Selina found out during her visit to Ghana and so wonderfully described in the book *You Eat What You Are*. The Spaniards start their day early with a small breakfast, have a big meal at noon, and then don't eat again until late in the evening. Indonesians and Southeast Asians eat rice at every meal with many light snacks such as rice cakes between meals. Hungarians have one large meal at noon with small meals and snacks throughout the day. The Chinese have small meals and snacks throughout the day with a big meal served in the evening. Indians have two main meals a day—at midmorning and in the evening with much snacking in between.

Likewise, breakfast traditions vary widely between cultures. Australians like a big "breaky" with lots of eggs, meat, and Vegemite, a yeast extract that is rarely appreciated by visitors, on their toast. *Akara* (Insert 3.8), a popular breakfast food in many African countries, is made from black-eyed pea meal and resembles a hushpuppy. South American breakfasts tend to be simple, consisting of

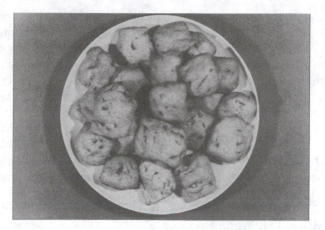

INSERT 3.8
Akara, a deep-fried product made from black-eyed pea flour and enjoyed by Africans. (From McWatters, K.H. and Brantley, B.B., *Food Technology* 36(1): 66, 1982. With permission.)

strong, sweet coffee with milk and breads or rolls with butter and jam. The Japanese wake up with an intensely sour red plum called an *umeboshi* to clear the head and cleanse the mouth, followed by a bowl of *misoshiru* made from fermented bean paste. An Israeli breakfast consists of a wide range of fresh vegetables mixed with meats, cheeses, or eggs and accompanied by hearty hot cereals. Like most Europeans, the Dutch like breads and rolls for breakfast with unsalted butter and jam, but many tend to drink tea instead of coffee.

Cereal grains and their products comprise the most widely consumed source of calories around the world. Wheat breads tend to be favored by most cultures because of their light, spongy texture. Croissants, brioches, and baguettes are French contributions to bread eaters of the world. Australians enjoy damper bread, which tastes like a big biscuit, because it can be easily prepared in the bush and baked over an open fire. *Lavash* is a thin, crisp bread popular in Middle Eastern countries such as Iran, and *flatbrod* is a crisp rye bread consumed in Norway. Italians consume their grains in the form of pasta. Bulgur, a coarse cracked wheat grain, is used in the preparation of many Turkish dishes. Rice flour is used to make noodles in Asian countries such as Vietnam.

Fruits and vegetables are great sources of fiber and many vitamins. Fresh berries and rhubarb, a sour red stem, are gathered and enjoyed in Iceland. Tropical fruits such as mangoes, bananas, and papayas are staples in many African countries. Dates and figs are enjoyed in Iran. The *durian* is a fruit enjoyed in Asia that has a sweet and enticing flesh for those who can get past a very offensive odor, so offensive that it is banned in hotel lobbies and on airplanes. Romanians like their fruits preserved in thick sugar syrup in a dish called *dulceata*, and Austrians consume many of their fruits in soups. Beets, cabbage, and potatoes are staples for Eastern European countries such as the Ukraine. Cauliflower is a staple in Finland. The *daikon*, a white radish that looks like a white carrot, is prized in Japan. Sauerkraut made by fermenting cabbage is a favorite vegetable dish among peoples of northeastern Europe such as Estonia and Latvia. Tomato sauce is an important ingredient in many Italian foods, and okra is the primary ingredient in African gumbos.

Meats and dairy products provide protein and essential minerals. *Asado* (beef grilled over red hot coals, without flames as shown in Insert 3.9) is a favorite meal in Argentina, pork is the most widely consumed meat in the Philippines, and lamb is the most popular meat in New Zealand. Hamburgers and fried chicken are America's gifts to the world. *Ceviche* is an uncooked fish popular in Caribbean countries that is "preserved" in lime juice and spices. Czechs prefer their meat cooked until tender and served with a sour cream topping. Bean curd or *tofu* is a meat substitute enjoyed in many Asian countries such as China and Japan.

The Danes enjoy specially prepared cheeses that have a nutty, buttery flavor. Cheese dumplings in a flavored milk sauce, known as *ras malai*, are widely consumed on the Indian subcontinent. Ricotta cheese, a mildly flavored white cheese, is eaten with sourdough bread in Malta. Yogurt and kefir are consumed as liquid beverages in many of the Slavic countries such as Croatia and Macedonia. *Mish*, a skim-milk cheese fermented in earthenware jars, is served with most Egyptian meals. Cottage cheese is a major component in blintzes and knishes.

Not all food is consumed for nutritional purposes. Sweets and fatty foods are enjoyed the world over by those who can afford them. The Greeks consume large quantities of *baklava*, a very sweet pastry usually containing nuts. Morocco boasts of its *makalhara*, a honey-dipped pretzel. Coconut pudding and sweet, sticky rice cakes are favorites of Indonesians. Canadians make delicious pies from pumpkin and rhubarb. Chocolate products are enjoyed

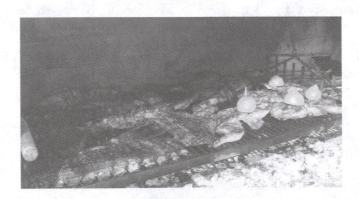

INSERT 3.9
Carne asada (barbequed beef) is an Argentine specialty shown here on an open hearth. (Photo courtesy of Dr. Carlos Margaria, United States Distilled Spirits.)

throughout the world, but the Belgians and the Swiss may be the biggest consumers. Toasted sunflower and pumpkin seeds are snacks enjoyed by Russians. The Dutch like to dip French fries in mayonnaise, but Americans prefer their fries with ketchup.

3.20 Selecting Healthy Foods

In Chapter 2, the principles for designing a nutritious diet were introduced. The point of this chapter is to show how many things can influence the choices of the foods we eat. Although many of us try to eat healthy, there are many temptations and influences that affect our health that we do not consciously consider. Selection of healthy foods should be done in the context of a healthy diet. If we are not at the weight we want to be, it is much better to develop a long-term plan to lose or gain weight a little at a time rather than through crash programs that might be more dangerous than our current condition. It may be harder to design a healthy diet from convenience foods than from whole foods and from fast foods than slow foods, but a careful study of food labels and restaurant websites can help us maintain our lifestyle without greatly damaging our health. Finally, we should be adventuresome and try foods from other cultures because we may be surprised at what we are missing!

3.21 Remember This!

- Although many of us try to eat healthy, there are many temptations and influences affecting our decisions that we do not consciously consider.
- Meal patterns vary widely across cultures.
- Pathogenic eating can extend to being overconcerned about healthiness leading to unhealthy habits.
- The main factor that distinguishes fast food from other restaurants is the speed of service.
- Advertising may play a bigger role in our food choices than many of us are willing to admit.
- Staples are foods that form the basis of a cuisine.
- A sensible exercise program combined with a sound diet is the most effective and healthiest way to lose weight.

- The healthiest diet is one in which adequate calories are balanced with proper levels of protein, vitamins, and minerals.
- No matter how nutritious, safe, and high quality a product is, if it does not taste good, we will not be very likely to choose it.
- It is not just the taste but the combination of all the sensory characteristics (i.e., flavor, appearance, and texture) that influence our choice of food.

3.22 Looking Ahead

This chapter was designed to provide an introduction to food choice. In future chapters, we will be introduced to the types of foods we eat and how they are manufactured for safety, a longer life, convenience, and a pleasant eating experience.

Testing Comprehension

1. Identify 10 personal food choices made today. Describe the three factors that were most influential in making those decisions. Describe ways these factors complemented each other and ways they contradicted each other. How could these choices have been improved if given more conscious thought?

2. Based on the Nutrition Facts statements in Insert 3.1, classify each product as healthy or unhealthy. On a separate list, based on the image on the name of that product as listed in the legend, classify each one as healthy and unhealthy. Explain any differences found between the two classifications.

3. Select a favorite food product and one that is not nearly as appealing. Identify the two most important sensory characteristics and the nutritional value of these products. How could each of these products be improved?

4. Provide an example of a food that could be heathy but not safe and one that could be safe but not healthy. How do the authors differentiate between healthy foods and safe foods? Critique their perspective.

5. Compare and contrast the challenges, dangers, and benefits of diets to lose weight and to gain weight. How effective are these diets? Why? What factors are involved in the obesity epidemic beyond diet and exercise?

6. Select the three most significant factors that influence students with respect to food choice before they even reach middle school. Analyze the power that these factors have over us as we make the transition into college life and how they affect our nutritional status and health. How can we modify our mindset to develop better eating patterns?

7. List and describe five recent food advertisements. Rank order from most effective to least effective. Why are some ads very effective and others not so much? Why does advertising affect others much more than it affects us?

8. Calculate the total amount of calories consumed by Ignacio, Selina, and Kyle at an ice-cream social. Ignacio chose a large bowl of the Snickers Vanilla flavor, Kyle a small bowl of all-natural Butter Pecan, and Selina a small bowl of no-sugar-added Peanut Butter Tracks. Selina's selection provided 35 calories per ounce, with Butter Pecan providing 140% of the calories per ounce of the Peanut Butter Tracks. Ignacio's selection contributed 5 more calories per ounce than Kyle's choice. One-half of a pound of ice cream was scooped into a large bowl with only 60% of that amount scooped into the smaller bowl. Selina went back for seconds and Kyle ate an organic, oatmeal cookie that had only 25% of the calories of his ice cream. Who consumed the most calories and who consumed the least? Did any of these three consume a food they would not normally consume at the social? Explain.

9. Identify an example of a food product that can be prepared and consumed quickly, one that requires a long time for preparation and consumption, and one that is intermediate in convenience. Compare and contrast the sensory characteristics and nutritional value of these three items. What are the main reasons for these differences? How does each one fit into the college lifestyle?

10. Select one meal each from three different foreign cultures. Describe the cultural significance of each meal. Compare and contrast these meals with respect to healthiness, safety, and sensory attributes. Which of these meals could be most easily developed as a processed food? a fast-food? a healthy snack? How would the development of each affect the cultural significance of the meal?

References

Barer-Stein, T., 1999. *You Eat What You Are*, Willowdale, ON, Canada: Firefly Books.
Bratman, S. and D. Knight, 2000. *Health Food Junkies: Orthorexia Nervosa—The Health Food Eating Disorder*, New York: Harmony Books.

European Food Information Council, 2014. The Determinants of Food Choice. Available at http://www.eufic.org/article/en/expid/review-food-choice/.

International Food Information Council Foundation, 2014. Food and Health Survey. Available at http://www.foodinsight.org/articles/2014-food-and-health-survey.

Kittler, P. G. and K. P. Sucher, 2000. *Cultural Foods*, Belmont, CA: Wadsworth/ Thomson Learning.

McWatters, K. H. and B. B. Brantley, 1982. Characteristics of akara prepared from cowpea paste and meal. *Food Technol.*, 36(1):66.

Rolls, B., 2005. *The Volumetrics Eating Plan*, New York: Harper-Collins.

Wansink, B., 2010. *Mindless Eating: Why We Eat More Than We Think*, New York: Bantam Books.

Further Reading

Herbst, R. and S. T. Herbst, 2013. *The New Food Lover's Companion*, 4th ed., Hauppauge, NY: Barron's Educational Series, Inc.

Litt, A. S., 2005. *The College Student's Guide to Eating Well on Campus*, 2nd ed., Bethesda, MD: Tulip Hill Press.

Petrini, C., 2006. *Slow Food Revolution: A New Culture for Eating and Living*, New York: Rizzoli.

Pfund, F., 2011. *Advertising for Children*, Norderstedt, Germany: GRIN *Verlag*.

Regenstein, J. M., M. M. Chaudry and C. E. Regenstein, 2003. The kosher and halal food laws. *Compr. Rev. Food Sci. Food Saf.*, 2:111.

Samour, P. Q. and K. King, 2011. *Pediatric Nutrition*, 4th ed., Sudbury, MA: Jones & Bartlett.

Spence, C. and B. Piqueras-Fiszman, 2014. *The Perfect Meal: The Multisensory Science of Food and Dining*, Oxford: John Wiley & Sons, Ltd.

Stuckey, B., 2012. *Taste What You Are Missing: The Passionate Eater's Guide to Why Good Food Tastes Good*, New York: Free Press.

U.S. Department of Health and Human Services, 2014. Keep Food Safe. Available at http://www.foodsafety.gov/.

Whitney, E. N. and S. R. Rolfes, 2012. *Understanding Nutrition*, 13th ed., Belmont, CA: Wadsworth/Cengage Learning.

Section II

Commercial Food Products

4

Processed Foods

Malik and Leah were given a class assignment to interview an older person (someone over 50) about what America was like in the 1960s and 1970s, particularly as it related to food. Malik interviewed his mom, who was born in 1965 and grew up in the late 1970s and early 1980s; Leah talked to her grandfather who was born just after World War II. Malik's mom told him that all the houses were small but tidy and the yards were well kept. All the moms stayed at home and cooked delicious meals, and all the fathers knew best. Politics seemed much simpler then, at least until the Vietnam War came along. Leah's grandfather commented on watching the World Series in the afternoon when everyone was at work, and there were not nearly as many football games on TV. They both said the music was much better back then; they could hum the melodies and understand the words. Malik's mom loved the K.C. and the Sunshine Band's music; Leah's grandfather preferred Simon and Garfunkel.

Life seemed simpler then. Gas was much cheaper, and cars were much bigger. Cruising around town was big. The drive-in restaurant and movie theaters were the places to hang out and make out. When eating fast food, Burger Chef and White Castle were more popular than McDonald's. Leah's grandfather was pleased the burgers were only 15 cents. Malik's mom pointed out that they were small and not very tasty. The French fries were larger and less crispy, and the serving size was smaller. There was no such thing as supersizing back then. They had to walk up to a window to order because there was no place to sit down and there were no drive-thrus. Eating out was something they did infrequently. Most meals were prepared and eaten in the home.

The "supermarkets" were very small, and most eating out was done at a family restaurant. They didn't include a deli, bakery, or meat counter. In fact, they usually got their meat at a separate store. There was little fresh produce unless it was in season, and there was a very small frozen food section. With the exception of canned goods, there were not as many packaged foods or as much variety as today. Fresh milk and bread were delivered to the home twice a week by truck. The TV dinners back then were not nearly as good. If they had to go back, they would miss the microwave oven.

Although the kitchens were much simpler back then, their moms would spend much of their time there preparing most of the family's meals every day. People did not seem to be very concerned about eating healthy. Breakfast was much bigger, with bacon and eggs featured almost every morning. Malik's mom was less tempted by chocolate or potato chips because they were much harder to get, but she did consume lots of whole milk and home-made cookies. Meat with lots of fat was the centerpiece for lunch and sup-per with lots of starches and vegetables. Almost every meal was completed with a dessert, usually cake, but sometimes only a can of fruit cocktail (not a favorite of Leah's grandfather).

Meals were important back then, with the whole family getting together and talking. No one would even think of watching TV or listening to music on the radio during meal times. Malik's mother and Leah's grand-father both said the family meal is what they missed the most about the good old days. Store-bought ice cream was not big back then, but Dairy Queen and Tastee Freez were great places to hang out and eat good soft-serve cones.

4.1 Looking Back

- Although many of us try to eat healthy, there are many temptations and influences affecting our decisions that we do not consciously consider.
- Meal patterns vary widely across cultures.
- Staples are foods that form the basis of a cuisine.
- No matter how nutritious, safe, and high quality a product is, if it does not taste good, we will not be very likely to choose it.
- Organic food production minimizes the input of fossil fuels and synthetic chemicals.
- There are few, if any, magical foods, but a balanced diet contributes to health and well-being, whereas a poor diet can lead to laziness, inattentiveness, and a bad attitude.
- Good nutrition requires adequate consumption of nutrients without consuming too many calories.
- Preservatives are food ingredients that slow spoilage and help pre-vent food-associated illnesses.
- A processed food should be designed to spoil before it becomes unsafe to make it less likely that someone will eat the unsafe food and become sick.
- Fresh foods are more likely to contain harmful microbes than pro-cessed products.

4.2 What Are Processed Foods and Why Are They Processed?

Processed foods are products that have been preserved so that they will not spoil as quickly as the fresh, whole foods (**raw materials**) they were made from. Most raw materials are perishable and require careful handling or processing to prevent losses. Foods fresh from the farm, ocean, pond, or other source are only available when they are in season, which can be inconvenient.

The primary reason for food processing is to reduce or eliminate harmful microbes from growing in foods. Some food processes sterilize the product, others kill but do not eliminate microbes, still others slow or prevent microbial growth. One type of food preservation actually encourages growth of beneficial microbes to prevent the growth of harmful ones. The major benefit of controlling microbes through processing is to decrease the chances of safety problems and to slow spoilage. Remember that we want foods to spoil before they become unsafe. Some processes allow us to store the product at room temperature. These foods are called shelf-stable.

Another reason for preserving foods is to stop the loss of nutrients. Many of these losses are attributed to the presence of active enzymes. The same factors that affect microbes affect enzymes. One reason food processes affect microbes is that the enzymes in the microbe are inactivated. Fresh foods lose their nutritional value as they spoil. Some types of food processing are damaging to vitamins and minerals, but the same conditions that ensure food safety also prevent further loss of nutrients. Examples of different types of processed foods are shown in Insert 4.1. This chapter introduces us to food processing, describing the types of processing steps used to manufacture foods and the consequences of processing on shelf life, nutrition, quality, and safety. It also introduces the importance of packaging in the manufacturing of foods.

4.3 Benefits of Processing

Advanced technology has given us many advantages not enjoyed by previous generations. Advances in any technology, including food technology, come with associated costs, many of which are not obvious. Food processing and preservation can increase shelf stability of a raw material usually at the cost of nutrition and quality. When we buy or eat a processed food, we are trading away a product that may be higher in nutrients and better in quality for one that is less perishable, safer, more convenient, and frequently lower

Commercially sterile

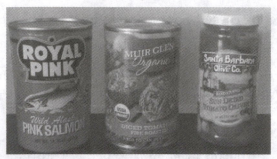

Canned salmon   Canned, diced tomatoes   Stuffed olives

Processed but not sterile

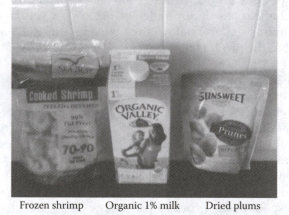

Frozen shrimp   Organic 1% milk   Dried plums

Fresh and whole

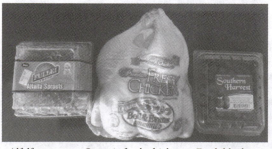

Alfalfa sprouts   Organic fresh chicken   Fresh blueberries

INSERT 4.1

Most of the foods we consume contain numerous microbes, and very few are sterile. Food processors can eliminate all pathogenic, spoilage, and fermentative microbes by a strong heat treatment. All fresh, unprocessed, whole foods contain microbes. (Photos courtesy of Robert Shewfelt.)

in price. Some other trade-offs that are made in food processing include the following:

- A processed food is more likely to be eaten because a fresh food is more likely to spoil.
- A shelf-stable food is ready to eat when we are, but we need to fit a fresh food into our plans before it spoils.
- Processed foods are more likely to maintain sensory and nutritional quality during storage than fresh foods.
- Some consumers like the flavor of processed foods better than fresh foods because that is what they get used to.
- Processed foods have less waste while fresh foods usually require trimming and are more likely to have cooking losses.
- Processed foods take more energy to produce but usually take less energy to store than fresh foods.

4.4 Processing Steps

Many steps occur in a food processing plant to convert raw materials into a processed food. Unit operations are distinct steps common to many food processes. These steps begin as the raw material is unloaded at the plant dock and continue until the packaged product is loaded up on another truck or railcar to the place we will buy it. Most raw materials are perishable and must be processed within a period of hours after arrival at the plant. Some common unit operations include materials handling (moving them from place to place in the processing plant), cleaning, separating, grading, pumping, mixing, heat exchanging (adding or removing heat), packaging, and controlling (making sure what is supposed to happen actually happens).

Food scientists need to know the unit operations of a process for a specific product. Each operation provides an opportunity for a problem to develop. An understanding of the potential problems that can occur provides ways to prevent them. The safety and quality of a food product are dependent on the processor's ability to control the individual steps and fit them together properly. The speed and capacity of a process are never greater than the speed and capacity of the slowest operation.

Minor variations in a process can result in major differences in a final product. Think of all of the different types of cheeses. The unit operations for all cheeses are very similar. The major differences between the types of cheese are attributed to addition, subtraction, modification, or rearrangement of a few unit operations and differences in starting materials. In some processes, the food is packaged before it is processed, while in others, packaging occurs at the end of the process. If careful attention is not paid to the order of operations, effects of late steps can undo positive aspects of early steps.

For example, there are many unit operations in the canning of green chilies. They are filled (in either the whole, cut, or diced form) into 4-ounce cans and sealed (capped) before being processed under pressure with steam. These operations include receiving, holding, washing, peeling, coring, grading, blanching, cutting, dicing, acidification, filling, exhausting, capping, heat processing, cooling, and packing the glass jars into cartons.

4.5 Types of Food Processes

As food scientists become more innovative with new products, the lines between fresh, processed, formulated, chilled, and prepared foods become blurred. Some foods fit into more than one category, but this separation into groups helps us understand how foods are manufactured. Raw agricultural materials (whole foods) are processed in many ways. Major types of processing include heating, freezing, drying, concentrating, curing, milling, extracting, and fermenting. Newer technologies are now being tested to preserve foods. Microwaves represent a technology introduced and widely accepted within the last two generations.

Irradiation is a controversial technology that can be used to either sterilize a food like canning or radurize (similar to pasteurize) certain products. Even more exotic processes are being developed that accomplish similar killing power as heat processes with little or no heat. These processes promise the quality and nutrition of fresh foods with the convenience and shelf stability of processed foods.

4.5.1 Heating

The purpose of heating foods is to kill microbes. The problem with heating is that it can also destroy nutrients and quality. Remember that raw foods are likely to harbor spoilage microbes and **pathogens** (microbes that can make us sick). Cooking kills both of these types of microbes but does not sterilize raw foods. **Blanching** is a short heat treatment in processing of raw fruits and vegetables to inactivate enzymes before other processing steps with minimal effect on microbes. **Pasteurization** involves a mild form of heating that kills all pathogens without killing all the spoilage microbes. Canning sterilizes the product in the container, usually under pressure. Aseptic processing and packaging sterilizes the product before putting it in the package.

Food engineers are responsible for designing safe food processes. If the heat process is not adequate to kill the harmful microbes, the food could spoil too quickly or, worse yet, become a safety hazard. If the process is too rigorous, the food could lose nutrients and quality. Processing techniques for a specific food are designed with an understanding of the potential microbes present and the properties of the food. For example, many pathogens are not able to grow in high-acid foods; hence, the heat treatment required to sterilize a high-acid food like tomatoes is not as great as that for a low-acid food like green beans. The design of a heat treatment relates to the temperature that will be applied and the time it will be processed. It must also consider the type of heat transfer in the product, the coldest point in the product, the length of time it takes to reach the selected temperature, and the length of time it takes the product to cool down.

In the early 1800s, Napoleon offered a prize to help feed his armies more efficiently. Nicolas Appert responded by developing the canning process to keep foods from spoiling rapidly. Meats, fruits, and vegetables that are found in cans or jars on supermarket shelves are canned. Raw materials are graded, sorted, and cut or formed before being placed in the container. Fruits and vegetables are usually blanched not only to inactivate enzymes that can hurt product quality but also to remove oxygen and decrease volume so that more product can fit in the container. The can or jar is then sealed and placed in a type of pressure cooker (called a retort). See the flow diagram in the process for diced pimiento peppers in glass jars in Insert 4.2.

Since some foods have acids (naturally occurring or added), they do not take as long to process as those that do not. Canning drives all of the oxygen

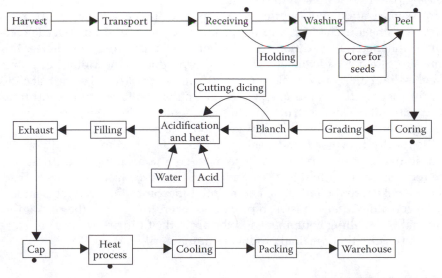

INSERT 4.2
Schematic of unit operations for dicing, packing in jars, and canning of pimiento peppers as illustrated by Virgil Esensee.

out of the container; thus, the microbes of concern are those that can live without oxygen. The most dangerous microbe that can survive in the absence of oxygen is *Clostridium botulinum*, the pathogen responsible for botulism. To test the adequacy of a canning process for a specific product, certain cans are inoculated with a microbe, such as *Bacillus stearothermophilus*, that is more resistant to heat than *C. botulinum*. If *B. stearothermophilus* cannot survive, then botulism is not a concern.

Heat energy is transferred by **conduction** (from one molecule to the next) in solid foods like tuna and puddings. It is transferred by **convection** in liquid foods like chicken broth or evaporated milk, which involves predictable patterns of swirling. Heat is transferred to the food on the outside of the container first and then into the center. The **cold spot** (last point in the container to reach the desired temperature) is the geometric center of the can in conduction heating and below the geometric center in convection heating. The length of time it takes for a process to be complete is based on the cold spot in the can.

Mixed foods like pork and beans and clam chowder contain **particulates** (chunks floating in thick sauces such that it is neither completely solid nor completely liquid). The presence of particulates makes it more difficult to predict heat-transfer patterns and the cold spot. The larger the container, the longer it takes to reach the proper temperature in the cold spot and the more nutrients and quality are lost in other parts of the container. One way to speed up the process is to agitate the containers by shaking them or moving them through the heat in a coiled track. Agitation provides a more even heating pattern throughout the container.

In pasteurization and **aseptic processing**, heating occurs outside the container in a heat exchanger, and the product is packaged into a sterile container under sterile conditions. The higher the temperature, the shorter the time is needed to adequately process the product. This time-shortening effect is dramatic. For example, it takes 30 minutes to pasteurize milk at 63°C (145°F) but only 15 seconds at 72°C (161°F). The high-temperature, short-time process results in less destruction to nutrients and quality. Pasteurized products are not sterile and require refrigeration to slow spoilage.

Aseptically processed and packaged products are commercially sterile and do not require refrigeration. The most common examples of these are the rectangular milk and juice cartons with the little plastic straw attached that we poke into the foil circle before imbibing. Since the product is added to the container after it has been processed, everything from the packaging material to the filling equipment and the air in the filling room must be sterilized to ensure that the final product remains sterile.

4.5.2 Freezing

Freezing is a milder form of preservation than heat treatment resulting in less loss of nutrients and quality than other processes. When we think of frozen foods, we tend to think of ice cream and frozen entrées, but many whole foods such as fruits, vegetables, meats, and seafood are found in the frozen food aisle. These items can also be shipped as ingredients for further processing into formulated foods as will be discussed in Chapter 5.

Freezing is also a type of heat exchange, but heat is removed from the product during freezing and not added to it as in canning. Freezing slows growth of microbes but does not sufficiently kill microbes to prevent spoilage or safety problems in thawed product that is not stored properly. The rate of freezing is affected by the processing equipment and the properties of the food. In general, the faster the method of freezing, the smaller the ice crystals formed in the product and the higher the level of quality. Although water freezes at 0°C (32°F), other foods have lower freezing temperatures. Sugars, salts, and other components can act as antifreeze. During freezing, water freezes first, concentrating the other components with freezing occurring from the outside in. The concentration of these components can lead to quality losses attributed to enzyme activity if the food does not freeze quickly. Vegetables are frequently blanched before freezing to prevent damage from enzymes.

The oldest and slowest way to freeze foods is in still air. It is also the technique most damaging to quality. A better way to freeze foods is to blow air at temperatures below minus 30°C with high forced air velocities to speed up the freezing process. A food or the package containing the food is placed in contact with a cold surface in indirect-contact freezing. The effectiveness of this type of freezing depends on how much contact is achieved between the food and the freezing unit.

Surface dehydration, known as **freezer-burn**, in frozen meats can be prevented by quick freezing and proper packaging. Scraped-surface freezers are used for liquids or slushes such as those available at the gas-and-go places at exits off the interstate highways. Individual quick freezing (IQF) of items such as French fries and onion rings involves the immersion of the product into liquid refrigerant. Since there is little contact of the product with air in IQF, there is less chance for oxidation or loss of moisture than in other freezing methods. Immersion in liquid nitrogen or other ultralow-temperature liquids (known as cryogenic freezing), the quickest and most expensive way to freeze foods, produces the highest-quality frozen foods.

Freezing is an excellent method of food processing in countries that have adequate home freezer/refrigerator units, but it places added responsibility on the consumer to handle the frozen food properly. Improper handling of defrosted foods can lead to a safety hazard. Defrosted foods should not be stored above 5°C (41°F) because microbes are free to grow after thawing. Quick defrosting in a microwave or slow thawing overnight in a refrigerator are the safest methods. Defrosted meat and dairy products represent a greater risk of hazard than bakery or other plant products as they are more likely to be contaminated and more likely to encourage the growth of microbes. Expiration dates for frozen foods assume that the product will be stored properly and are useless if it is not kept frozen. Another way of helping the consumer know if a product is still edible is the use of time/temperature indicators. These devices can be incorporated into the package by changing colors from green (good to consume) to yellow (consume soon) to red (discard and do not consume) to warn the consumer of temperature abuse.

4.5.3 Drying

Removal of water from foods such as drying of solid foods or concentrating of liquid/semisolid foods and beverages is another method of preserving foods. Microbes need water to grow. Microbial growth is slowed or halted in dried foods and concentrated beverages. There are many similarities between frozen and dried foods, as the act of freezing removes available water from the food by turning it into ice. Frozen, concentrated juices remove water both ways. Another type of product with less water and lower microbial growth is called an intermediate-moisture food. Intermediate-moisture foods like pepperoni and prunes are solid or semisolid foods that have less moisture (water) available to microbes but are not as dry as typical dried foods.

Dry foods are not as dry as they appear. Water is a very important component of most foods. Even dry flours contain as much as 10%–15% moisture. There are many ways to remove water from foods. The least sophisticated form of drying is leaving a harvested crop in the field to be dried by the sun such as raisins, dates, and tomatoes. Ovens at low relative humidity will also remove water but can leave a cooked flavor. By introducing a vacuum, the temperature required to remove water is lower to achieve the same effect with less cooked flavor. Increased air circulation in cabinets, tunnels, or other devices can also be used to obtain similar effects.

Spray drying forces a liquid like milk through a small nozzle to form a fine mist. The mist circulates in a large conical-shaped cabinet with circulating air (see diagram in Insert 4.3). The dried powder collects in a container.

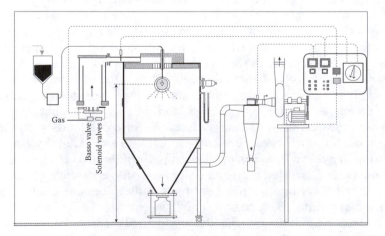

INSERT 4.3
Schematic diagram of a spray dryer as illustrated by Carlos Reyes-Rodriguez.

Drum drying involves the rotation of a warm drum or cylinder through a liquid food product. A thin film of the liquid becomes attached to the drum and dries as it is cooked on the drum. A knife blade scrapes the dried product off the surface of the drum into sheets, which are collected in a trough. Freeze drying involves freezing a solid or liquid food in a pan in a chamber. The chamber is then placed under vacuum to lower the pressure to a point that the ice is transformed directly into water vapor without becoming liquid water. This direct conversion from solid to gas is called sublimation rather than evaporation.

Different types of drying result in different types of final products. A property that is desirable for dried powders is its quickness at dissolving. Spray-dried products tend to be more readily soluble than other dry foods. Dried foods that contain sugars are usually hygroscopic, which means that they rapidly absorb water. Thus, they appear sticky to the touch. That is why we don't get a sticky mess when spilling a sugar-free beverage that we do with those that contain sugar. Packaging is critical in protecting a dried food from the moisture in the air.

4.5.4 Concentrating

The removal of water from a liquid food without changing it into a solid is concentration. We are most familiar with juice concentrates and syrups as concentrated foods. Most of these processes concentrate sugars, leading not only to increased sweetness but also to greater resistance to microbial growth. Many concentrated juices are susceptible to yeast spoilage or loss of flavor; thus, freezing is combined with concentrating to preserve quality. Another reason for concentrating liquids is to reduce the size of containers and thus reduce shipping costs. During the evaporation process, delicate flavors also evaporate, causing a loss of overall product flavor. These volatile components (known as essence) can be captured and added back to the product to give it a fuller flavor. Impurities in the water can add in off-flavors to reconstituted juice products.

4.5.5 Curing

Curing of meats is another way of decreasing the availability of moisture to microbes, thus decreasing microbial growth and producing convenient, ready-to-eat products. Curing is achieved by adding preservatives that bind water. The two most common water-binding preservatives are sucrose (sugar) and sodium chloride (salt). Other antimicrobial agents such as sodium nitrate and sodium nitrite are added, which also help maintain the red color. Salt and other preservatives can be added to a meat product by soaking the food in a brine (high-salt) solution. Sugar-curing of hams is achieved by hand rubbing the sugar into the meat. Some products, particularly salt-cured items, are also smoked, which adds flavor, contributes to drying, and can generate antimicrobial agents. Curing also results in typical flavor development in luncheon meats that many consumers like while others do not.

Curing of vegetables like onions and potatoes refers to the process of holding either in the field or a large ventilated room at high temperatures. Curing helps dry out the surface of the product and permits healing of wounds incurred during harvest. A cured onion or potato is less likely to spoil than one that has not been cured.

4.5.6 Milling

When we eat cereal grains, we are eating seeds. Few of us actually eat the whole seed as it is usually hard to digest. Many cereals are milled into flour to make it more digestible. Milling separates the seed into many fractions based on the structure of the seed. Flours are produced by dry milling, accomplished by adding of some water to swell the seed in preparing it for milling. A series of numerous grinding steps further separate fractions without damaging starch granules. Whole flour contains more fractions than white flour, which contains a higher percentage of starch and less fiber. Part of the milling process involves drying with most flours stabilized at 10%–15% moisture. Flours should be stored in dry conditions as they can absorb water and become susceptible to mold growth.

Wet-milling permits the combination of specific components of the grain like starch and protein. Large amounts of warm water are added to the grain, which is then soaked for longer than a day. The grain, now swollen with water, is then ground and components are separated by solubility properties. Products of wet-milling include cornstarch, wheat gluten, and other starch products.

4.5.7 Extracting

Many unit operations in food processes involve the removal of unwanted portions of a raw material. In addition to the removal of water, mentioned previously, some processes remove soil or other objectionable matter from the raw product, while others separate the edible from the inedible portions. Extraction involves the removal of part of a substance that is contained within it. Millions of consumers extract soluble components of crushed leaves or ground beans in their homes or offices each day to enjoy fresh cups of tea or coffee.

The liquid and associated solids of a fruit or vegetable are extracted to form a juice. The most commonly processed juice worldwide is orange juice. The flavor of a fresh fruit like an orange and its extracted juice can vary for many reasons such as cultivar (cultivated variety), growing area, season, and growing conditions. Since consumers want the same flavor experience each time they drink a specific beverage, juice processors blend juices from different sources to achieve the desired flavor. Juices from different fruits or vegetables can also be blended together to provide unique flavor and color sensations.

There are many fruit-flavored beverages on the market that have little juice and few associated nutrients. To make sure we are actually getting real fruit juices, we need to read the label carefully. Fresh juices are quite perishable. They need to be refrigerated or undergo further processing to be preserved. The type and length of the process (time/temperature relationships) and storage conditions affect shelf life as well as sensory and nutritional quality. Unit operations of juice manufacture are extraction, clarification, deaeration, pasteurization, concentration, essence addition, and canning, bottling, or freezing. Extraction yield can be improved by the use of pectic enzymes. A Willmes Press, used to extract juice from fruits including the preliminary steps in winemaking, is shown in Insert 4.4.

Oils, or liquid fats, are also extracted from plant parts to provide important ingredients for foods. Removal of edible oils from the rest of the plant material is usually achieved by physical pressure. After pressing, many unit operations are needed to convert the initial extract into a useable product. Refining and degumming remove unwanted substances from the oil to improve the stability of its flavor and color. Bleaching of the oil removes objectionable odors and colors while increasing its stability. Other deodorization steps improve its acceptability to the consumer. **Interesterification** rearranges the oil molecules to affect its melting temperature and thus its desirability as a food ingredient. Antioxidants are added to oils to prevent them from deteriorating rapidly.

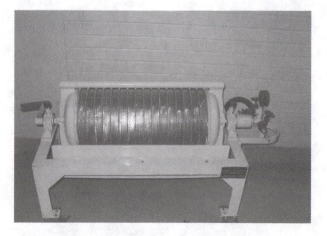

INSERT 4.4
Pilot-scale model of a Willmes Press. These presses are used to extract juices for juice and wine manufacture. Pilot-scale equipment is used to produce small batches of a prototype during the development of new products. (Photo courtesy of Katherine R. Herndon.)

4.5.8 Fermenting

Fermentation is the only primary method of food preservation that encourages multiplication of microbes. Among the earliest processed foods are those that were fermented, salted, sun-dried, or baked. Fermentation encourages the growth of beneficial microbes to outcompete spoilage and pathogenic microbes. To produce a fermented food, a starter culture of microbes is added to a perishable raw material to change it to a more stable food product. The stability of the product is attributed to the formation of a natural chemical preservative by the microbe. The most common preservatives generated are lactic acid and ethanol (see Insert 4.5 for chemical structures of these and other natural preservatives).

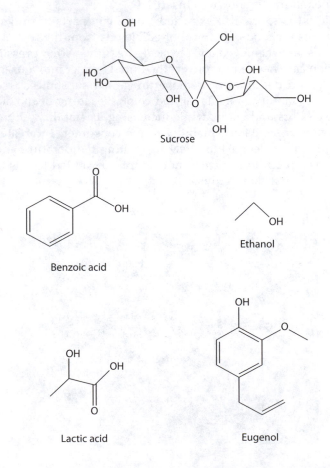

Sucrose

Benzoic acid

Ethanol

Lactic acid

Eugenol

INSERT 4.5
Chemical structures of natural preservatives. Sucrose or table sugar is found in sugar cane and sugar beets. Benzoic acid provides the tart taste of cranberry products. Ethanol is the alcohol in alcoholic beverages; lactic acid is in kimchi, sauerkraut, yogurt, and many other fermented products. Eugenol is the primary flavor of cloves.

The most common types of fermentation include the rising of dough before baking of bread as well as the production of alcoholic beverages and yogurt. Carbon dioxide is the chemical responsible for bread rising. Alcoholic beverages result from the production of ethanol. Yogurt production is a lactic acid fermentation. Other lactic acid fermentations include buttermilk, olives, pickles, salami, sauerkraut, sour cream, and vanilla. These lactic acid fermentations are conducted under strictly controlled conditions in commercial processing plants, but they can also be started by leaving the substrate (raw material) in the air or adding some of previously fermented product to the substrate. Genetic engineering of starter-culture microbes shows potential for more consistent quality of fermented products. Commercial fermentations can be disrupted by bacteriophages (bacterial viruses), which can attack starter cultures.

4.5.9 Irradiating

One of the most controversial forms of food preservation is the use of irradiation. Irradiation is a potent killer of microbes that can be used to preserve foods with little or no heat. It is also known as cold sterilization. The types of ionizing radiation used for foods have been selected because of their power to penetrate food tissue without making it radioactive. Chemical changes induced in foods by irradiation appear to be similar to those produced by other food preservation techniques. Radiation can be applied at high doses that will sterilize a product (imagine a raw steak stored in a plastic pouch safely in a cabinet at room temperature) or at a lower dose for **radurization**.

Irradiation kills microbes but does not inactivate toxins formed in the food before irradiation. Low-dose irradiation can be used to replace chemical fumigants to kill insects in imported foods, destroy vegetative (active) microbes, and inhibit sprouting in onions and potatoes. Bacteria tend to be more resistant to irradiation than yeasts and molds. The Food and Drug Administration has approved irradiation for bacon, preventing sprouting of potatoes and onions, spices, strawberries, poultry, ground beef, and pork. Although the most promising application of irradiation is to improve the safety of fresh meats, it can also be used to extend the shelf life of fresh fruits and vegetables.

Most food irradiation operations have relied on gamma rays to kill microbes. Gamma rays are also dangerous to human health; thus, elaborate safeguards are needed to protect workers in irradiation plants from stray rays. Processing large quantities of perishable foods means that either the raw material must be transported to a facility that specializes in irradiation or irradiators must be installed in a processing plant. An alternative technology, electron-beam radiation, can achieve similar results without the health risks associated with gamma irradiation. The electron beam does not penetrate the food as well as gamma rays; hence, greater doses of energy are required to achieve the same effect.

Opponents of food irradiation consider it to be a nonessential technology that encourages the food industry to cover up practices that encourage contamination. Proponents of the technology indicate that it could prevent numerous cases of food poisoning caused by inappropriate handling of foods in the home or foodservice operations. Part of the difference of opinion with regard to irradiation relates to their general belief of the safety of foods. Opponents of irradiation tend to believe that foods are inherently safe in their natural state and that they become unsafe when exposed to technology. Supporters of irradiation, including most food scientists, tend to believe that foods are inherently unsafe in their natural state and that a scientific under-standing of what causes safety problems leads to development of technology that provides safer foods.

4.5.10 Nonthermal Processing

While heat is the most effective means of killing microbes, the benefits are often achieved by sacrificing nutritional and sensory quality. Among the

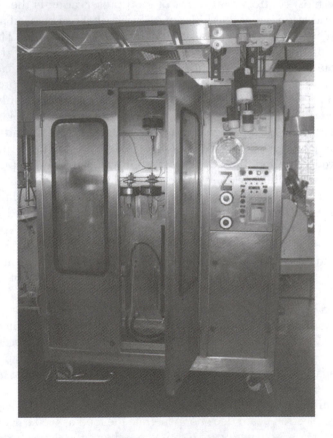

INSERT 4.6
Pilot-scale model of a continuous high-pressure throttling device that kills microorganisms in a liquid by implosion. (Photo courtesy of Katherine R. Herndon.)

alternatives to heat is high-pressure processing, which is currently used to pasteurize guacamole, salsa, and hummus. Microbes are killed in food products put under hydrostatic pressure. High-pressure processing is much milder than heat processing because the size and shape of the product are not important; thus, chunks (particulates) are not a problem.

High pressure can be applied in the container similar to canning or in bulk and then packaged like aseptic processing. High-pressure processing results in high-quality products, but it is a very expensive process. Another potential problem is that it does not always inactivate the enzymes that can decrease quality during storage. A pilot-scale high-pressure throttling device is shown in Insert 4.6. Although it will probably not replace conventional processing, it has potential for high-priced specialty products. Combination of heat treatment and high pressure can help take advantage of the benefits of both techniques.

4.6 Consequences of Processing

As indicated early in the chapter, foods are processed to keep them from spoiling. To achieve this end, there are some consequences that we must consider. Some operations are more severe than other processes. In general, the greater the benefit in extending shelf life and improving convenience derived by processing, the greater the chance of losing nutrients and quality. Not all these consequences are bad as some processes can destroy antinutrients present in foods or improve sensory quality. In this section, we will look at some of the trade-offs that result from food processing and how they vary by type of process.

4.6.1 Shelf Life

Put simply, shelf life is the length of time we can keep a product before we need to throw it away. From a more practical point of view, we want enough shelf life in a product so we don't have to rush to eat it before it spoils. While shelf life relates to the safety of a food product, it is most closely associated with spoilage. Since the primary cause of spoilage is microbial, the greater the destruction of microbes or inhibition of their growth, generally the greater the extension of shelf life. Other major causes of spoilage are enzyme activity and nonenzymic lipid oxidation.

Processing techniques that sterilize a product are the most likely ones to extend its shelf life. Canning, or commercial sterilization, is a very effective way of extending shelf life of foods. Canned foods last for years at ambient (typical room) temperatures or even in hot warehouses and shelters at much higher temperatures. It does not matter whether sterilization is done inside (canning) or outside (aseptic processing) the container. Theoretically, irradiation can also be used to sterilize foods, preserving raw foods for storage at room temperature, but it is not currently approved by governmental agencies for many applications. Note also that sterilization usually inactivates enzymes and excludes oxygen, greatly reducing other types of spoilage.

Processing techniques that inhibit microbial growth without sterilizing the food are also effective at extending shelf life of foods. Frozen foods are stable as long as they remain frozen, and dried foods remain stable as long as they do not become rehydrated. Some yeasts can grow in concentrated or intermediate moisture foods, but growth is usually slow. Combining two types of preservation such as concentrating and freezing can be very effective in extending shelf life. Chemical preservation either by curing or fermenting extends shelf life, but many of these products are held under refrigeration to prevent spoilage. While these techniques inhibit microbial growth, generally preventing microbial spoilage, other types of quality losses can occur.

Freezing and drying do not prevent enzyme activity, but they can slow it down. Blanching of vegetables can inactivate enzymes, but blanching is not usually performed with other raw materials. Even if enzyme activity is very slow, over a long period, damage can occur and the product can spoil. Concentration and fermentation can accelerate activity of some enzymes. Nonenzymic lipid oxidation proceeds slowly in foods containing fats. Few of these processing techniques inhibit this oxidation. Oxidation is actually accelerated in intermediate-moisture foods. If a frozen food is stored below its **glass-transition temperature** (point at which molecules in the food become immobile), enzyme degradation and oxidation are prevented.

Techniques such as pasteurization and radurization that kill pathogens but do not sterilize the product have less effect on shelf life. These products are considered perishable and usually require refrigeration. Microbes are the primary reason for spoilage, but loss of quality over time results from enzyme activity and lipid oxidation. Other techniques described in this chapter such as milling, extracting, and extruding do not generally preserve foods directly, but they are combined with other processing techniques to extend shelf life.

Shelf life is estimated by food engineers by determining the loss of a positive quality characteristic or the appearance of a negative characteristic. The end of the shelf life is when the product becomes unacceptable. In many processed foods, these changes occur in a predictable way that can be calculated using mathematical equations based on chemical kinetics.

4.6.2 Nutrition

Shelf-life extension is usually achieved by sacrificing something else. Frequently, nutritional value of foods is lost as a result of processing, with heat being one of the most destructive forces. Vitamins are lost during heat processing by changing them from active to inactive forms. Generally speaking, the higher the temperature with the shorter time needed to kill the intended microbes, the less the loss of nutrients that occurs. Once a food has been heat processed, however, vitamins or minerals are reasonably stable.

Minerals and water-soluble vitamins can be lost by leaching, which means that they dissolve in water during processing, become separated from the product, and are rarely consumed. Light and oxygen can also be very damaging to vitamins by inducing chemical reactions that break down vitamins. Fat-soluble vitamins tend to be more sensitive to the presence of light and oxygen because they tend to be more likely to become products of lipid oxidation. Some of the water-soluble B-vitamins are also quite susceptible to light-sensitive reactions. Irradiation tends to affect nutrients in ways similar to light. The stability of vitamins and minerals during storage of foods is also affected by pH.

Some processed foods are much less affected by nutrient loss than canned foods (see Insert 4.7). Freezing is a milder form of preservation than canning, but the blanching step (a heat process) will lead to leaching or inactivation. Drying is also milder than canning with nutrients affected by how much the raw materials are exposed to heat, light, and oxygen. Fermentation has little or no detrimental effect on the vitamins and minerals and can result in increased availability of these nutrients. Pre-fermentation steps, such as pasteurization of milk before yogurt production, will affect nutrient composition.

Exposure to light and oxygen is the most damaging aspect of curing, milling, and extraction. Milling and extraction can physically remove nutrients such as minerals, vitamins, and dietary fiber, while the presence of dietary fiber can bind minerals and vitamins, making them less available to us during digestion. While hydrogenation of oils improves the spreadability of margarine and other spreads, it results in the production of *trans* fatty acids. Partially hydrogenated oils are being phased out in American food products because of the health concerns about *trans* fats. In addition, packaging can be effectively used to keep light and oxygen away from the product.

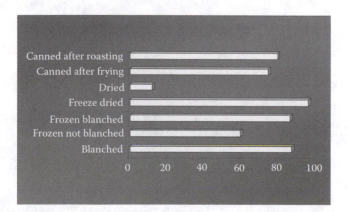

INSERT 4.7
Loss of vitamins in processed peppers. (Adapted from Martinez, S. et al., *International Journal of Food Science and Nutrition* 56: 45, 2005.)

Because vitamins and minerals are lost during processing, processed foods have a bad reputation for not being healthy or nutritious. When the nutritional value of processed foods is compared with that of the raw materials they come from, it is obvious that there are losses in most but not all cases and that losses vary by process and product (see Insert 4.8). Most consumers mistakenly believe that nutritional values of fresh foods never change. Food scientists believe that the poor reputation of processed foods is not deserved for the following reasons:

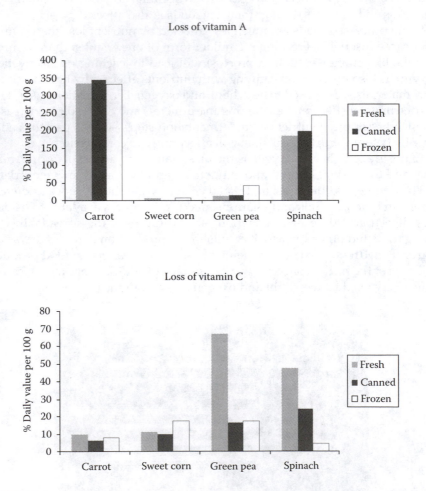

INSERT 4.8
Vitamins in fresh foods as affected by processing. (Calculated using data from the US Department of Agriculture National Nutrient Database for Standard Reference Release 20, 2007, http://www.nal.usda.gov/fnic/foodcomp/cgi-bin/list_nut_edit.pl; and the netrition.com website http://www.netrition.com/rdi_page.html.)

- Some processes are more destructive than others; thus, it is not fair to lump all processed foods together.
- Raw materials and fresh foods are more likely to lose nutrients during storage than processed foods.
- Cooking (a heat process), particularly boiling, is one of the most destructive processes for vitamins, with fresh foods more likely to be further cooked than processed foods.
- Fresh foods are more likely to spoil and be thrown away than processed ones.

Processed foods (even canned foods) do provide nutritional value. For example, canning modifies dietary fiber in fruit and vegetable products to improve its contribution to health. As we shall learn in Chapter 12, fiber is one of the most important reasons for consuming fruits and vegetables. In addition, heating of some products, carrots for example, increases the amount of some vitamins that are available to the body. Other processes can lower the levels of natural toxins and antinutrients present.

4.6.3 Quality

Sensory quality of foods such as appearance, flavor, and texture can also be lost during processing. Generally speaking, the conditions that affect nutritional value also affect sensory quality. We are all aware of the enticing odors resulting from roasting or cooking of our favorite foods. In many processes, however, heat destroys subtle flavors and can induce off-odors. Heat also tends to fade colors and can lead to unacceptable softening. Light causes oxidation of food components leading to loss of color and development of off-flavors. Oxygen and irradiation also lead to oxidation with a greater impact on flavor than on color. Texture is not as likely to be affected by light or oxygen as color or flavor.

As with nutritional value, the quality of some processed foods is much less affected than canned foods. One of the problems with canned foods is that the outside of the product becomes overprocessed before the cold spot in the can is properly processed. Techniques such as aseptic processing, microwaves, and more exotic processes such as **ohmic heating** are more even in their heating, providing a better-quality product. Freezing is also milder on sensory quality than canning, but enzymes can lead to quality losses during storage. Actually, blanching, because it inactivates enzymes, helps prevent quality losses during frozen storage. Very small changes attributed to enzymes that produce off-colors, -flavors, and -odors can make a big difference over the weeks and months of storage. Even if there is little loss of quality during freezing or storage, major losses can occur during thawing or holding of thawed product at room temperature before preparation.

Quality losses during drying or storage of dried foods vary by how much the raw materials or stored product are exposed to heat, light, and oxygen. Fermentation induces the flavor, appearance, and texture that we associate with a particular fermented food, with pasteurization of milk before yogurt production affecting some of the flavor of the raw milk. Exposure to light and oxygen are most damaging to quality during milling and extracting, but the oxidation of cured meats provides the characteristic flavor that those of us who like them crave. Part of this problem can be solved by adding flavor ingredients late in the barrel of the extruder. Packaging plays an effective role in protecting quality from damage caused by light and oxygen.

Processed foods also have the reputation of being poor in quality. Once again, food scientists think that this reputation is undeserved. Since the effect on quality varies by type of process, certain foods are much less likely to be low in quality than others. Comparisons should be made with other stored products and not freshly harvested crops. While it is impossible to observe the loss of nutrients during storage, the losses in flavor, appearance, and texture during spoilage in storage are obvious. As stated previously, microbes are the primary cause for spoilage of fresh foods, and enzymes are the next most likely cause. Prevention of spoilage is a major reason for processing raw materials (Insert 4.9).

Cooking induces changes in flavor, appearance, and texture, usually in desirable ways. Processed foods, even canned foods, do provide acceptable quality to some of us or they would never sell. Some people even prefer the flavor of processed foods to fresh or fresh-cooked products as the quality is what they expect.

Changes in climate and the environment combined with consumer demand to have exotic products the year round also hurt the quality of

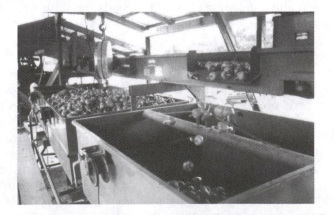

INSERT 4.9
Receiving of whole pimiento peppers into the processing plant. Quality monitoring starts at harvest in the field and continues until they are diced, packaged, canned, and shipped. (Photo courtesy of Virgil Esensee.)

processed foods as ingredients are sourced from around the world. The quality of many items, particularly those products containing garlic, lemons, egg whites, and seafood, is being adversely affected.

4.6.4 Safety

Safety is the most important consideration in the design of any food process. Raw materials should be handled in ways that minimize contamination and growth of microbes. Food is preserved to make it safer by reducing or eliminating harmful microbes and to extend its shelf life by reducing or eliminating spoilage microorganisms. Proper packaging prevents recontamination. No processing technique should be used as an excuse to avoid proper sanitary practices. A major criticism of irradiated foods is that the processor can pay less attention to proper sanitation than other preservation techniques. Such reasons are unacceptable for the proper preservation of foods.

Sterile products, like canned foods, are the safest foods we can eat, but they are not usually the most nutritious or highest-quality products. Safe foods are only as safe as handling and preparation. Once a canned food has been opened, it can become contaminated with microbes. If that microbe is a pathogen, and one that can grow in the food, it can grow without competition from other microbes with the food likely to become a safety hazard. Likewise, a frozen food that has become thawed or a dried food that has been rehydrated can support the growth of microbes that are already present, as these techniques slow growth of microbes with little or no killing. Fermented or cured foods may be safe under specified conditions (some require refrigeration), but they can become safety hazards if stored improperly. Milling and extraction have little effect on microbes, and thus they must be performed under sanitary conditions and further processed to prevent safety problems.

4.6.5 Packaging Considerations

We must remember that the preservation technique is only as good as the package that contains it. Although any preservation technique slows or stops spoilage, recontamination of processed foods can restart spoilage or introduce microbes, leading to food-borne illness. Food packages are designed to protect the food from microbes, insects, rodents, and physical impact. The main function of a package is to preserve the physical and chemical integrity of a product including preventing microbial or chemical contamination. Packaging also functions to keep in water, odors, and gases and keep out water, oxygen, odors, and light. A primary package is the one directly in touch with the food product. The secondary package contains the primary package(s). The tertiary package contains the secondary package(s), and so on. Any part of the primary package in touch with the food must be compatible with the food and must not be toxic.

In the design of a food process, the construction of the package must be carefully evaluated. Considerations include whether (1) the process occurs before or after packaging, (2) the packaging material can withstand the conditions of processing and distribution, and (3) the package is compatible with the product. Canning occurs inside the package, and some frozen product is packaged before freezing. Most other processes including aseptic processing, pasteurization, concentration, most freezing, dehydration, and fermentation occur before packaging. When packaging comes after processing, great care is needed to prevent recontamination.

Any product that is processed by heat in the package needs a package that can withstand the heat and usually water associated with the process. Any package that will be exposed to water, either in the processing plant or elsewhere, must not be damaged by water. The package must be able to withstand normal abuse that it could experience during its journey from the processing plant to the consumer. Most packages are designed with tamper-evident seals to prevent unscrupulous humans from deliberately contaminating a product without the consumer's knowledge. Consumers are also buying products that are convenient by offering the option to cook the package in a microwave oven, conventional oven, or both. Components of the food might interact with the package. Thus, possible interactions must be studied to ensure that no reactions occur that could result in a product hazard or unacceptable product.

Fresh, whole foods are important components in a healthy diet, but there are times when processed foods are much more appropriate. To meet the needs of impoverished members of a community, food banks stock and distribute processed foods that will not spoil rapidly. The first wave of supplies in response to natural disasters like earthquakes, hurricanes, tornadoes, and tsunamis include bottled water and highly nutritious processed foods. On military missions and when hiking or camping, processed foods provide quick energy that is both convenient and easy to carry. Formulated foods, the topic of Chapter 5, can provide highly nutritious items to malnourished children and nursing mothers in regions where modern conveniences are not available.

4.7 Remember This!

- The main function of a package is to preserve the physical and chemical integrity of a product including preventing microbial or chemical contamination.
- Food is preserved to make it safer by reducing or eliminating harmful microbes and to extend its shelf life by reducing or eliminating spoilage microorganisms.

- The conditions that affect nutritional value also affect sensory quality.
- The higher the temperature of a heat process with the shorter time needed to kill the intended microbes, the less the loss of nutrients.
- The greater the destruction of microbes or inhibition of their growth, generally the greater the extension of shelf life.
- Fermentation is the only primary method of food preservation that encourages multiplication of microbes.
- Processing techniques for a specific food are designed with an understanding of the potential microbes present and the properties of the food.
- Unit operations are distinct steps common to many food processes.
- Food processing and preservation increase the shelf stability of a raw material usually at the cost of nutrition and quality.
- Most raw materials are perishable and require careful handling or processing to prevent losses.

4.8 Looking Ahead

This chapter was designed to provide an introduction to food processes and the types of products that are produced with a special emphasis on those made directly from raw agricultural materials. Chapter 5 will introduce formulated foods, made from mixing ingredients. Chapter 6 will describe chilled and prepared foods. We will find how processed food is analyzed for quality and safety in Chapter 7. Chapter 12 explores the nutritional properties of plant products, animal products, and so-called junk foods. The basic principles behind food microbiology will be presented in Chapter 13 and those behind food engineering will be presented in Chapter 14.

Testing Comprehension

1. Identify the most probable causes of the obesity epidemic that started about the time Malik's mother was in high school.
2. Distinguish between the foods in Insert 4.1 that are sterile from those that are not sterile. Which of these foods is the safest, the healthiest, and the most appealing? Why?
3. Prepare a list of all the foods Leah should take with her in a backpack on a 3-day, 2-night camping trip in the woods. She will have no

access to any other supplies for a 60-hour period. Explain why these items were selected and any compromises she would need to make.

4. Identify three processed foods and three whole foods not mentioned in the chapter. List all the advantages and disadvantages of consuming each of these foods.

5. Compare and contrast two of the types of food processes described in the chapter. Identify the preservation principle for each of these two types of processes. Identify three raw materials that could be suitably preserved by both processes. For each of these raw materials, describe any personal preferences. Explain.

6. Outline the case either for or against the widespread distribution of irradiated foods during natural disasters or to impoverished regions. Should irradiated foods be clearly labeled? Why or why not?

7. Compare and contrast the rationale for blanching, pasteurizing, and canning. Provide examples of products that require each of these unit operations.

8. Food scientists are obsessed with shelf life of products. Discuss the benefits and detriments of extending the shelf life of fresh foods by processing.

9. Calculate the percentage of sugar in frozen orange juice concentrate that has had 70% of its water removed if the original juice was 10% sugar. If ten thousand 12-ounce cans of original juice concentrate are shipped from Florida to a local supermarket, how many gallons of water will not need to be shipped because of concentration? Do the environmental benefits of transporting less water make up for the effects of freezing and concentrating? Explain.

Reference

Martinez, S., M. Lopez, M. Gonzalez-Raurich and A. B. Alvarez, 2005. The effects of ripening stage and processing systems on vitamin C content in sweet peppers (*Capsicum annum* L.). *Int. J. Food Sci. Nutr.*, 56:45.

Further Reading

Ahmed, J., H. S. Ramaswamy, S. Kasapis and J. I. Boye, 2009. *Novel Food Processing: Effects on Rheological and Functional Properties*, Boca Raton, FL: CRC Press.
Clarke, S., S. Jung and B. Lamsal, 2014. *Food Processing: Principles and Applications*, 2nd ed., Ames, IA: Wiley.

Fellows, P. J., 2009. *Food Processing Technology: Principles and Practices*, 3rd ed., Cambridge: Woodhead Publishing.

Holdsworth, E. and R. Simpson, 2008. *Thermal Processing of Packaged Foods*, New York: Springer Science.

Potter, N. N. and J. H. Hotchkiss, 1999. *Food Science*, 5th ed., New York: Chapman & Hall.

Schaschke, C. J., 2013. *Food Processing*, http://bookboon.com, London: Davenport House.

Shewfelt, A. L., 1971. *Your Future in Food Science*, New York: Carlton Press.

Shi, J., 2007. *Functional Food Ingredients and Nutraceuticals: Processing Technologies*, Boca Raton, FL: CRC Press.

Sun, D. W., 2012. *Thermal Food Processing: New Technologies and Quality Issues*, 2nd ed., Boca Raton, FL: CRC Press.

5

Formulated Foods

Nil is always on the go. He doesn't have much time for meals, and he's now wary about hamburgers. He needs his food quick, and he needs it to be healthy. Fortunately for him, there are a wide range of products that are ready to eat and nutritious. He lives primarily on energy bars and energy drinks. He can't remember the last time he has eaten meat, bread, or vegetables. He just figures he is eating a balanced diet with lots of protein. He can read that right off the labels, when he has the time to read them. The other thing he likes about these products is that they come in lots of different flavors. His favorite bar is Crackling Chocolate Almond, and his favorite energy drink is Loca Moca, but he likes to mix it up, with at least half his meals in another flavor. The caffeine in the drinks keeps him active, but sometimes it interferes with a decent night's sleep.

Tiana does not like to cook, but she has heard that any packaged food with more than five ingredients is dangerous. She is also concerned that anything with gluten in it will make her sick or fat or both. As a result, her diet has become very restricted. She is pleased that there are lots more gluten-free products out there now, but most of them don't taste that good, and many of them have as many as 10 or 15 ingredients. She wonders why food companies can't make more products to suit her.

Leah is poor. She lives in a dorm. She doesn't have much in the way of kitchen appliances. She is not on the meal plan. Early in the month, when she has some money, she lives on macaroni and cheese; when money runs low, she switches to Ramen noodles. Both meals are satisfying without having too many calories. They are easy to prepare in her room: all that is needed is hot water. It is a good thing she likes the flavor of the macaroni and cheese and the noodles. They never seem to get old.

Nil and Leah have abandoned whole and natural foods for what are called formulated foods. The best way to tell what is in formulated foods is to read the ingredient statement. Many of us depend on formulated foods for our nutrients. Frequently, these foods are hard to fit into the guidelines in "ChooseMyPlate.gov." Tiana is restricted to mostly canned, dried, and frozen meals as most formulated foods have more than the five ingredients that some "healthy-food" advocates say are to be avoided.

5.1 Looking Back

Previous chapters focused on food issues we deal with daily. Some key points that were covered in those chapters help prepare us for understanding formulated foods:

- The main function of a package is to preserve the physical and chemical integrity of a product including preventing microbial or chemical contamination.

- Food is preserved to make it safer by reducing or eliminating harmful microbes and to extend its shelf life by reducing or eliminating spoilage microorganisms.

- Unit operations are distinct steps common to many food processes.

- Although many of us try to eat healthy diets, there are many temptations and influences affecting our decisions that we do not consciously consider.

- It is not just the taste but the combination of all the sensory properties (i.e., flavor, appearance, and texture) that influence our choice of food.

- The Nutrition Facts part of the label indicates the serving size, how many servings per container, calories per serving, and the fat calories per serving.

- Nutraceuticals are foods specifically designed to act as drugs.

- Good nutrition requires an adequate consumption of nutrients without consuming too many calories.

- Preservatives are food ingredients that slow spoilage and help prevent food-associated illnesses.

- An expiration date represents the food scientist's best guess about how long a food will last before it spoils.

This chapter focuses on the formulation of ingredients into food products. The previous chapter emphasized the operations that are used to process foods. Chapter 6 presents information on chilled foods (perishable and requiring refrigeration to maintain quality) and prepared foods (ready to eat with or without heating). These distinctions are made to help us understand how foods are made. Most of us don't think much about whether a food has been processed or formulated, chilled, or prepared. In many cases, these categories overlap. However, an understanding of how foods are formulated and their importance in modern diets is critical to understanding food science.

5.2 What Are Formulated Foods and Why Are They Formulated?

Formulated foods are products that are mixtures of ingredients. Unlike the processed foods described in Chapter 4, formulated foods are not directly recognizable as their original plant or animal sources. Formulated foods are not new. Products like bread, low-calorie frozen dinners, ice cream, and yogurt have been around for a long time, but never before has there been such a wide selection of formulated products.

Formulated foods provide us with flavorful combinations of ingredients in a convenient form, usually preserved or in a stable product. A world with just fresh and processed foods would be a very different one, and, for many of us, a much duller one. Most formulated foods have been preserved in some way to reduce or minimize microbial growth. Each of the ingredients is present to perform at least one specific function in that product. Ingredients may function to preserve the safety of the food, improve the nutritional value of the product, or enhance product quality.

5.2.1 Benefits and Consequences

Formulated foods that have been preserved in some manner have all of the advantages of processed foods. Like their processed counterparts, they tend to be shelf stable, safe, and convenient. In formulating a food, the food scientist faces fewer restrictions than during food processing. The trade-offs between nutrition and quality are not as significant in formulated foods as in processed foods. Any deficiencies in the nutrients of the raw materials or ingredients can be ignored to create a "fun" or "junk" food, or they can be overcome by adding nutrients to become a "health" or "functional" food. Likewise, ingredients can be added to improve the flavor, color, or texture of a product to enhance its appeal.

Formulated foods are frequently safer than processed ones because they contain preservatives. Although preservative has become a dirty word in our culture, preservatives function to reduce microbial growth, decrease food spoilage, and increase food safety. Thus, leftovers from formulated foods with preservatives are less likely to spoil than those from fresh or processed foods. Finally, many formulated foods fit in nicely with our fast-paced culture. They tend to be ready to eat or require minimal preparation. They can be eaten with our fingers on a slow walk or a fast ride, leaving little or no mess other than the package, which can be easily discarded.

There are problems with formulated foods, however, particularly from a nutritional standpoint. Three components in formulated foods that improve their flavor are salt, sugar, and fat. When consumed in moderation, each of these components makes a valuable contribution to our diet. However, when consumed in excess, they can be detrimental to our health and can decrease our desire to eat more nutrient-dense foods. Formulated foods that contain fruit or vegetable ingredients may convey the false idea that they provide the benefits of whole fruits and vegetables. Even the "health" or "functional" foods that Nil lives on tend to provide high levels of only a few nutrients and do not provide a balanced diet. Many of them also have high levels of salt, sugar, or fat.

Health-conscious consumers of formulated foods have an obligation to carefully read food labels to make sure they are indeed getting the vitamins and minerals they need. Although the food industry is frequently blamed for making processed foods "tasteless," it would appear the major problem with many formulated foods is that they are too tempting.

5.2.2 Formulation Steps

Many steps occur in a food manufacturing plant to mix ingredients and transform them into tempting foods and beverages. Just as in processed foods, there are distinct unit operations common to many types of food formulations. These steps begin as the ingredients are unloaded at the plant dock and continue until the packaged product is loaded onto another truck or railcar for transport out. Most ingredients are shelf stable, but many companies do not want the added expense of maintaining large warehouses for storing supplies. Some common unit operations include materials handling, pumping, mixing, heat exchanging, packaging, and controlling.

In the production of fruit-on-the-bottom yogurt, for example, there are many unit operations (see Insert 5.1). All ingredients must be received and properly stored. The milk must be standardized to the proper fat content. The fat content of the yogurt will be the same as the fat content of the milk because it will not change during fermentation. Pasteurization of the milk occurs after the addition of the dry ingredients (such as sugar). In the production of yogurt, pasteurization must be more vigorous than for regular milk because it must eliminate undesirable microbes that can compete with the starter culture that is added to produce the yogurt. The fruit is put into the bottom of the container with the pasteurized milk on top. As the product is incubated, the starter-culture organisms multiply and the liquid milk slowly develops a tart flavor and a thick consistency. When the incubation period is complete, the containers are chilled, ready for shipment to supermarkets or other points of sale.

5.2.3 Clean Labels

With the increased concern about food additives and a demand by consumers for natural ingredients, food manufacturers are looking for "cleaner" labels. A clean label is one that has only clearly recognizable ingredients,

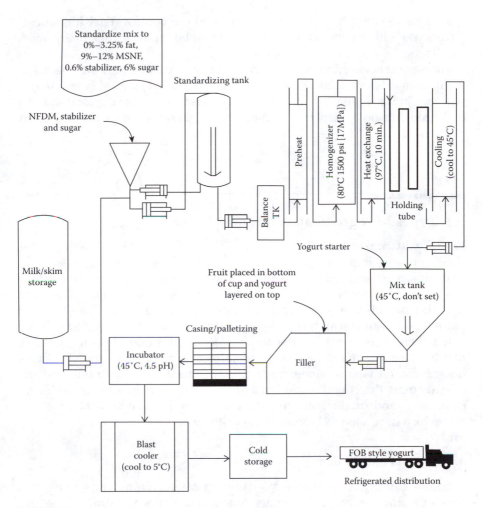

INSERT 5.1

Schematic for producing a fruit-on-the-bottom drinkable yogurt. (O'Rell, K.R. and Chandan, R.C.: Manufacture of various types of yogurt. In *Manufacturing of Yogurt and Fermented Milks*, 2nd ed., Chandan R.C. and Kilara, A. eds., Ames, IA: Wiley-Blackwell, Chapter 12, 2013. Copyright Wiley-VCH Verlag GmbH & Co. KGaA. Reproduced with permission.)

none of which sound like chemicals. The main emphasis has been on preservatives that inhibit growth of microbes, particularly mold. For example, clean ingredients to inhibit molds in baked goods include cinnamon and clove to disrupt cell membranes instead of adding the active compounds within these spices—cinnamaldehyde or eugenol. Raisin paste concentrate can be added instead of propionic or tartaric acids for mold inhibition and vinegar to replace acetic acid for reducing dough pH. Ingredients specifically targeted for removal are high-fructose corn syrup and monosodium glutamate. Some companies that removed these controversial ingredients have since added them back because of complaints from consumers about lost flavor.

Phrases/terms used to enhance products with clean labels include *naked*; *natural*; *no artificial colors, flavorings,* or *preservatives*; *pure*; *real*; and *simply*. Another initiative food companies have taken is to reduce the total number of ingredients on the label with an ultimate goal of five or less as desired by Tiana.

5.3 Types of Ingredients and Their Function

What really makes food formulation different from food processing is the wide range of ingredients that are used. In selecting the ingredients for a formulation, the food scientist must consider the quality of the food, its safety, its stability, and its cost. Ignoring any one of these aspects could doom it in the marketplace. When concerned about what is in our food, the best place to start our research is by looking at the label. All the ingredients are listed there. It is important not to jump to conclusions about ingredients. Just because one might have a weird-sounding or unpronounceable name doesn't mean that it is dangerous. Each ingredient has at least one, and frequently more than one, function in a product. Food scientists responsible for designing food products must understand how each ingredient functions and which ingredient is best for the specific product.

5.3.1 Flours and Grains

Worldwide, individuals take in more of their calories from flours and grains than any other source. The primary function of flours and grains is to provide calories. They are also critical in providing the basic structure and texture of a product. Flours and grains are the main ingredient in baked goods; however, they can also be found in soups, beverages, confections, and many other products.

Although the largest component of flour is carbohydrates, flour proteins are also important. Wheat flour is best for making bread. The protein complex, gluten, which is formed when water is added to the flour, is the reason wheat flour is superior to other flours. Gluten is elastic, which allows it to bend, expand, and stretch rather than break. Thus, the CO_2 gas bubbles produced by yeast or baking powder are trapped in pockets formed by the gluten network, creating the light, fluffy texture that bread lovers enjoy. Bread flour, particularly white flour, is rather bland; the delicate bread flavors form during baking. Unique bread flavors are the result of adding other flours like rye, potato, soy, oats, and others. Most of these breads contain only a small amount of the other flour for flavor, while maintaining a high level of wheat flour for a light, fluffy texture. In general, the less wheat flour, the coarser and heavier the texture. For instance, compare cornbread with wheat bread.

Whole-wheat flour contributes flavor but at the cost of lightness. The use of whole-wheat flour or addition of other whole grains such as rye increases the dietary fiber in a product but changes the product quality. Be careful not to judge a loaf of bread by its color. Some breads that appear to be whole wheat merely have caramel coloring added to turn them brown. To make sure, check the fiber content on the Nutrition Facts part of the label.

Whole grains include bulgur, rye, oats, buckwheat, amaranth, millet, barley, and many others. They make excellent cereals, or they can be ingredients in casseroles, soups, pasta dishes, and other products where grains are important in providing texture. Flours or meals can be produced from these grains, as well as corn, soy, peanut, potato, black-eyed pea, and others. Some of these grains are used sparingly in baked goods, and many are added as thickeners in products like soups, salad dressings, and beverages. Grains also serve as the fermentation substrate for many alcoholic beverages.

Starches extracted from flours are important ingredients in many products. Different starches have unique properties. Most are added to foods to provide the proper texture. Starches swell in the presence of water. Selection of the right starch is critical in product performance. They are primary components of flours in breads, cakes, cookies, breakfast cereals and other baked goods. They also show up on ingredient statements in salad dressings, gravies, soup mixes, puddings, and many other products. Some starches are stable when frozen and thawed; others are not. Most starches will gel after boiling, but some won't. Starches can be modified to cook and gel quickly (quick grits or oatmeal), which improves speed and convenience in food preparation.

The structural changes in starch during processing and cooking are shown in Insert 5.2. A main problem with cooked and cooled starches is

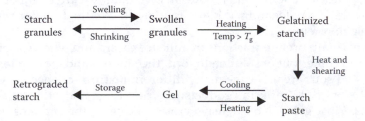

INSERT 5.2
Changes in the form of starch resulting in changes of textural properties in foods. (From Jane, J., Starch: Structure and Properties. In *Chemical and Functional Properties of Food Saccharides*, Tomasik, P., ed., Boca Raton, FL: CRC Press; Taylor & Francis Group, Chapter 7, 2004. With permission.)

retrogradation, which manifests itself as staling. Staling is the result of the starch separating from the water in the product. Staling produces off-flavors and poor texture.

5.3.2 Fruits and Vegetables

Fruits and vegetables are often eaten whole—fresh, frozen, canned, or dried. Fruits and vegetables are also necessary ingredients in many other products. Fruits form the fillings in many pies and baked goods; contribute to the flavor of many beverages, ice creams, and other desserts; serve as a topping for cereals; and appear in jams, jellies, preserves, and roll-ups. Vegetables are major components of many soups and frozen entrées, but they also appear in pies (pumpkin and sweet potato), cakes (carrot), and juices.

In addition to providing nutrition and flavor, fruits and vegetables add color and texture to products. Fruits, when used as ingredients, are usually accompanied by extra sugar. Although dietary fiber is an important nutritional component of fruits and vegetables, fiber is frequently removed to improve the functionality of the ingredient or its appeal to the consumer. Unfortunately, the clear juices that are more popular with students than those with pulp also have less dietary fiber. Fresh fruits and vegetables that will be used as ingredients are usually processed to keep them from spoiling. Fruits and vegetables can be processed into juice concentrates, preserved with sugar, canned, frozen, or dried until ready for use.

5.3.3 Dairy and Eggs

Dairy products are excellent sources of high-quality protein and calcium. They are also of great interest to food scientists because of their functional properties (contributing directly to a specific function of an ingredient in a food product). Many formulated foods were developed by taking advantage of the functional properties of milk and egg proteins. For example, yogurt, pudding, cheese, and fondue all owe their texture to milk proteins. The texture of omelet and meringue is attributed to the functional properties of egg proteins.

The two main protein fractions in milk are casein and whey. Casein coagulates and comes out of solution to form the smooth and creamy texture of yogurt and sour cream or the many different textures of cheeses. Gels are formed from fluid milk in products like puddings and other milk-based desserts. Most gels have extensive cross-linking of the proteins and will not reverse when reheated. Gelatin, derived from meat, will change back into liquid form upon reheating. Formation of protein gels that bind water is a very important component of the cooking technique called **molecular gastronomy**, which provides the customer with unique textural sensations.

These gels can be formed with egg white, milk, and certain plant and animal proteins. Egg yolk protein acts as an emulsifier, keeping water and fat from separating in products such as mayonnaise. Egg whites are known for their ability to foam, providing the light, fluffy texture of cakes, meringues, and shakes.

5.3.4 Plant Proteins

Although complete proteins come from animal products, many consumers get their proteins from plant sources. Plant proteins are not complete proteins. Plant proteins from one source, like corn, can be nutritious if they are balanced with complementary proteins from another source, like beans. For use as ingredients, plant proteins must first be isolated and purified. The isolation process separates the small quantities of protein in plant cells from the nonprotein material—the cell walls, carbohydrates, fats, and acids. Purification must be rigorous enough to remove all unwanted material for the protein to function properly yet mild enough to maintain the desired functional properties of the protein. Plant proteins can function as emulsifiers, water binders, and gelling agents.

Textured vegetable proteins replace meat protein in veggie burgers and other meat substitutes for the consumer who doesn't want to eat meat and doesn't want to give up some of their favorite products. Plant proteins can be modified by chemical, enzymatic, or physical processes to meet the ingredient's functional requirements. Sources of plant proteins include grains such as corn and oats and oil-rich seeds such as soybeans and peanuts.

Vegans and people wishing to cut down on their meat consumption may still want to consume products with the flavor and texture of meat. Food processors have designed meat analogs for these consumers. Meat analogs use plant proteins, particularly from soy, but can also be made from oat, rice, and wheat. Soy protein can be spun into fibers to form textured vegetable protein and with better texture than from other plant proteins. Quorn, a fungal protein, is also used in forming meat substitutes. Soy and almond are popular sources of protein for dairy substitutes.

5.3.5 Fats and Oils

Although many of us are trying to cut back on our fat and oil intake, they are still important ingredients in many of our favorite products. Fats and oils are extracted from plant and animal products and belong to a chemical group called lipids. Fats are solid and oils are liquid at room temperature. Rendering, pressing, extracting, refining, modifying, and forming are common unit operations for fat and oil products. Rendering melts an animal fat and separates it from other components. Pressing physically removes the oil from a plant seed. Organic solvents such as hexane are used to extract oils from water in the seed. Refining removes undesirable compounds, bleaching removes pigments, and deodorizing reduces off-odors and -flavors. Hydrogenation improves the functional properties of the fat or oil, but the process increases the level of *trans* fatty acids. More information on *trans* fatty acids is available in Chapters 6 and 11. Butter, chocolates, cooking oils, margarine, mayonnaise, peanut butter, and salad dressings are examples of products with fats and oils as primary ingredients.

So why do we want to put fats and oils into food products? First, there is the issue of satiety (feeling full). Fats and oils slow down the stomach-emptying time. The longer the stomach-emptying time, the longer it is before we become hungry again. Another reason for adding fats and oils is that they enrobe flavors and contribute to mouthfeel (how a food feels when it is in the mouth). Our food may not taste as good without the fat and oil because they can act as carriers of flavors. In addition, when fats and oils are heated, they turn liquid in the mouth and contribute to the juiciness of meats and other entrées, serving as lubricants in the mouth. Finally, fats and oils can either serve as flavor precursors or become oxidized. A precursor is a flavorless compound that changes form to either a desirable or an undesirable flavor during mixing, heating, or storage. Oxidation is a series of reactions that leads to off-flavors, generally described as tasting like cardboard or like fresh-mowed grass.

5.3.6 Sweeteners

Sugar can be a major source of calories for anyone with a sweet tooth. However, sugar is much more than a sweet source of calories. Sugars contribute to the color and texture of food products. Table sugar, or sucrose, can caramelize. Other sugars such as fructose (primary sweetener in honey), glucose (blood sugar), and lactose (milk sugar) are "reducing sugars" and can turn brown at lower temperatures. Sugars also provide bulk and contribute to mouthfeel. By taking away the sugar in a food that is 10% sugar, there is 10% less food than the food with sugar. In addition, the form of sugar (crystalline or noncrystalline) can affect the structure of a confection. Sugar has other functional properties relating to the sponginess of cakes and the creaminess of ice creams in addition to adding a sweet flavor to these products.

Artificial sweeteners can be used to replace sugars. There is a major reduction of calories when artificial sweeteners are used. For example, a 12-ounce can of regular cola contains 39 grams of sugar (196 calories). A sugar-free product with aspartame (NutraSweet) contains 1 calories. Other artificial sweeteners include saccharin (Sweet'n Low), sucralose (Splenda), sorbitol, and acesulfame K (Sunett). Each sweetener has its advantages and disadvantages. For example, aspartame breaks down when heated, making it

Neotame	8000
Alitame	2000
Sucralose	600
Saccharin	300–500
Steviol glycosides	300
Acesulfame potassium	200
Aspartame	180
Cyclamate	30
High fructose corn syrup	1
Sucrose	1
Maltitol	0.9
Sorbitol	0.6

INSERT 5.3

Sweetness of sugar substitutes relative to sucrose. (Adapted from Nabors, L.O., Alternative sweeteners: An overview. In *Alternative Sweeteners*, 4th ed., New York: Marcel Dekker, Inc., Chapter 1, 2012.)

unsuitable for baked goods; saccharin and acesulfame K have a bitter aftertaste; sorbitol works well in baked goods, but it can cause flatulence.

Sucralose is the only artificial sweetener that is a direct derivative of sucrose. Some of these problems can be overcome by mixing the alternative sweeteners. For clean labels, rebaudioside A (Truvia) is a purified natural extract from leaves of the *Stevia* genus. Most of these sweeteners are much sweeter than sucrose and may require a bulking agent like polydextrose or maltodextrin to provide the texture and volume of the missing sugar. For relative sweetness of low-calorie sweeteners, see Insert 5.3.

5.3.7 Fat Replacers

Replacing the fat in products is of even more interest than replacing the sugar. Unfortunately, individual fat replacers cannot perform all the functions of lipids. Flavor and mouthfeel are the two functions that are the most difficult to replace. Protein particles can produce a similar mouthfeel and reduce the calories by half; carbohydrates can increase the viscosity. Neither, however, is as stable to high-temperature frying and cooking. Sucrose esters (like Olestra) are chemically similar to fats and have similar stability but are not digested and absorbed by the body. The sucrose esters have the full lubricating properties in the mouth as real fats. Unfortunately, because they are not digestible, the lubricating properties can cause side effects such as diarrhea and abdominal cramping if consumed in excess. Another option to reduce caloric content is to simply remove the fat without adding a fat replacer, but such removal can have unexpected consequences. For example, most low-fat peanut butter products have more calories per serving than the full-fat versions.

Other fat replacers include gums and hydrocolloids, which are carbohydrates similar to dietary fiber. They provide similar textures to foods, while replacing the bulk of the fat; hence, the low-fat product contains fewer calories. The gums and hydrocolloids are either not absorbed by the body or absorbed at a much lower rate than the fats. Unfortunately, these ingredients do not provide the lubrication or the flavor properties of fat. Starch and protein-based products can provide bulk and some lubrication but not flavor. Many companies are working on synthetic fat replacers that will have all the advantages of fat without the problems, but none are currently approved by the Food and Drug Administration.

Although fat reduction is a good thing for most of us, there are difficulties. In general, many of the functional properties of a fat can be maintained even with the elimination or replacement of more than half of the fat in a product. Complete elimination of the fat, however, makes it difficult to match the flavor and texture of the full-fat product. Another potential problem with low-fat products is that consumers may eat more low-fat product to fill them up and thus still not reduce their calorie intake. See Insert 5.4 for more information on fat replacers.

Chemical base	Subtype	Composition	Functionality
Lipid	Sucrose fatty acid polyester (Olean and Olestra)	Transesterified and interesterified sucrose by fatty acids	Provides mouthfeel and lubrication of fats absorbed
	Sucrose fatty acid esters	Monoglycerides, diglycerides and triglycerides of	Excellent surfactants and emulsifiers
	Structured lipids	Mixed chain-length fatty acids	Specific applications
Protein	Simplesse	Microparticulated whey protein	Baked goods, salad dressings and mayonnaise
Carbohydrate	Gums	Negatively charged high-molecular weight polymers	Stabilizers, gelling agents, increases viscosity
	Starches	Varying sources	Slippery mouthfeel
	Maltodextrins	Polymer of mixed-length saccharides	Water binding, viscosity, smooth mouthfeel
	Polydextrose	Polymer of glucose, sorbitol, and citric or phosphoric acid	Bulking agent and texturizer
	Oatrim	Hydrolysis of oat hulls	Mimics fat mouthfeel

INSERT 5.4
Types of fat replacers found in foods. (Adapted from Akoh, C.C., *Food Technology* 52 (3): 47, 1998.)

5.3.8 Flavorants and Colorants

Flavor and color frequently make the difference between a food we enjoy and one we just won't eat. Some ingredients are added to foods to enhance the flavor and color. Most flavor ingredients that are added to food are colorless, yet color can influence perception of flavor as mentioned in Chapter 3.

As we will learn in greater detail in Chapters 7 and 15, flavor is the combination of the senses of taste and aroma. Most flavor ingredients (flavorants) are volatile (evaporate rapidly at room or body temperatures) compounds that contribute to the aroma of food products. Flavorants can be natural or synthetic. Early attempts at artificial flavoring were only suggestive of the real thing, but recent advances have been much more sophisticated. In many products, a flavor-impact compound is responsible for much of the characteristic aroma of that product; however, the aroma of most products is the combination of a wide range of aromatic compounds. Flavorants may provide or add to the flavor impact of a product, enhance or mask other flavors, or provide a background for other flavors present. Monosodium glutamate is a flavor enhancer that tends to bring out flavors not normally perceived by a consumer.

Makers of sports beverages, breakfast cereals, and other products know that many consumers are more likely to buy a product if it is brightly colored; thus, they add artificial colors to these products to enhance their appeal. These colorants are similar to those used in the home to color Easter eggs and cake icings. Natural colorants are isolated from fruits, vegetables, flowers, or insects and added to food products. Most food manufacturers prefer artificial colorants because they are brighter, more stable, and easier to handle than natural colorants. Natural colorants do not appear to be any safer than artificial ones, but they are required for a clean label.

5.3.9 Stabilizers

Stabilizers are added to formulated foods to keep them from breaking down. Peanut butter with the oil floating to the top of the jar and a milk-chocolate bar with an uneven white coating are examples of food breakdown that is not related to microbes. Stabilizers prevent the separation of food components and help maintain product structure.

One important group of stabilizers is the emulsifiers. Many formulated foods are emulsions such that oil is dispersed in water (sauces and soups) or water is dispersed in oil (margarine and mayonnaise). Ordinarily, water and oil don't mix, but emulsifiers can dissolve in both water and oil. With part of the emulsifier dissolved in water and the other part dissolved in oil, it can keep the water and oil bound together. Some natural peanut butters do not have added emulsifiers and are more likely to separate out, leaving an oily layer on top of the jar. Most peanut butter–like products are not really peanut butter as they don't contain the ingredients that the government recognizes in its Standard of Identity. Next time reaching for peanut butter on the shelf, look to see if it is really peanut butter or a peanut butter spread. Egg yolk contains lecithin, a natural emulsifier that helps keep mayonnaise together. Soy lecithin is used as a stabilizer in vegan products.

Gums represent another important type of stabilizer. Gums are water-soluble polysaccharides that help thicken liquid and semisolid foods. They thicken by binding water present and swelling up. Each gum possesses unique properties that are useful in formulating food products that we enjoy. For example, gum tragacanth is stable over a wide pH range, agar forms nice gels, guar gum is an excellent thickener at low concentrations, and alginate works well when combined with calcium as found in milk products.

5.3.10 Preservatives

In addition to being resistant to breakdown, formulated foods are also resistant to microbial spoilage. Preservatives are food additives that prevent or slow spoilage. An example of a product not protected by preservatives is shown in Insert 5.5.

Many spices are added to foods to prevent microbial growth and rancidity as well as to add flavor. Garlic, nutmeg, oregano, and thyme are known to protect foods from harmful microbes. Cloves, cumin, and sage slow the growth of molds; basil and rosemary serve as antioxidants. Chemical compounds added to foods to prevent the growth of molds and yeasts include sorbic, benzoic, and acetic acids or their salt forms. Sulfur dioxide, nitrates, and nitrites are used to prevent the growth of bacteria that can cause illness or spoilage. Natural antioxidants such as vitamins A, C, and E or synthetic antioxidants such as BHA (butylated hydroxyanisole) and

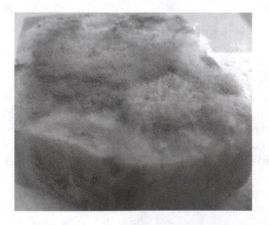

INSERT 5.5
The deterioration of a preservative-free food—moldy cheese. (Photo courtesy of Robert Shewfelt.)

BHT (butylated hydroxytoluene) prevent fatty foods and oils from developing rancidity.

5.4 Formulated Products

5.4.1 Baked Goods

Think of the vast array of breads, cookies, crackers, cakes, and specialty items such as chocolate éclairs that are available in the marketplace today. All are baked goods. The differences in these products are the result of the ingredients that provide unique colors, flavors, and textural sensations during eating. Some of these sensations are a direct result of the ingredient, but others develop during the heating process known as baking.

Most baked goods rise using a leavening agent. Breads and baked goods rise from carbon dioxide (CO_2) bubbles producing a light, fluffy texture. There are two ways of generating CO_2 gas in baked goods—microbially or chemically. Yeast produces CO_2 microbially; baking soda or baking powder produces it chemically. The most dramatic action during baking is the rising of the flour, which begins before heating and is caused by the expansion of CO_2 gas. In addition to gas expansion, baking results in coagulation of proteins, gelatinization of starch, and evaporation of the water. All these changes contribute to how a baked product feels in our mouths. Other actions that are occurring during baking are the development of the flavors, hardening of the crust, and darkening of the color.

Many factors affect the quality of baked goods. The most important factors are temperature and time. As little as 15 seconds can make a noticeable difference in flavor and texture. Other factors affecting the quality of the finished product include the size, the shape, mixing time and method, the heat transmission properties of the baking pan, and the evenness of the temperature in the oven.

5.4.2 Pasta and Noodles

Pasta and noodle products have become staples of the American college student diet like Leah's. Popular for their ease of preparation, low cost, and satisfying quality, these products are the food of choice for many. Noodles and pasta provide good nutrition at a low price. They are high in carbohydrates and reasonably low in fats; however, they do not supply a complete, balanced diet unless supplemented with protein, minerals, and fiber.

By American regulations, noodles must have at least 5.5% egg solids, but pasta is generally made from flour and water only. To make pasta, the granules are then made into a paste by adding water, and the paste is formed into dough. The dough is extruded into the desired shape and dried to approximately 12% moisture. Instant noodles (the kind that Leah and many of her friends turn to at the end of the month) are prepared by frying the noodle dough after it has been steamed.

Noodles and pasta vary by size, shape, color, and light transmission. Pastas are typically manufactured by extrusion, which is a complex food process that involves mixing and kneading to force the formulated food through an orifice under pressure to a desired size and shape. During extrusion, the hot dough rapidly expands, causing rapid evaporation of moisture and a puffing of the product. The key to maintaining quality and retarding spoilage is in controlled drying. Most noodle and pasta products Americans are familiar with are hard and dry; noodles from certain Asian countries are more commonly fresh, refrigerated products. Although pasta and noodle products require little preparation, timing is of utmost importance. When not cooked long enough, pasta and noodle products are tough, but overcooking leads to stickiness. Once again, as little as 15 seconds can lead to a noticeable loss in quality. The popular instant (Ramen) noodles have been cut, waved, steam-cooked, portioned, and fried before packaging. During the frying process, they lose moisture and pick up fat.

5.4.3 Gluten-Free Products

These products are a triumph of modern food technology as gluten is a protein that has superior functional properties of elasticity, extensibility, gas holding capacity, and mixing tolerance to proteins from other grains. Gluten is the reason that biscuits, breads, cakes, croissants, and other baked goods are so light and fluffy. The gluten network formed during mixing can withstand the kneading process. A gluten-free label excludes grains from barley, rye, and related grains in addition to wheat. Flavor and cost are critical quality attributes.

Loaf volumes of gluten-free breads are smaller than those made from wheat flour as shown in Insert 5.6. Starches from buckwheat, corn, rice, and sorghum are gluten-free but feel dry and sandy in the mouth with a starchy aroma. By adding egg, milk, and soy proteins as well as hydrocolloids such as agarose, guar gum, psyllium, or hydroxymethylpropylcellulose, product developers can enhance flavor and mouthfeel. Beer brewed from either barley or wheat also contains gluten, but gluten-free or low-gluten (<20 ppm) beers can be made from buckwheat, corn, millet, rice, rye, and sorghum.

Despite consumer concerns about gluten, it is neither toxic nor fattening. Celiac disease results from an abnormal response of the immune system to cereal proteins most closely associated with wheat gluten. Classical symptoms include abdominal swelling, diarrhea, and weight loss, but some celiacs have few clearly defined symptoms. Diets containing gluten are more likely to provide the nutrients we need than gluten-free diets. Most gluten-free products have lower mineral **bioavailability** and are deficient in B vitamins, dietary fiber, and protein. Grains in gluten-free products are not usually enriched and thus gluten-free diets tend to be nutritionally inferior

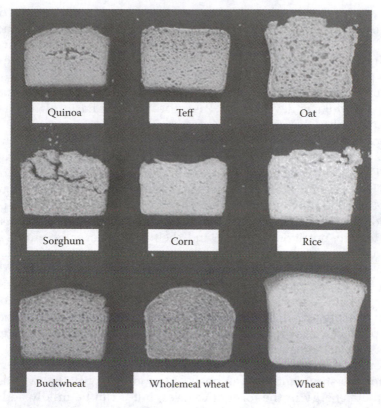

INSERT 5.6
Appearance of slices cut from wheat and gluten-free breads. (From Hager, A.-S. et al., *European Food Research & Technology* 235: 338, 2012. With permission.)

to diets containing gluten. Although Tiana thinks that her diet is a healthy one, she is probably depriving herself of important nutrients.

5.4.4 Beverages

Beverages are considered as liquid foods, and water is the major component in beverages. One of the most important nutrient requirements is water. We are urged to drink six glasses of water daily. Although most of us consume large quantities of liquid refreshment, many of us look to other sources than tap or bottled water to supply this nutrient. The problem with getting water from beverages is that many contain caffeine or alcohol, which are diuretic (induce urination), causing elimination of more water than one would anticipate.

Juices are considered to be healthy beverages because they contain some vitamins and minerals from the original fruit. The unit operations of juice manufacture are extraction, clarification, deaeration, pasteurization, concentration, essence addition, and canning, bottling, or freezing. The liquid portion of the fruit is removed from the solid part during extraction. Extraction yield increases by the addition of pectic enzymes, which release more of the liquid portion of the fruit. Clarification removes the pulp to make a clear juice, but it lowers dietary fiber. Deaeration removes the air to reduce the chances of off-flavor development. Pasteurization kills harmful microbes but does not sterilize the juice.

Concentration involves the removal of water so that the nutrients, colors, and flavors can be put into a smaller container, making it easier to ship and store. During the concentration process, some of the delicate aromas evaporate. These gaseous aromas, known as essence, can be captured, liquefied, and returned to the concentrated juice to give it a fuller flavor. The type and duration of the juicing process and the conditions of storage affect flavor, color, texture, nutritional quality, and shelf life. A beverage with a fruity name and fruity properties doesn't always contain juice. Many fruit-flavored beverages have little juice, ample amounts of added sugars, and few nutrients; others have more vitamins and minerals than fresh-squeezed juice. Once again, it is important to read the label to know what is in the product.

Energy drinks are one of the fastest growing categories of food and beverage products. They may or may not be carbonated and are likely to contain high levels of calories and caffeine. A sugar-free energy drink is an oxymoron as it is the calories from sugar that provide the body with energy. Caffeine is a stimulant that can push us to more activity that will help us burn more energy in the form of calories, but it can be mildly addictive. Many carbonated beverages are caffeine-free, but most so-called energy drinks feature caffeine as a primary ingredient. Energy drinks also feature one or more B vitamins to enhance the nutritional image of the product with those vitamins carefully selected because they do not contribute to off-odors or -flavors.

Caffeine and some acidulants in popular beverages can interfere with calcium absorption. The acidulant of most concern is phosphoric acid. A frequent drinker of caffeinated beverages who drinks no milk, consumes few dairy products, and does not take a calcium supplement should be concerned. We can tell if our favorite beverage contains phosphoric acid by checking the ingredient statement. Consumption of carbonated and energy beverages as a part of an overall balanced diet should present no major nutritional problems. Nil's overreliance on energy drinks for his nutritional needs, however, is likely to induce nutritional imbalances and potential long-term health problems.

5.4.5 Confections

Confections are sweet, tempting treats that offer more satisfaction than nutrition. Confections are based either in chocolate or in sugar. In both types of confections, sugars are important ingredients. Minor differences in the unit operations can result in major differences in the final product. One of the most important variables is whether the sugar is in the crystalline form or not. Those confections containing crystalline sugar include rock candy and fudge; those with noncrystalline sugar include caramels, gumdrops, hard candy, jelly beans, marshmallows, peanut brittle, and taffy. It is difficult to appreciate that the flexibility of a single ingredient, sugar, can be the principal factor in the texture of these diverse candy products.

Manufacturing chocolate is a complex process that begins with the raw white to pale purple cacao bean. Raw beans are fermented to remove the pulp, kill the germ, and modify both color and flavor. Fermented beans are then cleaned, roasted, winnowed, milled, and ground to form the chocolate liquor. Winnowing removes the outer coating of the bean and separates the germ from the rest of the seed. The chocolate liquor is more than half fat. Although most people associate chocolate with caffeine, it actually contains very little. Removal of the fat (cocoa butter) from the liquor leaves cocoa powder. White chocolate is made using the cocoa butter with no cocoa powder.

The unit operations in the manufacturing of chocolate include the combining of ingredients, mixing, refining, conching, tempering, and molding or enrobing. Conching is a very slow mixing process that changes the very grainy cocoa mixture into a fine smooth-textured mixture. Tempering involves stirring and heating to permit fat crystallization. Although many consumers think chocolate is sweet, it is actually very bitter because of the presence of tannins and theobromine (a molecule that is similar in structure to caffeine but without its stimulating properties). Another secret to chocolate's success as an ingredient is that it melts at body temperature. This melt-in-the-mouth property adds to the overall enjoyment of chocolate confections.

Many baked goods, because of their high sugar content, are also considered confections: cakes, cookies, éclairs, and recently the decadent cronut, a cross between a croissant and a donut. The mixing technique is important and strongly influences the texture of the final product. During mixing, air is incorporated into the cake batter to help provide a light, fluffy texture. In some cakes, air is pumped directly into the batter using a high-speed mixer. The processing schematic for manufacturing of Graham crackers, a key component of smores, is shown in Insert 5.7.

Commercial boxed mixes contain **surfactants** (chemical compounds that disrupt surface tension of a liquid) to allow the added water to combine with the shortening present in the mix. Ready-to-eat cakes can require several mixing steps including creaming in which the sugar and fat are mixed before adding water. The primary reason for creaming is to incorporate air into the batter. Baking powder is added as a chemical leavening agent. Full flavor development occurs during baking. Cookie batter is made from soft wheat and is either molded or cut after extrusion. The proper mixing of air into the batter, as with cakes, is essential for a proper cookie texture. Creaming is usually part of the cookie process. Commercial cookie baking

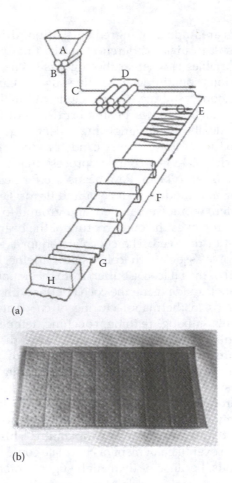

(a)

(b)

INSERT 5.7

(a) Cracker dough processing consisting of (A) dough hopper, (B) forming roll, (C) dough web, (D) reduction rolls, (E) lapper, (F) final reduction, (G) relaxing curl, and (H) cutter-docker. (b) Cracker dough after cutting and docking. (From Hoseney, R.C., *Principles of Cereal Science and Technology*, 2nd ed., St. Paul, MN: American Association of Cereal Chemists, Inc., 1994. With permission.)

occurs in long ovens on a slow-moving conveyor belt. Baking melts the shortening, fully dissolves the sugar, and can gelatinize the starch.

5.4.6 Sausages

Many of us associate sausages with breakfast; however, sausages are much more than breakfast products. They include the pepperoni on our pizza, the frankfurter in our hot dog, and the salami in our sandwich. Most of these products originated in Europe, where they remain a staple of European diets. They come in fermented or unfermented forms.

Probably the most popular form of sausage in America is the frankfurter or wiener. The unit operations of wiener production include forming a batter, filling, twisting, heating, smoking, cooking, peeling, and packaging. To form the batter, cuts of meat, water, and curing salts are blended together in a huge grinder until smooth. The comminuted (ground) meat, which is mushier than raw hamburger, is then stuffed into a casing and allowed to gel and become solid. Twisting forms the individual frankfurters. Heating, smoking, and cooking are the primary preservation methods for this product and also give it its characteristic flavor. Once cooked, the artificial casing is peeled off.

Unit operations for link sausage are similar to those of wieners, except the casing is left on the sausage. Wieners and link sausage originated as a salvage operation to use up as much of the slaughtered hog as possible. The sausage stuffing was meat that could not be recovered as distinct cuts, and the cleaned intestine was used for the casing. Today, artificial casings have replaced natural intestine casings, but persistent shoppers can still find natural sausages. Wieners were originally exclusively hog products, but beef, chicken, and turkey have been added to replace all or part of the pork meat, primarily to reduce the fat content.

5.4.7 Frozen Desserts and Entrées

The frozen food aisle is the favorite location in the supermarket for consumers who are more interested in convenience and quality than price. The frozen food aisle has something for almost everyone. The entrées provide balanced meals that are convenient, tasty, and low in calories. Even with all the choices available, these meals can still become boring after a while. Besides, 300 calories at a single meal is probably not enough to sustain a healthy diet over a long period. One concern with many of these products is that they tend to be high in salt. Several frozen foods are low in salt, but many consumers complain about the lost flavor in low-salt products. They turn either to higher-salt alternative or adding salt just before they consume the items.

Frozen entrées, whether they are of the low-calorie or full-fat variety, are complex foods with many ingredients and components. Many are full formulations of ingredients that are completely mixed together, but others have several components that are prepared separately and then placed into the package. Most of these items have been at least partially prepared, and most are designed to be heated before consumption. The packaging usually is designed with the idea that the product will be heated in a microwave oven. There are even foil shields, particularly for frozen pizza, that direct the microwaves to a particular location to provide better crisping. Some packages are dual-ovenable, meaning they can be heated in a microwave or a conventional oven. Before we try placing a container in either a microwave or conventional oven, we should read the directions carefully. Some ingredient statements for formulated foods including a frozen entrée are shown in Insert 5.8.

Ice cream is an American favorite. The unit operations of ice cream start with pasteurizing and homogenizing the milk, followed by mixing the ingredients, aging, whipping air into the mix, freezing, and hardening. Ice cream is a frozen foam, that is, a gas dispersed in a liquid. The gas is air; the liquid is cream. The incorporation of air into the mix is the step that gives ice cream its smooth and creamy texture. This step increases the volume of the original mix; the extra volume is called **overrun**. Without the air, the ice cream would be hard and grainy. When churning homemade ice cream, air is being incorporated into it. The Italian version of ice cream, gelato, is developing a following around the world. Gelato tends to be lower in fat than ice cream as it uses less cream and

---

R. ingredients: cooked brown rice, vegetables (mushrooms, onions), water, rolled oats, mozzarella cheese (pasteurized milk, cultures, salt enzymes), nonfat milk, cornstarch, natural flavors, anatto (vegetable color), bulghur wheat-hydrated, cheddar cheese (pasteurized milk, cheese culture, salt enzymes), soy protein concentrate contains less than 2% of salt, parsley, vegetable gum, autolyzed yeast extract, wheat gluten, dried garlic, milkfat, apocarotenal (vegetable color) spices, citric acid, natural flavors, barley malt, natural butter flavor, anatto (vegetable color), dried onion, dried mushrooms

---

S. ingredients: cultured pasteurized nonfat milk, cream, live and active cultures: *S. thermophilus*, *L. bulgaris*, *L. acidophilus*, bifidius, and *L. casei*, passion fruit puree, evaporated cane juice, pectin, natural flavor, locust bean gum

---

T. ingredients: enriched flour (wheat flour, malted barley flour, niacin, reduced iron, thiamine mononitrate, riboflavin, folic acid), low moisture mozzarella cheese (cultured pasteurized milk, salt enzymes), skim milk, tomatoes (tomatoes, water, tomato paste), margarine (partially hydrogenated soybean and cottonseed oils, water, salt, vegetable mono and diglycerides, nonfat dry milk solids, soy lecithin, artificial flavor beta carotene, vitamin a palmitate), water, modified food starch, smoked flavored provolone cheese (cultured pasteurized milk, salt, enzymes and natural smoke flavor), asiago cheese (pasteurized cultured milk, salt enzymes), sugar, yeast, contains 1% or less of parmesan cheese (pasteurized cultured part skim milk, salt, enzymes), romano cheese (pasteurized cultured cow's milk, salt enzymes), dough conditioner (diacetyl, tartaric acid, guar gum, active malt flour, calcium pyrophosphate, soy lecithin, ascorbic acid, enzyme), dried whole egg, shortening (partially hydrogenated soybean and cottonseed oils) salt, dextrose, butter powder (butter, cream, salt, anatto extract), nonfat dry milk, maltodextrin, buttermilk, partially hydrogenated soybean oil, salt, sour cream (cultured cream, nonfat dry milk), disodium phosphate, natural and artificial flavors, lactic acid, citric acid, color), dehydrated sweet cream (sweet cream, nonfat milk, and lecithin), corn starch, butter powder (butter, nonfat milk solids, sodium caseinate, bht added to improve stability) sodium acid pyrophosphate, sodium bicarbonate, dehydrated parsley, dough conditioner (wheat starch, L-cysteine hydrochloride, ammonium sulfate), spices

---

U. ingredients: whole grain oats, sugar, canola oil, peanut butter (peanuts, salt), yellow corn flour, brown sugar syrup, soy flour, salt, soy lecithin, baking soda
contains peanut, soy; may contain almond and pecan ingredients

---

INSERT 5.8

Ingredient statements for formulated foods. R, Gardenburger Original; S, Chobani Greek Yogurt Passion Fruit Low-Fat yogurt; T, Red Baron Stuffed Pizza Slices Singles 2 Supreme Pizzas; U, Nature Valley Peanut Butter Crunchy granola bar.

more whole milk than ice cream. Less overrun is found in gelato, making it denser than ice cream. Ice cream is usually served frozen, but gelato is served at a higher temperature. All these differences tend to give gelato a mouthfeel that is distinct from its American counterpart.

5.4.8 Functional Foods

The terms *functional foods* and *nutraceuticals* tend to be used interchangeably, but there are some important differences. Functional foods have been described by Dr. Rotimi Aluko as foods that "apart from supplying nutrients can reduce the risk of chronic diseases such as cancer, hypertension, kidney malfunction etc." He further goes on to describe nutraceuticals as "health-promoting compounds or products that have been isolated or purified from food sources and they are generally sold in a medicinal (usually a pill) form". Other disease targets of functional foods and nutraceuticals include cancer, diabetes, heart disease, immune diseases, and obesity.

Functional foods can be traditional items such as fish, milk, tea, and tomato or formulated products like energy bars and beverages, soy burgers, and yogurt with added probiotics. Examples of nutraceuticals include fish oil capsules, glucosamine/chondroitin pills, and isoflavone extracts from soybeans. Added nutrients frequently found in formulated functional foods and other fortified foods are calcium, B vitamins, ascorbic acid, and antioxidant vitamins. Ingredients designed to give an energy burst include caffeine, L-carnitine, ginseng, guarana, and taurine. Although some of these ingredients provide health benefits at certain levels, the levels in functional foods or nutraceuticals may be too low to offer any benefit.

When levels of the bioactive compound are high enough to provide the benefit, the food or beverage may not be palatable, posing challenges to product developers. Some of the concerns facing the developers of these products are bioactivity, customization, expense, health claims, packaging requirements, quality control measures, sensory characteristics, and stability. **Bioactivity** means that the ingredient actually works at the level and form within the product; customization means that it is compatible with the other ingredients in the product. Bioactive compounds in foods include specific carbohydrates, carotenoids, fats, polyphenols, and protein peptides.

5.5 Remember This!

- Minor differences in the unit operations can result in major differences in the final product.

- Diets containing gluten are more likely to provide the nutrients we need than gluten-free diets.
- Noodles and pasta provide good nutrition at a low price.
- Stabilizers are added to formulated foods to keep them from breaking down.
- Individual fat replacers cannot perform all functions of lipids.
- Fats and oils are extracted from plant and animal products and belong to a chemical group called lipids.
- The protein complex, gluten, which is formed when water is added to the flour, is the reason wheat flour is superior to other flours.
- In selecting the ingredients for a formulation, the food scientist must consider the quality of the food, its safety, its stability, and its cost.
- A clean label is one that has only clearly recognizable ingredients, none of which sound like chemicals.
- Formulated foods are products that are mixtures of ingredients.

5.6 Looking Ahead

This chapter was designed to provide an introduction to formulated foods, made from mixing ingredients. Chapter 6 will describe chilled and prepared foods. Chapter 7 explores the role of food scientists in measuring foods for quality and safety. Chapter 8 describes the design of food products.

Testing Comprehension

1. What is the difference between a formulated food and a processed food? Name five processed products that are not formulated foods and five processed foods that are formulated.
2. Compare and contrast the beneficial and detrimental aspects of a chocolate brownie and one that is gluten-free.
3. Diagram the manufacturing process of a low-salt pretzel.
4. Select a favorite formulated food product not mentioned in the chapter. List the ingredients and the likely unit operations of the process and draw a simple flow diagram of the process.
5. Compare and contrast the benefits and limitations of functional and natural beverages.

6. Critique the argument that foods with five or less ingredients are healthier than those with more than five ingredients. Provide an example of a healthy food that has more than five ingredients and an unhealthy one that has five or less ingredients.

7. A product developer of cured meat products is asked by the boss to eliminate nitrates from all company products by using celery salt as an alternative. The developer finds that although celery salt provides a cleaner label, it has much more natural nitrate in it than if sodium nitrate was added directly. What are the developer's responsibilities to the boss and the company? What are the company's obligations to their consumers?

8. Calculate the calorie reduction that could be achieved if the 40 grams of added sugar in a piña colada smoothie were replaced with 10 grams of honey (8 grams sugar). Before the formulation change to a no-sugar-added version, there were 490 total calories in the smoothie with 54 calories coming from fat and 36 calories from protein. How much sugar remains in the no-sugar-added product?

References

Akoh, C. C., 1998. Fat replacers: A scientific status summary. *Food Technol.*, 52(3):47.

Aluko, R. E., 2012. *Functional Foods and Nutraceuticals*, New York: Springer.

Hager, A.-S., A. Wolter, M. Czerny, J. Bez, E. Zannini, E. Arendt and M. Czerny, 2012. Investigation of product quality, sensory profile and ultrastructure of breads made from a range of commercial gluten-free flours compared to their wheat counterparts. *Eur. Food Res. Technol.*, 235:333.

Hoseney, R. C., 1994. *Principles of Cereal Science and Technology*, 2nd ed., St. Paul, MN: American Association of Cereal Chemists, Inc.

Jane, J., 2004. Starch: Structure and properties, Chapter 7, in *Chemical and Functional Properties of Food Saccharides*, Tomasik, P., Ed., Boca Raton, FL: CRC Press.

Nabors, L. O., 2012. Alternative sweeteners: An overview, Chapter 1, in *Alternative Sweeteners*, 4th ed., Nabors, L. O., Ed., New York: Marcel Dekker, Inc.

O'Rell, K. R. and R. C. Chandan, 2013. Manufacture of various types of yogurt, Chapter 12, in *Manufacturing of Yogurt and Fermented Milks*, 2nd ed., Chandan, R. C. and Kilara, A., Eds., Ames, IA: Wiley-Blackwell.

Further Reading

Akoh, C. C., 2008. Fat-based fat substitutes, Chapter 17, in *Fatty Acids in Foods and Their Health Implications*, 3rd ed., Chow, C. K., Ed., Boca Raton, FL: CRC Press.

Albers-Nelson, R., 2010. Clean Label Mold Inhibitors for Baking. Oklahoma State University Cooperative Extension Food & Agricultural Products Center Food Technology Fact Sheet-173. Available at http://osufacts.okstate.edu/docushare /dsweb/Get/Document-7328/FAPC-173web.pdf.

Damodaran, S., K. L. Parkin and O. R. Fennema, 2007. *Fennema's Food Chemistry*, 4th ed., Boca Raton, FL: CRC Press.

Fellows, P. J., 2009. *Food Processing Technology: Principles and Practices*, 3rd ed., Boca Raton, FL: CRC Press.

Katz, B. and L. A. Williams, 2011. Cleaning up processed foods. *Food Technol.*, 65(12):33.

Lindhorst, T. K., 2007. *Essentials of Carbohydrate Chemistry and Biochemistry*, 3rd ed., Weinheim, Germany: Wiley VCH.

Man, D. and A. Jones, 2000. *Shelf-Life Evaluation of Foods*, Gaithersberg, MD: Aspen Publications, Inc.

Ohr, L. M., 2011. A fresh look at food safety: The call for clean labels has prompted food processors to seek "natural" antimicrobials and shelf life extenders. *Prepared Foods*, 169(5):51.

Pollan, M., 2009. *Food Rules: An Eater's Manual*, New York: Penguin Books.

Smith, S. J. and Y. H. Hui, 2005. *Food Processing: Principles and Applications*, Ames, IA: Blackwell Publishing.

This, H., 2006. *Molecular Gastronomy: Exploring the Science of Flavor*, New York: Columbia University Press.

6

Chilled and Prepared Foods

Garrett loves to shop, particularly for food. Shopping is a social occasion for him. He knows most of the employees at the supermarket by their first names and has been known to kill a couple of hours shopping for food for the week. He particularly likes the perimeter of the store because that is where the good stuff is. He likes fresh produce, high-quality meats, and chilled and frozen foods. The middle aisles are particularly boring with all those cans, boxes, and cartons. He knows the food on the perimeter is more expensive, but he is very selective and usually gets good value for his money.

Tiana's grandparents had four peach trees in their backyard. When she visited them in the summer, she had delicious fresh peaches and loved them. She can't understand why anyone would buy a fresh peach at a supermarket because the flavor is so lame. She also can't understand why anyone would buy cut-up fruits and vegetables. They aren't anywhere near the quality of the ones her grandparents grew and prepared. If she can't have the best, she doesn't want the rest.

Selina is concerned about her weight. She avoids most food on campus and all fast foods but still finds herself gaining weight. She is very busy and does not have a lot of time to cook and needs something that is quick, easy, and filling. She's big on prepared sandwiches from the supermarket deli and frozen dinners although most of them have more than five ingredients. She has tried many diets, but they either have unappealing foods or don't fill her up. She wishes there were some magic pills that would do the trick.

Garrett, Tiana, and Selina are familiar with chilled and prepared foods. Garrett takes time shopping and gives his selections thought and attention. Some up-front time helps him save time later while still eating a healthy, satisfying diet. Tiana is more demanding in her standards for fresh fruits and vegetables, and she does without them many times. She is not willing to sacrifice quality for convenience. Selina is interested in convenience and does not think about her food selections enough to eat healthy and maintain her weight. Chilled and prepared foods can help us design healthy diets, but we must evaluate them just like any other food.

6.1 Looking Back

Previous chapters focused on food issues we deal with daily. Some key points that were covered in those chapters help prepare us for understanding chilled and prepared foods:

- The protein complex, gluten, which is formed when water is added to the flour, is the reason wheat flour is superior to other flours.
- Minor differences in the unit operations can result in major differences in the final product.
- Food is preserved to make it safer by reducing or eliminating harmful microbes and to extend its shelf life by reducing or eliminating spoilage microorganisms.
- Unit operations are distinct steps common to many food processes.
- Most raw materials are perishable and require careful handling or processing to prevent losses.
- The main factor that distinguishes fast food from other restaurants is the speed of service.
- The Nutrition Facts part of the label indicates the serving size, how many servings per container, calories per serving, and the fat calories per serving.
- Good nutrition requires an adequate consumption of nutrients without consuming too many calories.
- Preservatives are food ingredients that slow spoilage and help prevent food-associated illnesses.
- An expiration date represents the food scientist's best guess about how long a food will last before it spoils.

6.2 What Are Chilled and Prepared Foods? Why Are They Important?

As the pace of society increases, most consumers are looking for ways to reduce the times it takes to fix a meal and increase convenience. Chilled and prepared foods are part of the food industry's answer to meet these desires. Chilled foods tend to be fresh and perishable, requiring refrigeration. Prepared foods are those that are ready-to-eat or ready-to-heat then eat. Prepared foods can come in commercial packages, or they can be purchased and consumed at a retail outlet such as a cafeteria or restaurant. Because chilled and prepared foods have generally been exposed to less harsh preservation measures than their processed counterparts, they have a reputation for being of a higher quality. The cost of higher quality and increased convenience may be an increased safety risk.

Chilled and prepared foods are perishable. They deteriorate along the path from where they are produced to when they are consumed. Fresh meats deteriorate much more rapidly than fresh carrots, but both items last longer at refrigerated temperatures than at ambient temperature. Since chilled foods tend to be minimally processed raw materials, handling of these raw materials before packaging must also be carefully controlled. Although many chilled foods may be consumed without heating, many prepared foods are heated either shortly before or after purchase. Such heating may serve to decrease microbial load, increasing the safety of the product, but it may also provide a false sense of security to the consumer. We will cover how foods are distributed in much greater detail in Chapter 9.

6.3 Chilled Foods

As we walk around a modern supermarket, we notice that the higher-value items tend to be located around the perimeter with the lower value staples located in the internal aisles. Chilled foods tend to be higher value items. If we take a walk around Garrett's favorite supermarket, we will find the produce section as he enters the store. At the back of the store are the fish and meat coolers, the area for meat cut to order, sushi bar, and around the corner are the dairy product cases. See Insert 6.1 for the layout of a typical supermarket.

6.3.1 Whole Fresh Fruits and Vegetables

For pure eating pleasure, it is hard to beat a fresh mango or watermelon at the peak of the growing season. Unfortunately, it may be difficult to find a ripe one in the supermarket that will deliver on flavor. It may have been harvested locally or it may have been shipped from as far away as Argentina or New Zealand. Fresh produce is picked live and continues to live and respire through the handling system.

The plant and its detached fruit undergo trauma during harvest, releasing ethylene from the wound. **Climacteric fruits** like apples and bananas will continue to ripen off the plant by producing the plant hormone ethylene. These fruits are harvested typically before they reach full ripeness because they deteriorate rapidly after being detached from the plant and are unlikely to withstand shipment if picked when fully ripe. If picked early, they can be ripened by treating them with ethylene to control the ripening process.

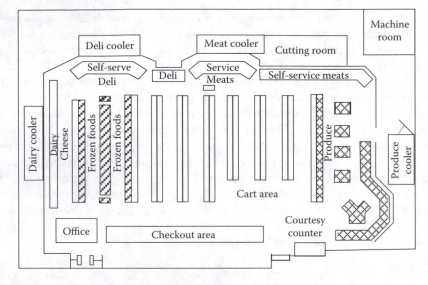

INSERT 6.1

Layout of a typical modern supermarket. (From Bahman, A. et al., *Applied Energy* 98: 11, 2012. With permission.)

Nonclimacteric fruits like blueberries and oranges must be allowed to ripen on the plant and tend to be harvested closer to their peak level of ripeness. Fresh fruits are sorted and graded in a packinghouse before shipment to market. These two types of fruits should be stored and shipped separately from each other as the ethylene generated by climacteric fruits can induce disorders in nonclimacteric fruit.

Many fresh fruits such as cherries and strawberries are shipped in refrigerated conditions to slow respiration, decay and ultimate spoilage. Most tropical fruits like bananas and papayas are not refrigerated because storage at low temperatures reduces flavor and accelerates decay. Some fresh fruits such as apples and pears are stored in controlled atmospheres (high carbon dioxide, low oxygen) to slow ripening so they can be shipped year round. The complexity of fruit handling is shown in Insert 6.2.

Fresh vegetables undergo many of the same biological processes as fresh fruits and are preserved by similar techniques. Some consumers believe that tomatoes and squash are vegetables, but they are considered fruits by plant scientists. Tomatoes ripen off the vine and should not be refrigerated; squash do not ripen after harvest and need refrigeration. During handling, fresh fruits and vegetables are loaded and unloaded many times from harvest to the retail store. Any rough handling will cause bruising and lower the quality at purchase and consumption. The marketing system tends to value appearance and shipping stability over flavor, which may be why Tiana is

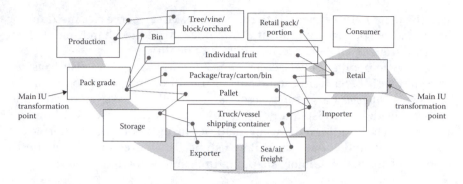

INSERT 6.2
Schematic demonstrating the complexity of postharvest handling systems with emphasis on identifiable units (IU). (From Bollen, A.F. et al., *Biosystems Engineering* 98: 391, 2007. With permission.)

frequently disappointed in the flavor of the fresh peaches that look so good in the supermarket.

6.3.2 Packaged Salad Vegetables and Cut Fruits

One of the objections to fresh fruits and vegetables is that they take so long to prepare. Fresh-cut items make them more convenient to consumers who want to eat healthy but are always on the run. Cutting involves wounding of the plant tissue. As at harvest, ethylene is generated and wound healing begins. In cut lettuce, the wound scar may not be noticeable, but the white blush of cut carrots and brown ends of cut green beans are objectionable to consumers. It is usually more difficult to preserve the flavor of cut-up produce than whole produce.

Since cut fruits and vegetables are usually more perishable than their whole counterparts, they are usually shipped whole from the growing area intact then cut and packaged closer to large metropolitan areas. **Modified atmosphere packaging** (MAP), which is low in oxygen and high in nitrogen or carbon dioxide, slows the deterioration process. Once the consumer opens the package, however, any benefits of the MAP are lost. Refrigeration of cut products is critical to slow spoilage.

6.3.3 Fresh Fish and Seafood

Fresh fish and seafood are very perishable. A fresh-caught fish has little or no aroma, but foul aromas can develop in a relatively short period because of the breakdown of amines and related compounds in the muscle tissue. Immediate chilling, preferably close to the freezing point of water, helps preserve fish flavor. MAP in nitrogen atmospheres can slow unpleasant aroma development, but it can also enhance the chances of botulism. Because most refrigeration systems are not kept at the freezing point, storage on ice helps keep the temperature down. At the same time, ice can serve as a medium for the spread of spoilage and harmful microbes. Expedited handling of fresh foods minimizes safety concerns and loss of quality.

Contrary to popular belief, *sushi* means "with rice," not "raw fish." *Sashimi* refers to raw fish. Sashimi can be part of the filling in a sushi roll in one of four forms: *futomaki* (large rolls), *hosomaki* (thin rolls), *temaki* (hand rolls), and *uramaki* (inside-out rolls). Many other ingredients can serve as fillings for sushi rolls. The basic ingredients in sushi rice include nori sheets, short-grain rice, soy sauce, and wasabi paste. Raw fish used as ingredients in sushi rolls include eel, mackerel, salmon, snapper, tuna, and yellowtail.

6.3.4 Fresh Meats

Fresh meats are also called muscle foods because the edible portion of most meat, including fish, is from the muscle tissue of the animal. Unlike fresh fruits and vegetables, which are living tissue, meat is dying tissue. Study of the reactions involved in the conversion of muscle to meat is called post-mortem physiology. A series of these complex reactions proceeds to rigor, which produces tough meat from larger animals. Thus, for most meats, rigor needs to be resolved before the meat can be marketed and sold. Textural problems, known as cold shortening, can develop in beef, lamb, and pork if the carcass is cooled too rapidly after harvest. Beef and pork carcasses are hung on hooks at low temperatures to allow for the resolution of rigor and the development of flavor.

Red meats are actually purple right after harvest. It is only in the presence of oxygen that the meat becomes the bright red color associated with fresh hamburger and steak. Inappropriate lighting in a retail case causes quality loss owing to undesirable wavelengths and increased temperatures. Although many supermarkets are equipped to produce the appropriate cuts from partial carcasses, some chains prefer "case-ready" meats. Case-ready cuts are prepared and packaged at a central processing facility and then shipped to the store for display.

Food scientists are wary of consuming raw meat because any harvest operation is likely to contaminate the surface of the meat. In nondiseased animals, the inside of the muscle is assumed to be sterile; however, if the surface is contaminated, any cutting, grinding, or puncturing of the surface will contaminate the inside of the muscle. Meats spoil rapidly even when refrigerated. Spoilage is characterized by the development of off-odors, dull colors, and slime. Shelf life of meats is affected by the initial numbers of microbes in the meat, storage temperature, and relative humidity. Use of MAP in meats can slow the spoilage process considerably and thus extend the shelf life. Drip, the release of liquid from the tissue, is also a major problem with chilled meats because drip supports more rapid microbial growth than tissue. Quick cooling the meat and holding it at low temperatures reduces drip but can lead to cold shortening. Absorbent materials in the bottom of retail packages, known in the trade as *diapers*, help reduce the level of visible drip in the package.

6.3.5 Deli Meats

Fresh meat cuts can serve as either raw materials for processed deli meats such as smoked turkey, cured ham, and roast beef or ingredients in formulated products such as luncheon meats. In general, these products have been cooked and are sold as cold cuts in ready-to-eat form. In the processed products, the original texture of the muscle structure is obvious, but in formulated products, the meat is usually comminuted (finely ground) and then restructured. Some of these products like salami are fermented to provide unique flavors, colors, and textures. The distinct color of frankfurters is attributed to the addition of nitrites, which stabilize the myoglobin in the meat. Nitrites also protect the product from the growth of *Clostridium botulinum*, the microbe responsible for botulism. Deli meats are usually packaged in atmospheres of little or no oxygen to slow the growth of spoilage microbes; however, *C. botulinum* is only able to grow in the absence of oxygen.

In recent years, there has been some concern expressed about the consumption of deli meats because they contain nitrosamines and *Listeria monocytogenes*. Nitrosamines, which are carcinogens, are formed by the interaction of nitrites with free amines in the meat. Nitrites can be found naturally in many items, including lettuce and other vegetables. Listeriosis is primarily a concern for the immunocompromised (the young, elderly, pregnant, or people with AIDS). Moderate consumption of deli meats is unlikely to increase the risk of developing cancer. The United States Department of Agriculture recommends that luncheon meats and hot dogs be cooked before they are served for anyone who may be immunocompromised. Maintaining adequate refrigeration of perishable products like deli meats is necessary, and expiration dates should be strictly observed.

During wholesale delivery to retail outlets, deli meats are reasonably stable if they are kept refrigerated. Once the package has been opened, however, the protection offered from the low-to-no-oxygen environment is lost and the meats will spoil fairly rapidly. It is generally best not to keep freshly opened products more than 5 to 7 days at refrigerated temperatures. Leftovers can be kept for longer periods if properly packaged and frozen, but freezing can change the texture of the meat product and decrease its desirability.

6.3.6 Milk and Its Alternatives

Milk is collected on dairy farms under sanitary conditions and pumped into a tanker truck. A sample of the milk is collected from each farm before it is pumped into the truck. Once the truck arrives at the processing plant, a sample of the milk is collected and tested for added hormones, antibiotics, pesticides, and other undesirable compounds. If the milk passes the test, it is pumped into large refrigerated holding tanks until ready for further processing. If the milk sample fails, the load is rejected. Samples from each individual farm are then tested and the farm that is responsible for the rejection is billed for the cost of the lost milk.

Milk is filtered to remove undesirable components. Then, it is centrifuged to separate out the fat, which is then added back to produce 0%, 1%, 2%, and whole milk. Pasteurization by heat, as we learned earlier, kills all harmful microbes but not all the spoilage microbes. Homogenization breaks the fat globules into very small droplets to prevent the fat from separating from the milk during refrigerated storage. Thickeners can be added to 0% milk to improve its acceptability. Extra fat can be used for cream or half-and-half products. Milk is pumped into sterile containers. In many manufacturing plants, plastic containers are formed on-site just before being filled. Dairy companies have designed more user-friendly packages, making them easier to open, pour, and put in drink holders. A display case for milk and alternatives is shown in Insert 6.3.

Many people are lactose intolerant. Lactose is the primary sugar in milk and is found in many other dairy products. A lactose-intolerant person experiences bloating, gas production, diarrhea, and other intestinal discomfort when consuming too much lactose. One way to avoid this discomfort is to avoid products containing milk, but dairy products are among the best sources of calcium. Alternatives include consumption of low-lactose milk or consumption of an enzyme called β-galactosidase (found in products such as Beano) just before a meal. Other possibilities include low-lactose dairy products like yogurt and many cheeses or a dairy substitute such as soy, almond, coconut, flaxseed, and rice milks.

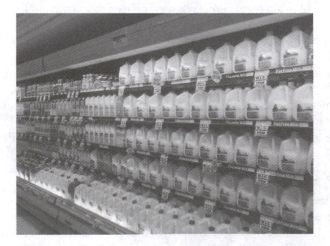

INSERT 6.3
A milk display case in a supermarket. (Photo courtesy of Robert Shewfelt.)

Soy and almond milks are made by water extracts of proteins and fats through a complex process. These items are high in protein with no lactose. Some consumers like the flavors of these alternatives, but many consumers do not. For this reason, they are usually flavored with vanilla or chocolate to help mask the strong soy or almond flavor.

6.3.7 Spreads

Our favorite bread products are usually enhanced by butter or margarine. Although the flavor of a hot muffin is tempting, it can become dry in the mouth and hard to swallow without a little of our favorite spread. Just like oil in an engine, the fat in the spread helps lubricate the biscuit to make chewing and swallowing a more pleasant experience. Butter is a by-product of milk production and is composed primarily of milk fat. Margarine is made from vegetable oil and contains an emulsifier to mix the oil and water. By definition, fats are solid at room temperature, and oils are liquid at room temperature. Spreadability is a critical quality factor for a spread. Since butter is perishable at room temperature, it must be refrigerated. When removed from the refrigerator butter may not spread well because of the predominance of saturated fats that are more solid. Newer butter products, however, have been restructured to improve their spreadability.

Vegetable oils are liquid because they are more unsaturated than the fats in butter. To achieve a better texture in margarine, the oils can be hydrogenated. **Hydrogenation** adds hydrogen to the unsaturated double bonds in the oil to produce a margarine that is solid, but it is not as solid as butter and spreads easily. Margarine provides excellent spreadability, but there are problems associated with the manufacturing process. Hydrogenation produces *trans* fats, which may contribute to heart disease as much or more than saturated fats. Regulations require a product label to display the *trans* fat content in addition to total and saturated fats. Food scientists have been successful in lowering the levels of hydrogenated oils and *trans* fats in margarines, similar spreads, and popular snack-food products.

In addition to spreadability, color and flavor of spreads are important functional properties. Without added color, margarines are generally not acceptable to consumers. The colorant of choice in margarines is usually β-carotene (pro-vitamin A). Butter has a distinctive character that is hard to duplicate in margarine. Butter flavor can be greatly influenced by the feed of the cows producing the milk; thus, butter flavor may vary by season.

In a desire for low- or no-fat foods, the fat content has been lowered or eliminated in many spreads. These spreads may perform well when applied to a bread product, but they may not have certain functional properties we have come to expect. During storage, the biggest problem with spreads is development of rancidity. The fatty acids in fats and oils oxidize and the flavor becomes unacceptable. Unsaturated fatty acids are susceptible to lipid oxidation, but saturated fatty acids do not oxidize. Since margarines are higher in unsaturated fatty acids than butter, margarines are more susceptible to oxidative rancidity. Adding antioxidants such as butylated hydroxyanisole and butylated hydroxytoluene helps slow the development of off-flavors owing to oxidative rancidity. Butter tends to be more susceptible to hydrolytic rancidity by the release of short-chain fatty acids or spoilage by microbes. Maintaining low temperatures during handling and storage can slow the development of rancid off flavors in margarines and butter.

6.3.8 Prepared Foods

Prepared foods are ready-to-eat or ready-to-heat then eat. In our fast-paced society, many of us want convenience and we want it now. Generally, we do not consider a fresh, whole fruit as a prepared food even if it is ready to eat. Some consumers see prepared foods as an answer to the drudgery of meal preparation; others see them as a technological blight on consumption of healthy, flavorful foods. A growing trend in companies that manufacture packaged, prepared foods is to employ product developers with a culinary background to upgrade the quality of these products. A person with formal training in the culinary arts and a food science program can become certified as a **Research Chef** (http://www.culinology.com/certification) through the Research Chef's Association.

6.3.9 Salads and Sandwiches

Prepared salads can be found in the produce or deli section of many supermarkets. Unlike the fresh-cut products described earlier in the chapter, these salads are ready to eat right out of the package. Fresh fruits and vegetables deteriorate rapidly as they decay, die, and exude fluids. In salads with mixed items, the items exuding the fluids become limp or wilted, and those absorbing the fluids become soggy. Cutting accelerates deterioration and leakage. Because of the lack of proteins, fresh-cut fruits are not as susceptible to the growth of harmful microbes as other products but they are still likely to spoil. They can become contaminated during preparation, particularly if the preparation area of the fruits and vegetables is not separated from the preparation area of the raw meats. Proper hygiene is critical as human contact with foods during preparation is a leading cause of contamination.

Contamination of fresh fruit and vegetable salads with harmful microbes is very serious because these products are rarely heated to kill the harmful organisms. Some salads contain other ingredients such as liquid dressings, croutons, cooked meat or seafood, or eggs and mayonnaise. Salads tend to be mixtures of distinct ingredients in a product rather than a blending of ingredients into a continuous, homogeneous product. The more distinct the ingredients in a salad are, the greater the possibility for ingredient interactions and deterioration. In addition, different ingredients have different storage requirements, leading to quality problems. One way to handle such problems is to have separate packages for particular ingredients inside the larger package. This approach sacrifices some convenience for better stability and quality. Although most consumers are afraid of products containing mayonnaise, believing it can increase the chances of food poisoning, mayonnaise actually inhibits the growth of microbes. It is important, however, that any salad with high-protein ingredients such as eggs, milk, or meats be kept refrigerated.

Sandwiches come in many shapes and sizes, but they are all characterized by the presence of a filling in a bread product. Refrigerated sandwiches have a short shelf life and are usually prepared daily. Refrigeration helps prevent growth of harmful microbes, but it promotes bread staling. Thus, there is usually a trade-off between safety and quality. Long-term storage of sandwiches in refrigerated vending machines sacrifices quality to provide safety. Kiosks that sell sandwiches without refrigeration sacrifice safety to provide quality.

6.3.10 Pasta Products

Refrigerated food sections of most supermarkets feature fresh pasta. These products are vacuum packaged to preserve freshness. Of particular concern is the migration of moisture from the high-moisture product such as the sauce to the low-moisture product, the pasta, because it leads to soggy pasta. One way to avoid this problem is to keep the pasta separated from the sauce. Because pastas are intermediate-moisture products, they are not susceptible to most microbes except molds. The low- or no-oxygen package environment (vacuum package) prevents the mold growth. Fresh pasta, however, is susceptible to staling. The shelf life of fresh pastas is approximately 2 to 3 weeks. Marinara, cheese, and meat sauces have specific storage requirements.

6.3.11 Prepared Entrées

Prepared entrées are available at most supermarkets and many specialty shops. They tend to be high in protein and fats from meats, eggs, and cheeses. As such, they are usually very perishable because of microbial growth. They need to be kept hot or cold, outside the temperature growth range for microbes (10°C–40°C). Prepared entrées that are held at warm temperatures on steam tables tend to dry out and lose valuable nutrients, particularly vitamins. Consumers who purchase prepared entrées and hold them at room temperatures for extended periods (more than 90 minutes) are increasing their chances of food poisoning. When entrées are packaged with other components, the best conditions for one component may not be the best for the others. For example, breads or rolls generally do not store well at the refrigerated temperatures required for casseroles or other perishable items.

6.4 Food Service

Food service provides meals or meal components for consumption on-site. Among the various types of food service outlets are fine-dining, casual-dining, cafeterias, and other campus outlets, fast food, catering, and vending machines.

6.4.1 Fine-Dining Restaurants

Dining out has become an adventure that has led to a "foodie" culture. Driven largely by a desire for unique dining sensations, the evolution of celebrity chefs, and a growing number of consumers with high-disposable income, fine-dining establishments are growing in numbers. The ideal is that all entrées are prepared from fresh ingredients of local origin and in season purchased on the day of preparation by chefs who prepare each entrée between ordering and presentation to the diner. Sauces, stocks, mousses, and even some meat dishes are generally prepared ahead of time to prevent long waits by the customer. A preference for natural, organic ingredients has been a key component of modern fine-dining cuisine, although exotic ingredients from distant lands are also popular.

Molecular gastronomy has been developed in Europe to merge food science with the culinary arts to better understand the chemical and physical changes that food materials undergo during cooking processes (see Insert 6.4). While not a cuisine as such, molecular gastronomy has given chefs new tools to attract the "foodie" clientele with a new set of culinary sensations. The application of the principles of molecular gastronomy to food

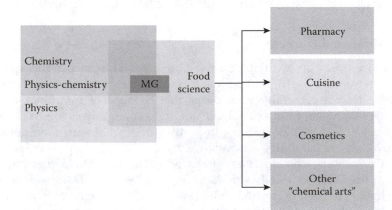

INSERT 6.4
Placement of Molecular gastronomy (MG) as it overlaps the basic sciences and food science. (From This, H., *Journal of Culinary Science and Technology* 9: 140, 2011. With permission.)

preparation referred to as molecular cooking or note-by-note cuisine emphasizes the use of individual compounds, extracts from food materials, and food gels to achieve unique flavors, colors, and textures. Extensive use of hydrocolloids provides the unique textures that attract adventurous customers. Whether molecular gastronomy will greatly change the cuisines of Europe and the Americas is not clear, but the scientific studies it inspires could have a profound effect on food science.

6.4.2 Casual-Dining Restaurants

Restaurant chains provide convenience by saving food preparation but not by saving time. Most consumers assume that the meals are prepared on-site from scratch, but many items may have been prepared elsewhere and heated or poured out of containers before serving. These items, from appetizers to main entrées to desserts, are prepared in processing plants under carefully controlled conditions and delivered to the restaurant. Many manufactured items are delivered frozen. Restaurants find the advantages of frozen products are their stability and safety. Although there may be some sacrifice in flavor or other quality characteristics, returning consumers are sufficiently pleased with the product's quality. Safety problems can come from items that are prepared on-site in any restaurant from improper employee hygiene, inadequate sanitation, items that are insufficiently cooked, or cross-contamination of uncooked foods with raw meats. A congenial atmosphere and flair in placement of the item on the plate enhances the eating experience. Many foreigners complain that most American restaurants have large portion sizes, which encourage overeating.

6.4.3 Campus Dining

In a sense, cafeterias were the first fast-food restaurants because ordering occurs at the same time as service. The prepared foods are displayed with hot foods kept on steam tables. Cafeterias are still part of the traditional food options on campus, but they are being supplemented by many other choices. Care must be taken when choosing foods on campus as calories can add up quickly, but cutting back on calories can lead to inadequate consumption of important vitamins and minerals (see Insert 6.5).

The unlimited supply of food in college dining halls and other facilities on campus is frequently cited as a major cause of the Freshman Fifteen, particularly by first-year women students. *Eating Well on Campus* offers some suggestions to help overcome the temptations of dining on campus by

- Scoping out all the choices before making selections will give us a better chance for healthier choices
- Selecting and consuming at least one fruit each lunch and supper

	Ethan		Garrett		Tiana		Selina	
Student	Ethan		Garrett		Tiana		Selina	
Entrée	Greek gyro		Italian sub		Turkey/avocado wrap		California roll	
Side	Side salad		Black bean hummus		Berry cup		Fruit salad	
Beverage	Soy milk		Small cappuccino		Mango peach smoothie		Coffee venti	
	Amount	%DV	Amount	%DV	Amount	%DV	Amount	%DV
Calories	710		1310		990		400	
Carbs	60 g	20	110 g	36	132 g	45	81 g	27
Sugars	28 g		34 g		65 g		36 g	
Protein	37 g		60 g		41 g		10 g	
Fat	37 g	56	72 g	110	35 g	56	5 g	8
Cholesterol	125 mg	41	135 mg	46	90 mg	31	5 mg	2
Sodium	2170 mg	91	4630 mg	193	1870 mg	78	370 mg	15
Vitamin A		14		156		117		4
Vitamin C		80		142		325		326
Calcium		70		48		31		4
Iron		101		110		39		40

INSERT 6.5

Ethan, Garrett, Tiana, and Selina met for lunch on campus to plan a class project. Ethan had a Greek gyro with a chef salad and soy milk to drink. Garrett went with the Italian hero, black bean hummus, and a small cappuccino. Tiana decided to eat healthy so she ordered a turkey wrap with a berry cup and a strawberry-banana smoothie. Selina didn't really want to get anything, but she opted for a California roll with a fruit salad and a huge coffee so she could keep awake in her afternoon classes. These values were calculated from the website http://urds.osu.edu/NetNutrition/Home.aspx.

- Choosing a wider range of foods that represent all the food groups
- Avoiding casseroles and stews for more plain foods
- Saving dessert for the end of the meal since we might be full and more likely to pass it by

6.4.4 Fast Foods

Fast foods have become America's scapegoat for its obesity problem. Fast food offers the opportunity to get a high-calorie meal in a short time, but a judicious consumer does not necessarily need to avoid fast foods to eat a healthy diet (for some options, see Insert 6.6). Fast-food menus are centered on a limited selection of items, but many chains are branching out with lower-calorie alternatives to hamburgers, fried chicken, and fries. Unlike most casual-dining restaurants, their fast-food counterparts usually offer a form of portion control. Most chains prefer to have all the ingredients preserved or prepared outside of the restaurant with heating, assembling, and servicing the major activities. Different strategies are employed to keep prepared meals hot and include made-to-order preparation, limited holding times, and hot-food cabinets.

Packaging serves many important functions in fast-food restaurants, including maintaining temperature, unitization, marketing, item identification, and spill prevention.

Fast-food restaurants get blamed for food poisoning outbreaks, but many of these reports are unfounded. A primary reason for blaming restaurants is that most people blame the last meal that they consumed for a stomach illness as we learned in Chapter 1. Most food-associated illnesses, particularly those that would be associated with fast foods, take 12–24 hours to develop. Fast-food restaurants employ many minimum-wage workers, but they have excellent systems to maintain sanitation and safety. Since they serve so many meals, however, when a serious mistake is made, many consumers are likely to become ill.

6.4.5 Catering

Food catering businesses have the same challenges as other food service outlets plus the added challenge of needing to transport the food from the place of preparation to the place of consumption. The major safety concern is keeping hot foods hot and cold foods cold. Some of the conditions that maintain safety can degrade quality, particularly in keeping hot foods hot. Shelf-stable foods such as breads, cakes, and cookies present little problem, but main entrées and frozen desserts can also present a challenge. Caterers want to present the food at top quality at the proper time.

Traffic delays, setup time by personnel at the consumption location, and long-winded speakers at pre-banquet meetings are all factors that caterers must take into consideration with respect to serving times. Facilities for

Store	Chick-fil-A®		Chipotle Mexican Grill		McDonald's®		Subway®	
Entrée	Deluxe Chicken Sandwich		Chicken burrito		Big Mac		Veggie sandwich	
Side	Cole Slaw		Chips with salsa		Medium fries		Veggie salad	
Beverage	Medium sweet iced tea		Water		Medium cola		Fruit punch	
	Amount	%DV	Amount	%DV	Amount	%DV	Amount	%DV
Calories	990		1330		1130		310	
Carbs	95 g	32	48 g	16	111 g	37	63 g	21
Sugars	55 g		14 g		65 g		29 g	
Vitamin C	57 g	95	11 mg	18	9 mg	15	99 mg	165
Iron	3 mg	19	8 mg	43	5 mg	30	4 mg	22
Fiber	6 g	24	22 g	88	8 g	32	7 g	28
Protein	33 g	66	58 g	116	30 g	60	9 g	18
Fat	54 g	83	54 g	83	48 g	74	3 g	5
Cholesterol	90 mg	30	155 mg	52	75 mg	25	0 mg	0
Calcium	260 mg	26	380 mg	38	300 mg	30	360 mg	36
Sodium	1800 mg	75	2600 mg	108	1240 mg	52	290 mg	12

INSERT 6.6

Listed are four fast-food meals calculated from nutritional information on websites for Chick-fil-A (http://www.chick-fil-a.com/Food/Menu), Chipotle Mexican Grill (http://www.chipotle.com/en-us/menu/nutrition_calculator/nutrition_calculator.aspx), McDonald's (http://www.mcdonalds.com/us/en/full_menu_explorer.html), and Subway (http://www.subway.com/nutrition/NutritionList.aspx?id=salad&Countrycode=USA). Selections made were the Deluxe Chicken Sandwich, Cole Slaw, and a medium iced tea-sweet at Chick-fil-A; a soft flour tortilla burrito with chicken, black beans, fresh tomato salsa, and sour cream, chips with fresh tomato salsa, and water at Chipotle Mexican Grill; a Big Mac, medium world famous fries, and medium Coca-Cola at McDonalds; and a Veggie Delite sandwich, Veggie Delite salad, and Minute-Maid Fruit Punch (100% juice) at Subway. There are many possible selections at these restaurants and the meal selected is not necessarily representative of each chain.

heating/reheating, short-term storage, and meal assembly at the consumption location must also be considered. Food must be secured properly in the transportation vehicle to provide proper presentation to the consumers. In a sense, home-delivery systems such as for pizza or Meals on Wheels are also catering businesses. These delivery systems use specialized, hot-food containers to keep the meals from getting cold.

6.4.6 Vending Machines

It seems we are never very far away from a vending machine in America. Some vending machines have become very sophisticated, dispensing hot coffee, meals, fresh fruit, cold sandwiches, and exotic ice cream. Carbonated beverages, sugared snacks, and their salted counterparts are ideal for vending machines because they are well packaged, not very perishable, and require no preparation before eating. Furthermore, they are easily consumed right out of the package.

Minimally processed juices, fruit cups, sandwiches, and entrées with meat are perishable and require refrigeration. Failure of the refrigerated vending equipment can lead to rapid growth of microbes, compromising the quality and safety of the product. Some of these items may be heated in the vending machine or in a microwave oven. Improper heating of foods that have not been properly refrigerated can give the purchaser a false sense of security about its safety. Frozen items require even more monitoring for proper temperature conditions than refrigerated products. Thawing and refreezing will damage the quality of the product before it threatens its safety.

6.5 Remember This!

- The unlimited supply of food in college dining halls and other facilities on campus is frequently cited as a major cause of the Freshman Fifteen.
- Molecular gastronomy has been developed in Europe to merge food science with the culinary arts to better understand the chemical and physical changes that food materials undergo during cooking processes.
- Food service provides meals or meal components for consumption on-site.
- Fresh fruits and vegetables deteriorate rapidly as they decay, die, and exude fluids.
- Maintaining adequate refrigeration of perishable products like deli meats is necessary, and expiration dates should be strictly observed.

- Expedited handling of fresh foods minimizes safety concerns and loss of quality.

- Food scientists are wary of consuming raw meat because any harvest operation is likely to contaminate the surface of the meat.

- MAP, which is low in oxygen and high in nitrogen or carbon dioxide, slows the deterioration process of perishable items.

- Prepared foods are those foods that are ready-to-eat or ready-to-heat then eat.

- As the pace of society increases, most consumers are looking for ways to reduce the time it takes to fix a meal and increase convenience.

6.6 Looking Ahead

This chapter was designed to provide an introduction to food processes and the types of products that are produced, with special emphasis on those made directly from raw agricultural materials. Chapters 7 through 10 cover how food scientists ensure the quality and safety of food products, design new products and processes, improve sustainability during handling, work in government to regulate foods and beverages, and perform research on foods.

Testing Comprehension

1. Distinguish the differences between chilled and prepared foods. Name five chilled foods that are not prepared foods and five prepared foods that are not chilled.

2. Describe the differences between fruits and vegetables. What are the nutritional benefits and limitations of each of them?

3. Identify the major challenges to safety presented by handling chilled foods, distributing prepared foods, and preparing foods for a food-service operation.

4. Select a favorite prepared food product not mentioned in the chapter. List the ingredients and the likely unit operations of the process. Then, draw a simple flow diagram of the process.

5. Compare and contrast the benefits and limitations of fine-dining, casual-dining, and fast-food restaurants.

6. Illustrate the challenges that a caterer would face in supplying lunch to a sanitation workshop of employees of local restaurants. The workshop would be held by members of the Food Science faculty in the current classroom on a Saturday from 9:00 a.m. to 5:00 p.m. The lunch break is scheduled to be 45 minutes and must be held in the same building.

7. Using any of the websites in Insert 6.5 or 6.6 or similar types of websites, design a meal that provides at least 30% of the daily value for vitamin C, iron, calcium, and fiber without going over 600 calories and 30% of the daily value for fat or sodium.

8. Fast-food chains have a reputation for being major contributors to obesity. Go on a website of a major chain and identify at least five steps it can take to promote healthier eating in its restaurants. Identify the impact that this chain could make on the health of Americans, its reputation with the American public, its workers, and its bottom line. How long would it take to implement this plan? How likely would it be to be successful?

References

Bahman, A., L. Rosario and M. M. Rahman, 2012. Analysis of energy saving in a supermarket refrigeration/HVAC system. *Appl. Energy*, 98:11.

Bollen, A. F., C. P. Riden and N. R. Cox, 2007. Agricultural supply system traceability, Part I: Role of packing procedures and effects of fruit mixing. *Biosystems Engineering*, 98:391.

Litt, A. S., 2005. *The College Student's Guide to Eating Well on Campus*, 2nd ed., Bethesda, MD: Tulip Hill Press.

This, H., 2011. Molecular gastronomy in France. *J. Culinary Sci. Technol.*, 9:140.

Further Reading

Florkowski, W. J., R. L. Shewfelt, B. Breuckner and S. E. Prussia, 2014. *Postharvest Handling: A Systems Approach*, 3rd ed., San Diego: Academic Press/Elsevier.

James, S. J. and C. James, 2002. *Meat Refrigeration*, Boca Raton, FL: CRC Press, Taylor & Francis Group.

Kays, S. J. and R. E. Paull, 2004. *Postharvest Biology*, Athens, GA: Exon Press.

Kerry, J., J. Kerry and D. Ledward, 2002. *Meat Processing: Improving Quality*, Cambridge, UK: Woodhead Publishing Limited.

Lamikanra, O., ed. 2002. *Fresh Cut Fruits and Vegetables*, Boca Raton, FL: CRC Press, Taylor & Francis Group.

Myhrvold, N., C. Young and M. Bilet, 2011. *Modernist Cuisine: The Art and Science of Cooking*, Bellevue, WA: The Cooking Lab.

Stringer, M. and C. Dennis, 2008. *Chilled Foods—A Comprehensive Guide*, 3rd ed., Boca Raton, FL: CRC Press, Taylor & Francis Group.

This, H., 2006. *Molecular Gastronomy: Exploring the Science of Flavor*, New York: Columbia University Press.

Section III

Functions of Food Scientists

7

Quality Assurance

Ignacio grew up in the city and thought it would be cool to spend Spring Break with his friend Garrett on his dairy farm. At first, he enjoyed the drive through the countryside, the fresh air, and the fresh, home-cooked meals. He thought it was pretty dull in the evenings though, and he wasn't real eager to get up so early to milk cows. Garrett's dad urged him to try some raw milk, assuring him that there was "nothing like it for flavor and nutrition!" Garrett seemed to enjoy it, so although he resisted at first, Ignacio finally got up his courage late in the week and drank a whole glass. It was rich and full-flavored. It sure didn't taste like any kind of milk he had ever tried before. The next morning, he was sick with stomach cramps, nausea, vomiting, diarrhea, and a fever. He was sure it was the milk, but Garrett and his dad insisted that all that talk about the only safe milk being pasteurized milk was hogwash. They had been drinking raw milk all their lives and they never got sick! It took Ignacio approximately 3 days to recover. He now knew what it was like to live on a farm. It might be OK for others, but it was definitely not for him. He'd also steer clear of raw milk, regardless of what Garrett said.

Alice bought her favorite chocolate bar at the snack shop on her way to chemistry class. It was the last bar in the box. She was running late, so she threw it into her book bag for later. She forgot all about the candy bar, but later, while looking for a highlighter, she rediscovered the treat. She had not had lunch and was incredibly hungry. She tore off part of the wrapper and bit in. Instead of the usual great flavor she was expecting, this bar took her taste buds to a new level. It was awesome! Somehow it was sweeter but not too sweet and the chocolate was more chocolaty. The flavors exploded in her mouth, sending her into spasms of delight. She had never tasted anything quite like it. Was she hallucinating? She took a second bite. It was as good as or better than the first! She closed her eyes and savored every little sensation. She thought about sharing it with a friend, but it was so tempting, so satisfying, and so delicious. She could not resist eating the whole thing. After a quick look to see if anyone was looking, she licked the wrapper clean.

The next day, Alice bought the same kind of chocolate bar at the same place. It was the first bar in a brand new box. She threw it into the same book bag and waited until the same time she had eaten the candy bar the day before. She could hardly wait for the first bite! When she ripped open the wrapper and took the first bite, she was bitterly disappointed. It was nothing like what she had the day before. Thinking back, it was probably as good as it usually was, but it was still disappointing. She bought several bars of the same brand

| Name | Serving size | Calories/ serving | Fat cals/ serving | Sugars/ serving | % Daily values/serving | | | | | |
					Vitamin A	Vitamin C	Calcium	Iron	Sodium
Peter Pan Creamy Peanut Butter	2 tbsp (30 g)	210	150	3 g	0	0	0	2	6
Roasted Honey Nut Skippy® Super Chunk Peanut Butter	2 tbsp (32 g)	190	140	3 g	0	0	0	4	5
Jif® Extra Crunch Peanut Butter	2 tbsp (32 g)	190	130	3 g	0	0	0	4	5
Trader Joe's Organic Creamy Peanut Butter Unsalted Naturally Sweet	2 tbsp (32 g)	190	130	1 g	0	2	0	4	0
1/3 Less Sodium & Sugar Skippy® Natural Creamy Peanut Butter Spread	2 tbsp (32 g)	210	150	2 g	0	0	0	4	3
Reduced Fat Jif® Extra Crunch Peanut Butter 60% Peanuts	2 tbsp (32 g)	190	100	4 g	0	0	2	4	3

INSERT 7.1

Comparison of nutritional value for selected peanut butter products.

at several different places, but it was never as good as the one on that magical day. She has just about stopped eating that bar because it just can't compete with perfection. Every now and then, she buys one but is still disappointed.

Jennifer likes peanut butter. She eats some almost every day because she has read on the Internet that anything with nuts in it is healthy or something like that. She usually buys what is cheapest. Then she learned from a friend that peanut butter is high in fat and sugar. She decided to do her own investigation to find the peanut butter that is the healthiest. She went on the Internet to find the best peanut butter and narrowed it down to six products (see Insert 7.1 for the comparison). She finally chose the reduced fat extra crunchy product. Did she choose wisely? Why or why not?

Ignacio, Alice, and Jennifer are interested in the safety and quality of their food. Food scientists employed by food companies are responsible for ensuring that the products are safe and the quality is consistent. They work in the Quality Department to design and oversee laboratory tests to make sure that Ignacio's milk has been properly pasteurized, Alice's chocolate bars are consistent in quality, and that Jennifer's peanut butter meets quality standards. In this chapter, we will see what is involved in measuring the quality and ensuring the safety of commercial food products.

7.1 Looking Back

Previous chapters focused on food issues we encounter in our daily lives and with the types of food products we encounter in the marketplace. The following key points that were covered in those chapters help prepare us to understand quality assurance:

- Fresh fruits and vegetables deteriorate rapidly as they decay, die, and exude fluids.
- Expedited handling of fresh foods minimizes safety concerns and loss of quality.
- Food scientists are wary of consuming raw meat because any harvest operation is likely to contaminate the surface of the meat.
- Food processing and preservation increase the shelf stability of a raw material usually at the cost of nutrition and quality.
- Most raw materials are perishable and require careful handling or processing to prevent losses.
- Sensory properties include color, flavor, and texture.
- The Nutrition Facts part of the label indicates the serving size, how many servings per container, calories per serving, and the fat calories per serving.

- Spoilage is not a good indicator of a safety risk.
- An expiration date represents the food scientist's best guess about how long a food will last before it spoils.
- Fresh foods are more likely to contain harmful microbes than processed products.

7.2 What Is Quality and Why Does Anybody Care?

Perhaps the most important function of a food scientist is achieving and maintaining the quality of a product. Many authors have tried to define quality for products and services, but it is difficult to find one definition to meet all needs. The simplest definition, "an absence of defects," may be good for a laptop, lamp, or textbook, but we want more information when shelling out big bucks for a sound system, set of wheels, or a gourmet meal on a hot date.

When it comes to food, defects include blemished apples, bruised peaches, mushy bananas, green eggs, iridescent ham, slimy wieners, stale cereal, lumpy mashed potatoes, and crunchy macaroni and cheese. Truly fine dining is the intertwining of pleasant flavors and textures with an excellent presentation. Quality is thus more than the absence of the bad; it is also the presence of good to great to exquisite. Even that description oversimplifies the situation because different foods and flavors appeal to different people. What one consumer might consider good quality, another might reject: some like their salsa mild, others like it hot.

To help make sense of this complex situation, we can place the factors involving individual preference into a category called **consumer acceptability** and the factors involving price into a category called **value**. That leaves **quality** to describe properties of food that can be measured by food scientists. A favorable experience in the mouth leads to consumer acceptability, while quality or acceptability at a given price relates to value. This chapter will define quality, describe how it is measured by food scientists, explain what is done in the food industry to ensure safety and consistent quality, and relate quality to acceptability and value.

7.3 Quality Characteristics

Quality has been described as meeting or exceeding the expectations of the consumer. A more detailed definition involves properties of a food that distinguish it from similar foods and affect its preference by consumers. Thus, the quality of a given product is defined by characteristics that vary from one brand to another within a category (differentiation) and that make a difference to consumers (degree of preference or acceptability).

Quality includes sensory characteristics that can be readily detected by the five senses and hidden characteristics that are not readily detectable by consumers. Hidden characteristics include safety and nutrition. The package also contributes to maintaining the quality of the food and its acceptability to the consumer. We assume that all commercial products we buy or meals we order out are safe. Much of the rest of this chapter will focus on the work food companies and foodservice institutions do to make sure that their products are safe for the consumer. The consumer can use the safety and nutritional quality information on a product label to decide whether or not to buy it.

We use all five senses when evaluating the sensory quality of our foods, but food scientists tend to reduce sensory quality to three types of characteristics: flavor, appearance, and texture. As indicated previously, flavor combines the senses of taste and smell. Appearance involves the sense of sight. Texture involves the sense of touch, both with our hands and in our mouth. Finally, through our sense of hearing, we can experience the sizzle of a steak, the crunch of a raw vegetable, and the snap, crackle, and pop of a famous breakfast cereal.

When we say we taste a food, we are actually evaluating its flavor. The five main tastes are bitter, sweet, salty, sour, and umami. There may be other taste sensations, but these five are the most easily identifiable. Flavor includes both aroma and taste. We perceive aroma in two ways: directly through the nose (orthonasally) before we put food into our mouth and through the back of our mouth (retronasally) while we are chewing. To take full advantage of the retronasal contribution of flavor, we must have proper airflow through our mouth and nose. That is why when we have a cold, pinch our nose, or eat with our mouth tightly closed, we say the food does not taste as good, but aroma not taste is what is affected. Much of what most of us think of as food quality is how we perceive its flavor. Would we be tempted to eat so much chocolate, fatty meat products, potato chips, fresh-squeezed juice, or other treats if they did not emanate an enticing aroma and follow it up with a pleasant taste?

Most consumers think that color is overrated as a quality characteristic, indicating that they are willing to give up appearance for flavor. In reality, color tends to be the most important factor in deciding what is purchased and consumed. Although we now know that appearance is not a good indicator of a safety hazard, most of us are unwilling to eat food that just doesn't look right. For example, many consumers refuse to eat bananas that have brown spots. Meat cooked in a microwave oven is not as popular as when it is cooked in a conventional oven because the meat is not as likely to turn brown in the microwave. Food manufacturers add artificial colors to breakfast cereals, beverages, candies, and maraschino cherries because bright colors sell and dull colors do not. Color does not usually get the respect it deserves as a quality characteristic.

Texture is another characteristic that is generally underrated, but many consumers will refuse to eat a food strictly on the basis of its texture. Raw oysters are rejected by many consumers because they have a tendency to be slimy. One reason consumers reject bananas with brown spots is that they find them too mushy although they are sweeter than those without the spots. Most of us prefer our carrots and apples crunchy and our peaches and cherries soft. We don't like lumps in our mashed potatoes or grits or soft spots on our peaches or fried chicken. We don't want our maple syrup or orange juice to be too thin and watery or our milk to be thick. We also have textural sensations known as chemical feeling factors, for example, pungency (onions), heat (peppers), cool (menthol), and astringency (green tea or red wine). All of these textures that we feel, whether with our hands or in our mouths, affect our perception of quality.

As mentioned before, safety and nutrition factors cannot be readily detected by the consumer. However, they play a part in helping the consumer make a decision as to whether or not they will buy or eat a product. Without a sophisticated analytical laboratory, consumers must take the word of the manufacturer or the preparer that the product is safe and nutritious. All quality characteristics, whether they are sensory or hidden, must be measurable and must be measured within the context of a quality system. The Quality Department within a processing plant has a responsibility to do everything possible to provide safe, nutritious, and wholesome foods.

7.4 Measuring Quality

Measurement of sensory and hidden quality characteristics is not as easy as we might think. In this section, only a brief overview will be provided. Later chapters will provide greater detail. For a quality measurement to be useful, it must be accurate, precise, sensitive, and relevant. Many measurements are made using instruments. Thus, the reliability and precision of the instrument must also be considered. Measurements are only estimates of reality. **Accuracy** of a measurement is how close the estimate is to the real value. **Precision** is how close estimates are to each other each time a measurement is made on the same sample. **Sensitivity** of the estimate is how effective it is at detecting very small amounts. Sensitivity is easy to determine by diluting the sample until the characteristic can no longer be detected. **Relevance** is how important the measurement is in relation to consumer acceptability. This property is the most difficult to determine because measuring consumer acceptability is difficult.

Reliability of the instrument refers to the consistency of measurements over time. Food scientists can easily determine the precision of a measurement by measuring the same characteristic of the same product numerous times. Reliability of the instrument needs to be checked periodically by trained personnel. Installation, competence of the operator, proper calibration, and proper equipment maintenance can affect day-to-day readings. Sometimes, the most meaningful measurements are performed by an expert tester. Small defects in flavor, appearance, or texture can be detected by someone with extensive experience with a specific product.

Measuring the safety of a product is done primarily by microbiological testing and analysis to determine the number and types of microbes present in a select sample. To ensure the safety of a product, the presence of pathogens (microbes that cause food poisoning) must be determined. Thorough knowledge of the product, such as how it will be stored and prepared before consumption and the types of pathogens likely to be present, aids food scientists in deciding what further testing must be done.

Nutritional labels must be accurate at the time the food is consumed. Since all nutrients are chemical, analyses are done to determine the chemical composition. Vitamins and minerals must be estimated and translated into the percentage of daily values. A food scientist must be able to measure the nutritional composition of a food and allow for possible changes or deterioration during its shelf life (handling and storage). Although processing, particularly canning, is detrimental to nutritional quality, fully processed foods maintain most of their nutrients during storage. Thus, measuring the nutritional composition of processed foods is not difficult. However, it is much more difficult to estimate the projected vitamin and mineral content, at the time of consumption, of highly perishable items such as fresh meat, fruits, and vegetables. It is not enough to determine how much of a nutrient is present. Food scientists must also consider the bioavailability of a nutrient, which is how much of it is absorbed through the intestinal tract and actually reaches the bloodstream in the proper form that the body can use.

Sensory quality of foods can be measured by physical, chemical, or sensory testing. Many of these quality tests are performed in the laboratory. When possible, manufacturing plants are using nondestructive measuring systems such as sensors or visual systems to sort out defective items before they are added to the finished product. Color is best measured by an instrument called a colorimeter or spectrophotometer (see Insert 7.2a) that measures the physical properties of reflected light and translates those readings into values that can be related to consumer perception of color. Visual defects in foods can be detected by using machine vision systems with video cameras.

Textural properties such as viscosity of beverages and semisolid foods as well as gumminess, hardness, adhesiveness, chewiness, and fracturability of solid foods can be determined using other physical measurements. Versatile instruments are available like the one shown in Insert 7.2b to measure many different textural characteristics. Nondestructive visual techniques are being developed for texture as well. Taste is defined using chemical processes to

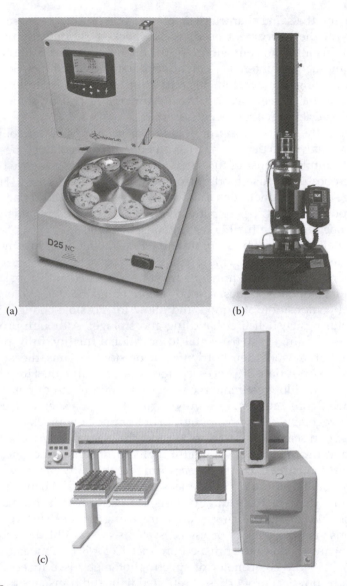

(a)

(b)

(c)

INSERT 7.2

(a) Example of an instrument used to measure color of a food—HunterLab D25 NC Spectrophotometer. (b) Example of an instrument used to measure texture of a food—5944 electromechanical testing system. (c) Example of an instrument used to measure aromatic properties of a food—Alpha MOS Heracles II Flash Gas Chromatography Electric Nose. ([a] Image provided by HunterLab. [b] Photo courtesy of Instron. [c] Image provided by Alpha MOS.)

measure sugar concentration for sweetness, acid concentration for sourness, sodium chloride for saltiness, and specific bitter compounds such as caffeine.

The aromatic part of flavor can be separated out of the volatile compounds using chromatographs. A liquid extract is injected into a gas or high-pressure liquid chromatograph that separates individual molecules by retention time based on properties like molecular weight. In some cases, a simple physical or chemical method can give a very good estimate of the sensory quality of food that is accurate, precise, and sensitive. Electronic noses (see Insert 7.2c) can help determine how similar products on a line are to each other or to a standard.

With respect to flavor, it is difficult to use an instrumental measurement to relate to consumer perception. There are many types of sensory tests to satisfy all of the taste quality specifications of a product. They range from determining if there is a difference between two brands, to finding the best formulation (a scientific version of a recipe). Tests may also make comparisons between competitors' products or between experimental formulations.

It is important to use human beings to actually "taste" the product. These types of sensory tests have trained panelists that are much more aware of and sensitive to specific tastes and aromas than a typical consumer. A unique method, known as a preference test, involves finding out which is the "best" product. The panelists here are typical consumers. We'll learn more about these sensory tests in Chapter 15.

Package integrity is another type of quality measurement that is performed. It is critical that a sealed package remain sealed, because without an intact package, the quality and safety of the product are compromised. Can seams are evaluated every hour on every line in every canning plant. Glass container seals are evaluated. Tamper protection devices are checked. Gas permeability and water vapor transmission rates of plastic/film packages help maintain the desired conditions inside the package. Packages that will be subjected to rough handling between leaving the processing plant and being purchased in the supermarket are tested for burst strength. In addition, Quality Department personnel check net weights to ensure that they are within a certain range. A net weight that is below what is stated on the package violates federal weight regulations. A net weight that is above the stated amount costs the company money.

7.5 Evolution of Quality Management

Quality has always been important for food products. Before mass production and distribution, chances are consumers knew where their food came from and could complain directly to the provider. Whether the person was a member of the family, a next door neighbor, or someone from the nearest town, their reputation and ability to earn a living were at risk; therefore, it was necessary to be careful. As food production becomes more mechanized and less personal, it is necessary to develop ways of making sure that each product is of good quality.

Quality Control (QC) was developed to make sure that a product is safe, wholesome, and of good quality. Consistent quality is achieved by inspecting the final product. Because inspecting every item (opening the can or package) is not only impossible but impractical, only some of the finished items are statistically sampled. A Quality Control Manager usually runs the QC programs, which are composed of activities focused on identifying and correcting defects in finished products or a more reactive approach to quality. **Statistical Quality Control** was incorporated into **Quality Assurance** (QA), which considers all parts of the process. QA programs are composed of activities for ensuring quality in the process to prevent defects from occurring or a more proactive approach to quality. The idea is that if the process is done correctly, then the final product will be safe and of good quality. A Director of QA is responsible for a QA program.

Quality Management (QM) takes this idea one step further in that it looks at what the consumer wants and needs (including changes in consumer preferences) and modifies the process accordingly. **Total Quality Management** (TQM) encompasses the entire company and is the responsibility of the Chief Executive Officer of that company. Each change in the way food companies viewed and managed quality has affected the type of products available to us in the supermarket.

7.5.1 Monitoring Quality in a Processing Plant

Nearly every piece of fresh fruit on a grading table is sorted by humans or machines, and every carcass of fresh meat in a slaughterhouse is evaluated by United States Department of Agriculture (USDA) inspectors. To ensure that fresh fruit in the supermarket is edible and reasonably consistent in quality, fruit graders remove fruit that are underripe, overripe, bruised, damaged, or unsightly. A USDA inspector visibly checks every carcass and marks for removal any that have visible signs of disease. Inspectors can stop a production line for a closer look, if necessary, by using a bell or buzzer. Diseased carcasses cannot be sold to an American consumer in any way (whole, cut-up, or further processed). Laws and regulations cover all aspects of food processing, from farm production to waste disposal at the processing plant.

Quality is more than what we can see. As mentioned earlier, many food quality measurements require destruction of an item. Since no food company can make money if its entire product is destroyed, statistical sampling is conducted to help determine the quality of the raw material and the finished product. Raw materials that do not meet the specifications of the processing plant are either rejected or sold at a reduced price. Tables and sampling schemes show the QC Manager how many samples are required to assess quality at a determined confidence interval. Then, the quality of the samples is compared to a specification or standard to ensure acceptability.

QA considers the whole process when evaluating quality with the emphasis on "getting it right the first time." By keeping the process operating correctly, the product should consistently be of good quality. Testing is still important in QA, but the testing occurs at various points in the plant to make sure the operations are working. As we read earlier, the Director of QA is responsible for the administration of quality testing and reporting; however, everyone working in the food processing plant also has a responsibility for product quality. QA begins when receiving raw materials and ingredients and continues through every unit operation during processing. Then, it extends beyond the plant through distribution and other activities of the company that can make a difference in final product quality. A constant study of the whole process by QA personnel and the people who operate the machinery leads to continuous improvement of product quality.

While QC and QA focus on the characteristics of the product that define quality, QM defines quality in terms of consumer acceptability. QM incorporates everything in QA, but it develops standards on the basis of what consumers want. Understanding the consumer is difficult; therefore, many techniques are necessary to gather information. Approaches involve use of the Marketing and Sales Departments to identify consumer wants and needs. These characteristics of the product are typically referred to as Key Quality Attributes or KQAs. Consumer profiles and KQAs are then incorporated into the quality measurements adopted by the company and monitored by the Quality Department. For the 14 basic principles of one highly respected version, see Insert 7.3.

QM is being recognized by organizations around the world. Standards have been developed by the International Organization for Standardization

1. Develop a realistic statement of objectives and purpose for the organization.
2. Learn the new philosophy.
3. Understand the purpose of inspection.
4. End the practice of basing decisions solely on the lowest price.
5. Constantly improve the system of service and production.
6. Institute training.
7. Teach and institute leadership.
8. Eliminate fear. Foster trust. Provide an environment that encourages innovation.
9. Optimize all activities toward the objectives and purpose of the organization.
10. Eliminate slogans and gimmicks. Treat employees as integral parts of the organization.
11. Eliminate quotas for production and management by objectives. Learn how to improve the systems.
12. Remove barriers that compete with pride of workmanship.
13. Encourage education and self-improvement for all members of the organization.
14. Implement all changes to transform the organization.

INSERT 7.3
Basic principles of Deming. (Adapted from Deming, W.E., *Out of the Crisis*, Cambridge, MA: MIT Press, 2000.)

(ISO). ISO provides a standardized approach to quality systems and auditing to compare companies and products globally. ISO 9000 incorporates many guidelines for specific processes to ensure uniform quality and safety of products and ensure that products are produced according to Good Manufacturing Practices. A company can become ISO certified by properly modifying its operation and facility and going through a thorough inspection. ISO 22000 specifically addresses food safety. Many companies will only buy ingredients for their products from ISO-certified manufacturers. Inspections of plant facilities of ingredient suppliers by a company not affiliated with either the supplier or user of that ingredient are known as third-party audits. These audits help maintain trust between supplier and manufacturer, but they do not relieve the manufacturer from the responsibility of maintaining quality and safety of the finished product.

7.5.2 Quality Department

Whether a manufacturing plant adopts QC, QA, QM, TQM, or a combination of any of these systems, the operation is monitored by a manager and employees of a Quality Department. This department has many responsibilities, including

- Developing all specifications for ingredients; procedures for sampling; guidelines for sanitation, process control, and worker safety; forms for inspection; and standards of quality for each finished product
- Testing incoming ingredients and packaging materials to ensure that they meet specifications
- Producing a Hazard Analysis and Critical Control Point (HACCP) plan for each product and keeping records to ensure that it is being followed
- Training of all personnel with respect to quality maintenance and proper sanitation practices within process operations
- Ensuring that the plant is complying with all local, state, and federal regulations
- Inspecting the entire plant for adherence to sanitation guidelines before the beginning of any shift
- Monitoring all operations within the plant
- Troubleshooting any quality issues that come up within plant operations
- Ensuring the safety of finished products
- Maintaining consistency and quality of the finished products
- Hosting and cooperating fully with any outside inspectors involved in supplier certification, third-party audits, or government regulation

- Responding to any consumer complaints or management concerns with respect to safety or other quality issues
- Handling any recalls, should they happen, determining their cause, and developing solutions to make sure they never happen again

Any successful processing facility must have buy-in from all personnel to make quality a priority. However, there is frequently a built-in tension between Manufacturing, which is rewarded for the amount of product produced daily, and the Quality Department, which is rewarded for maintaining a record of safe products of consistent quality.

7.6 Statistical Process Control

An essential element of QA and QM is Statistical Process Control (SPC). SPC involves the measurement of the effectiveness of a process or unit operation based on the idea that, by doing everything right in each operation of the process, the final product will be good. Measurements are made on the product at the end of a process to ensure that it is operating within guidelines. Statistical sampling techniques provide the number and frequency of measurements needed for a particular operation. A Shewhart Control Chart provides an operator with a visual indication of whether the process is "in control" or not (see Insert 7.4). A trend of points, either up or down, indicates if a process is about to go "out of control." Adjustments to the operation can then be made to prevent problems before they occur. When all operations

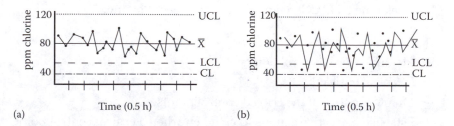

INSERT 7.4
Shewhart Control charts for monitoring chlorine concentration in a fresh-cut produce operation. (a) An operation that is in control, with all values falling between the upper control limit (UCL) and lower control limit (LCL). (b) An operation that is out of control as four values fall below the LCL, but no value falls below the critical limit (CL). (From Hurst, W.C., Safety aspects of fresh-cut fruits and vegetables. In *Fresh-Cut Fruits and Vegetables*, O. Lamikanra, ed., Boca Raton, FL: CRC Press LLC, Chapter 4, 2002. With permission.)

are in control, less inspection of the final product is needed. Thus, quality is assured for QA and QM through SPC.

Advances in technology have led to the development of in-line sensors. Such sensors measure physical characteristics of the product like color, viscosity, or temperature. They may also measure chemical composition such as percent sugars, percent acids, or percent salt. Technology is moving rapidly in improving accuracy, precision, and sensitivity of these measurements. Long-term reliability of a sensor is sometimes a problem, and the types of measurements easily made by sensors should be relevant to the consumer acceptability of the product. These systems can automatically create SPC charts and alert operators when a system is trending out of control.

7.7 Hazard Analysis and Critical Control Point

The HACCP system is a means of ensuring food safety of a food product. It started out as a way to meet the challenges of providing foods for astronauts in space and has been adapted to programs back here on earth. HACCP seeks to (1) destroy, eliminate, or reduce hazards; (2) prevent recontamination; and (3) inhibit growth of harmful microbes and limit toxin production. Hazard analysis identifies anything that could be harmful in a product. Types of hazards include biological (microbes or insects), chemical (pesticides or toxins), nutrition related (antinutrients), or physical (stones, metal, or glass). Hazards are classified as either severe or moderate. Unit operations have critical control points that are monitored and controlled to prevent hazards (see Insert 7.5 for a decision tree in designing a HACCP plan). HACCP is mandatory for juices, meat and poultry products, and seafood.

In developing a HACCP plan, we must do the following:

- Assess all hazards
- Identify critical control points
- Establish critical limits
- Monitor control of the critical control points
- Establish corrective actions to be taken when a critical control point is in noncompliance
- Develop a verification system
- Develop an effective documentation and record-keeping system

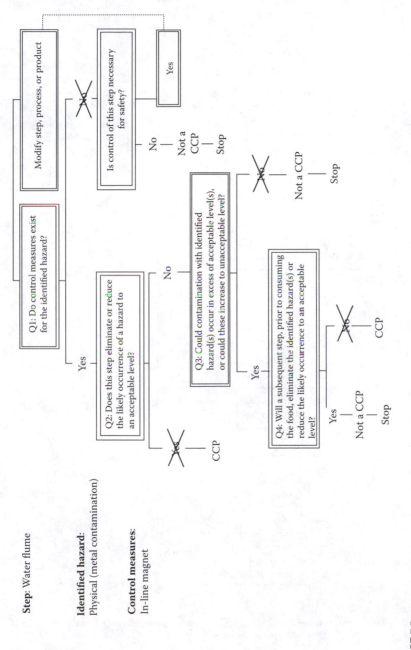

INSERT 7.5

Decision tree for applying HACCP to determine critical control points for a fresh-cut produce operation. (From Hurst, W.C., Safety aspects of fresh-cut fruits and vegetables. In *Fresh-Cut Fruits and Vegetables*, O. Lamikanra, ed., Boca Raton, FL: CRC Press LLC, Chapter 4, 2002. With permission.)

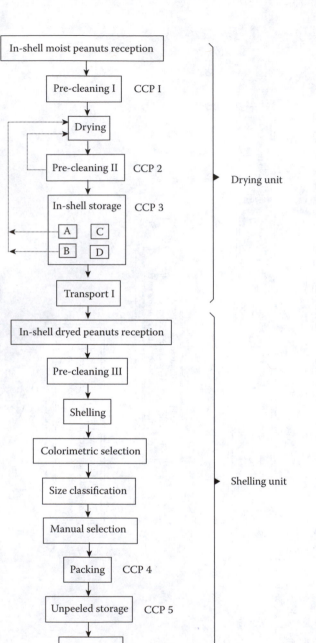

INSERT 7.6
HACCP plan for the prevention of aflatoxin during peanut processing. (From Gorayeb, T.C.C. et al., *Food Control* 20: 671, 2009. With permission.)

Because HACCP focuses on where safety problems are most likely to occur, it can reduce the need for extensive inspection and sampling. It can be applied to both small and large food processing operations as well as in a foodservice environment. HACCP works in conjunction with Prerequisite Programs (PRPs) and Standard Sanitation Operating Procedures (SSOPs), but it does not replace them. For a flowchart of a peanut processing operation with the critical control points shown, see Insert 7.6.

HACCP has been so successful in identifying and minimizing hazards in processed foods that advocates have proposed it be extended to sensory quality as well. Some scientists insist that it should be reserved for safety problems only. HACCP involves a systems approach to safety. Systems approaches characterize related operations within a process, view the whole process as a series of integrated steps, and study how the steps interrelate with respect to their fundamental properties. Quality measurements within a QA or QM system benefit greatly from a systems approach similar to HACCP with regard to quality characteristics.

7.8 Sanitation

One of the major obstacles to food quality and safety is product contamination either from microorganisms or from chemicals. Food processors must be careful to prevent contamination, beginning with the raw materials and on through every unit operation, using sanitation as the key to preventing contamination. Sanitation, in short, is keeping things clean. Sanitation begins with the production of the raw materials, before anything ever gets to the processing plant. Although it may be impossible to keep plants and animals completely free from microbes, any procedure that reduces the contact of raw materials with soil or animal feces will reduce the presence of microbes. Growing of plants on plastic minimizes contact with soil and pathogens associated with organic fertilizers. Efforts that minimize the opportunity for animals to roll in dirt or excrement reduce chances of contamination. Keeping harvested plant parts and live animals in clean environments during transport to and storage at the plant before processing are also major steps in limiting contamination.

In the processing plant, many things need to be done to keep it clean. Control of pests such as insects and rats in warehouses and processing areas is very important. There is a constant need to keep floors, horizontal surfaces, and food contact surfaces clean and free of dust and debris. Employees who handle food must be sure their hands and clothes are clean.

Most processing plants operate for 14 to 18 hours and then are completely cleaned and sanitized before the next day, when operations begin again. However, there are some industries, like chocolate, where standard sanitation

FRM 001 | **DAILY SANITATION CHECK SHEET**

Plant	Date & Time of Inspection									Inspected by
Rating Symbols: S – Satisfactory, NI – Needs Improvement; U–Unsatisfactory	S	NI	U	S	NI	U	S	NI	U	Explanation
1.0 PREMISES										
1.1 Outside areas										
1.2 Waste disposal										
1.3 Building repair										
2.0 RECEIVING										
2.1 Boxes										
2.2 Storage										
2.3 Dumpers & conveyors										
2.4 Floors, gutters & walls										
3.0 PREPARATION										
3.1 Washers & flumes										
3.2 Belts & elevators										
3.3 Graders										
3.4 Cutters & slicers										
3.5 Blanchers										
3.6 Pulpers & finisher										
3.7 Floors, gutters & walls										
4.0 CANNING										
4.1 Belts										
4.2 Fillers & can tables										
4.3 Floors, gutters & walls										
5.0 COOK ROOM										
5.1 Exhaust box										
5.2 Syrupers										
5.3 Seamers										
5.4 Floors, gutters & walls										
6.0 SYRUP & EVAPORATION										
6.1 Tanks & pipes										
6.2 Vacuum pans										
6.3 Floors, gutters & walls										
7.0 WAREHOUSE & STORAGE										
7.1 General housekeeping										
7.2 Stacks										
8.0 RESTROOMS										
8.1 Supplies										
8.2 Wash basins										
8.3 Toilets & urinals										
8.4 Floors & walls										
9.0 PERSONNEL										
9.1 Cleanliness & handwashing										
9.2 Head/beard covering										
9.3 Smocks & gloves										
9.4 Smoking										
OVERALL RATING										

Plant Inspector _____

INSERT 7.7
Template for a daily sanitation inspection log for a food processing plant. Note that this sheet would need to be adapted to the specific operations of the processing plant and be compatible with the company HACCP plan. (Courtesy of the University of Georgia Extension Food Science Outreach program.)

practices are not possible. These environments require even stricter controls on human and equipment sanitation. Some equipment can be cleaned by circulating chlorinated water or some other sanitizing solution through it by means of a Clean in Place system. Other equipment must be completely broken down, scrubbed with warm soapy water, rinsed, sanitized, and reassembled by means of a Clean out of Place system. Thorough inspections are conducted to ensure that everything meets exacting standards of cleanliness before the plant is allowed to operate. An example of a daily sanitation inspection sheet is shown in Insert 7.7.

Governmental guidelines such as PRPs and SSOPs are useful in maintaining adequate sanitation in processing plants. PRPs are overseen by the Food and Drug Administration, while SSOPs are guidelines of the USDA. The latter are required for all meat plants. Each company must develop specific procedures that are in compliance with these regulations from the receipt of raw materials, to clean-up and sanitizing of all processing equipment, monitoring of chlorine usage, and management of wastewater generated by the plant.

Food processing plants generate large amounts of waste. Governmental regulations impose certain requirements on the quality of the water and air leaving the plant. The Quality Department is responsible for ensuring that these standards are met. Whenever possible, waste from food processing operations is turned into usable products (by-products), such as exotic items for foreign markets (chicken feet), animal feed (fruits and vegetables not fit for human consumption), or fertilizer.

Sanitation is not limited to the food processing plant. It is also essential in every operation of a restaurant. Strict guidelines are provided for all foodservice operations from locally owned and operated restaurants to major food chains. Restaurant chains develop extensive guidelines and have company inspectors who check each unit to make sure they are operating appropriately. In many places, the local health board inspects a restaurant within its community. The types of things inspectors check that are considered critical violations were described in Chapter 1 (see Insert 1.6). Restaurants are required to post their health rating in a prominent place.

7.9 Consumer Acceptability

The ultimate goal in ensuring product quality is customer satisfaction. Although quality focuses on the characteristics of the product, acceptability must consider the attitudes of the consumer. Consumer acceptability is defined as the willingness to buy and eat a product.

While quality characteristics can be measured with accuracy and precision, it is much more difficult to measure consumer attitudes. Food processors using QC or QA systems don't become unduly concerned about measuring consumer acceptability. Ownership for consumer acceptability usually lies within the Research and Development department as they develop and validate new products. Production facilities ensure that they produce a consistent product, make it available to the public, and advertise. If consumers buy a product, and like it, they are likely to buy it again. As long as sales meet or exceed the company's expectations for purchases and profits, the item will continue to be produced. Companies who take a QM approach will attempt to learn what it is that current and potential consumers want and need.

Some consumers like their peanut butter creamy, and others like it crunchy. Within the creamy peanut butter category, there are subcategories. In consumer preference tests, University of Georgia students favored the leading peanut butter brand every time although the samples were not identified by brand. This company has developed their product to appeal to a segment constituting a majority of peanut butter lovers. It is hard to imagine that any company will develop a better peanut butter that will match or exceed the preferred brand. Since there are some consumers who do not like that brand, developers of a new product might be better trying to appeal to a segment that does not prefer the leading brand. Being the leader, however, doesn't always mean that consumers like it best. In other blind tests we've done in classes, most students cannot tell the difference between the two leading cola beverages, and a less popular brand frequently wins these preference tests. In this case, marketing is apparently a better determinant of success than actual consumer preferences.

When determining consumer acceptability, it is necessary to look at potential consumers of a product as well as current consumers. If companies only look at current peanut butter consumers or cola drinkers, they may miss an opportunity to get more people to consume their product. For example, the person who first cut big carrots into small ones, put them in a package, and sold them as baby carrots opened the product to many people not willing to take the time to clean, peel, and cut the big ones.

Measuring acceptability is a difficult task. First, we must determine the segment or segments of the population interested in that product. Then, we need to develop a test that presents consumers with one or more similar products and ask them if they like it or not. We must be careful not to get too complicated with the test questions, as normal consumers are not trained to measure specific quality characteristics. Frequently, this type of information can be inaccurate. However, consumers are the only ones who can let us know if they like it or not. Some research scientists present consumers with a sample and ask them if it "tastes great," is "acceptable," or is "unacceptable." Most sensory scientists use a nine-point scale that ranges from "like extremely" to "dislike extremely." See Insert 7.8 for some examples of scales used in consumer preference tests.

Smiley face	Acceptability	Willingness to purchase	Hedonic
😊	3—Tastes great	5—Definitely would purchase	9—Like extremely
			8—Like very much
		4—Probably would purchase	7—Like moderately
			6—Like slightly
😐	2—Acceptable	3—Might or might not purchase	5—Neither like nor dislike
			4—Dislike slightly
		2—Probably would not purchase	3—Dislike moderately
			2—Dislike very much
☹️	1—Unacceptable	1—Definitely would not purchase	1—Dislike extremely

INSERT 7.8
Selected scales used in consumer tests.

7.10 Remember This!

- Although quality focuses on the characteristics of the product, acceptability considers the attitudes of the consumer.

- Food processors must be careful to prevent contamination, beginning with the raw materials and on through every unit operation, using sanitation as the key to preventing contamination.

- The HACCP system is a means of ensuring microbial safety of a product.

- SPC involves the measurement of the effectiveness of a process or unit operation based on the idea that, by doing everything right in each operation of the process, the final product will be good.

- QM defines quality in terms of consumer acceptability.

- QA considers the whole process when evaluating quality with the emphasis on "getting it right the first time."

- As food production becomes more mechanized and less personal, it is necessary to develop ways of making sure that each product is of good quality.

- For a quality measurement to be useful, it must be accurate, precise, sensitive, and relevant.

- Quality includes sensory characteristics that can be readily detected by the five senses and hidden characteristics that are not readily detectable by consumers.

- Perhaps the most important function of a food scientist is achieving and maintaining the quality of a product.

7.11 Looking Ahead

This chapter introduced us to how food scientists define quality, measure it, and ensure that foods are safe and of consistent quality. Chapter 8 will describe how new food products are developed for the marketplace, and Chapter 9 will describe how we can maintain quality sustainably. Chapter 10 will describe the government's role in developing regulations to ensure safety and quality of food products. Chapter 11 will address the chemical basis of food quality. Chapter 12 will describe the nutritional basis of food quality, and Chapter 13 will present microbiological aspects of quality. Food engineering will be the subject of Chapter 14, and in Chapter 15, sensory studies (actual tasting of products) will be covered.

Testing Comprehension

1. Identify the cause of Ignacio's illness. Was the unpasteurized milk responsible or something else he consumed? How could a definitive diagnosis be made? If it was the milk, why didn't Garrett and his dad get sick?

2. Describe the importance of maintaining consistency of quality in a food product. Contrast the drawback of having 1% of the items of a particular product below the standard with that of having 1% of it above the standard. Are there any potential problems associated with too rigid an emphasis on consistency of quality?

3. Observe the sanitation scores at a local restaurant. How difficult was it to locate the form? What did the sheet indicate about the safety of the food? Should the sanitation score be checked every visit? Why or why not?

4. Choose a line of food products to manufacture. Identify the most important quality characteristics in this line of products. Determine the types of measurements needed to develop for testing the quality of these products. Should QC, QA, or QM be used in this plant? Why?

5. Diagram the process operations for the line of products in the previous question. Identify the critical control points in the process.

6. Construct a job description for the head of the Quality Department for the company described in the two previous questions. Include the title, a list of responsibilities, and the required qualifications.

7. Compare and contrast the importance of each of the four properties of a measurement within QC, QA, and QM.

8. Outline the approaches to establishing a quality program for fresh, frozen, and formulated chowders for either clams or corn. What are the unique challenges posed by managing quality programs for fresh, processed, and formulated products?

9. Calculate the number of grams of fat and the calories from sugar for each of the peanut butter brands in Insert 7.1. If Jif made a low-fat peanut butter to deliver only 40 calories of fat per serving, how many total calories would we expect this product to contain per serving? How would the other values in the table be affected? What other effects might we expect in this product when the fat was reduced?

References

Deming, W. E., 2000. *Out of the Crisis*, Cambridge, MA: MIT Press.

Gorayeb, T. C. C., F. P. Casciatori, V. L. D. Bianchi and J. C. Thomeo, 2009. HACCP plan proposal for a typical Brazilian peanut processing company. *Food Control*, 20:671.

Hurst, W. C., 2002. Safety aspects of fresh-cut fruits and vegetables, in *Fresh-Cut Fruits and Vegetables*, Lamikanra, O., Ed., Boca Raton, FL: CRC Press, Taylor & Francis Group.

Further Reading

Alli, I., 2004. *Food Quality Assurance: Principles and Practices*, Boca Raton, FL: CRC Press, Taylor & Francis Group.

Clute, M., 2009. *Food Industry Quality Control Systems*, Boca Raton, FL: CRC Press, Taylor & Francis Group.

Florkowski, W. J., R. L. Shewfelt, B. Brueckner and S. E. Prussia, Eds., 2014. *Postharvest Handling: A Systems Approach*, 3rd ed., New York: Academic Press, Elsevier.

Heredia, N. L., I. V. Wesley and J. S. Garcia, 2009. *Microbiologically Safe Food*, Hoboken, NJ: Wiley-Blackwell.

Hough, G., 2010. *Sensory Shelf-Life Estimation of Food Products*, Boca Raton, FL: CRC Press, Taylor & Francis Group.

Irudayaraj, J. and C. Reh, Eds., 2008. *Nondestructive Testing of Food Quality*, Ames, IA: IFT Press/Blackwell Publishing.

ISO, 2008. *How to Use ISO 22000—Food Safety Management Systems*, St. Louis, MO: Bizmanuelz.

Lyon, D. H., M. A. Francombe and T. A. Hasdell, 2012. *Guidelines for Sensory Analysis in Food Product Development and Quality Control*, 3rd ed., New York: Springer Science.

Marriot, N. G. and R. B. Gravani, 2010. *Principles of Microbiological Troubleshooting in the Industrial Food Processing Environment (Food Microbiology and Food Safety)*, New York: Springer Science.

Mortimore, S. and C. Wallace, Eds., 2013. *HACCP: A Practical Approach*, New York: Springer.

Petrozzi, S., 2013. *Practical Instrumental Analysis: Methods, Quality Assurance and Laboratory Management*, Weinheim, Germany: Wiley-VCH Verlag & Co.

Vasconcellos, J. A., 2007. *Quality Assurance for the Food Industry: A Practical Approach*, Boca Raton, FL: CRC Press, Taylor & Francis Group.

8

Product and Process Development

A group assignment in Jennifer's Food Science class required them to come up with a fantasy food product not currently available and create a marketing plan. After much debate, her group decided to develop a 1-calorie beer. The students designed a nice looking package and a clever marketing campaign aimed at NASCAR fans. The slogan was "The Buzz without the Calories!" They made sure to include a public service campaign to discourage drinking and driving. Jennifer and her team were very disappointed to receive a C minus. Written in green ink next to the grade they read, "TECHNICALLY IMPOSSIBLE." "Hey, if they can make a 1-calorie can of cola, why not beer? A whole lot more people have a beer gut than a cola gut!"

As part of a national food product development competition sponsored by the Institute of Food Technologists, Malik led a project to design a nutritious food without all those artificial colors, sugars, fats, preservatives, and stabilizers. Malik's particular interest was in soy. The problem with soy was that once we get past tofu, there are not that many products available, and most of them taste terrible. After working on his project for a while, the team began to understand the difficult challenge soy posed to product developers. Soy lipids easily and rapidly oxidize during storage. The oxidation produces strong beany and cardboard flavors. One of their biggest dilemmas was figuring out how to design a product with good flavor and shelf stability using only ingredients that qualified for a clean label. While their project did not win the IFT prize, Malik considered his experience to be one of the most satisfying and rewarding ones during his college days.

For her graduate research project sponsored by an industry trade organization, Alice developed a gluten-free energy bar. The main ingredients in the bar were oats, pecans and rice. Gluten-free products tend to be criticized because they either have too much sugar and salt or they don't have much flavor. She kept her energy bar low in salt and sugar, but the toughest problem was to keep the texture from being either too gooey or too mushy. Nobody wants their food sticking to the roof of their mouth! She had to use knowledge she gained in most of her courses to complete her project. She needed to understand the chemistry of ingredient interactions, microbiology to ensure product safety, engineering to design her process, and nutrition to make sure that it met written specifications. Then there were the endless training and test sessions for sensory evaluation of her prototypes. Alice's experiences in this project helped her land a job with a major manufacturer of gluten-free baked goods.

These three students tasted both the thrill and the disappointment of new product development. Product and process development allow food scientists the opportunity to use both creative and technical skills. Creativity is important in designing a product or process that results in something many consumers will enjoy eating and come back for more. Technical knowledge is essential to be able to separate the ideas that are possible from those that are not and to extend development beyond trial and error to one of skill and logic. This chapter will provide some insight into how food scientists work with others in the food industry to create new processes and products that feed our insatiable desires for variety in the supermarket. Product development is perhaps the most interesting and challenging activity that a food scientist performs as a professional.

8.1 Looking Back

Previous chapters focused on food issues we deal with in our daily lives and with the types of products we encounter in the marketplace. Some key points that were covered in those chapters help prepare us for understanding product and process development and are as follows:

- Quality includes sensory characteristics that can be readily detected by the five senses and hidden characteristics that are not readily detectable by consumers.

- Individual fat replacers cannot perform all functions of lipids.

- In selecting the ingredients for a formulation, the food scientist must consider the quality of the food, its safety, its stability, and its cost.

- A clean label is one that has only clearly recognizable ingredients that do not sound like chemicals.

- The main function of a package is to preserve the physical and chemical integrity of a product including preventing microbial or chemical contamination.

- No matter how nutritious, safe, and high quality a product is, if it does not taste good, we will not be very likely to choose it.

- Although not a true allergic reaction, celiac disease is an autoimmune disorder in which microvilli in the intestinal tract react with gliadin, a component of gluten found in wheat and other grains.

- Preservatives are food ingredients that slow spoilage and help prevent food-associated illnesses.

- A processed food should be designed to spoil before it becomes unsafe to make it less likely that someone will eat the unsafe food and become sick.

- An expiration date represents the food scientist's best guess of how long a food will last before it spoils.

8.2 Proliferation of Food Products

A look around the supermarket reveals a wide variety of products. Each one of these products was developed by a food scientist, probably as part of a research team. Some of these products are truly new products, something very different from anything we've ever seen before. Others may be a "new and improved" product or a line extension, such as a new flavor. Sometimes, one company brings out an alternative to a best-selling brand. All of these items provide us with a number of choices. For example, Alice was in her local supermarket the other day and counted 149 different brands/flavors/sizes/types of ice-cream products. Despite all of her choices, they didn't have her favorite "no sugar added" flavor—chocolate marshmallow.

It has been estimated that less than 10% of the products developed each year make it to supermarket shelves. Of those, most do not last a year before they are pulled by the manufacturer. The ones that remain are survivors in a very competitive marketplace. That is why we may find a great new product and enjoy it for a short time only to be disappointed when it is no longer available. Perhaps others didn't like it as well as we did or maybe they just didn't find out about it in time. Unless enough consumers buy the product, it will not survive. See Insert 8.1 for the story of an early product developer.

Supermarkets are not the only place we can find new products. Fast-food and casual-dining restaurants also introduce them to their customers. While we might think that these items are made from scratch in the back of the restaurant, it is usually not the case. Most fast-food products are processed or formulated in a food manufacturing plant and shipped to a central warehouse and then to the individual location where the products are prepared and assembled for sale. Even those delicious entrées and desserts at those upscale chains are frequently prepared elsewhere, divided into individual servings, frozen, and shipped to the restaurant for our dining pleasure. These products may be developed by food scientists working for the restaurant chain, a supplier (like a chicken processor for chicken sandwiches), or a team composed of scientists from both companies. In the continuing emphasis on high-quality products, many companies are hiring developers with a culinary background.

Early in his life Milt, like his father Henry, failed at everything he did. When he was out of money after another failure, he was working in Denver for a caramel maker. He learned that adding milk instead of paraffin to caramels improved the flavor and texture of the candy. He returned to Pennsylvania, added more milk to his caramels to make them easier to chew and more buttery, found a wholesale distributor, and made a small fortune. Instead of retiring on his fortune, he plowed his profits into a new idea—milk chocolate.

Milt found that it was much more difficult to incorporate milk into chocolate than it was to incorporate it into caramels. He moved close to the dairy farms in Pennsylvania, and worked by trial and error to come up with the right combination of ingredients. He found that the water of the milk and the fats in the chocolate did not mix well, so he needed to boil most of the water from the milk. He encountered many other difficulties before he was able to succeed, making the milk chocolate that Americans love.

Milt was not well educated. He never completed grade school, but he was part of a generation of entrepreneurs who designed their own products and manufactured them. He is actually credited with introducing mass production just a few years before Henry Ford. Ironically, Milt was never very interested in the business side of chocolate. Fortunately, he developed a partnership with William Murrie who handled all of the business aspects while Milt focused on product design and manufacturing. Although his chocolate was a success, many other products, such as onion-flavored ice cream, were not. It is thought that his cigar-smoking habit may have dulled his ability to perceive flavor.

Today, people who design products require a sound technical education. Products are not usually developed by a single individual now. Rather, they are designed by a team generally led by a food scientist and composed of several other employees such as those with a background in plant operations, quality and safety testing, package engineering, graphic design, product distribution, accounting, marketing, and sales. Some products may require a nutritionist, process engineer, lawyer or other expert on the team.

INSERT 8.1
Chocolate science.

8.3 Generating New Food Product Ideas

Before a product is developed, someone must come up with an idea. A concept then develops from the idea (like 1-calorie beer of Jennifer's team). Maybe somebody likes a product but has a suggestion to make it better. Maybe someone else has experimented at home and combines two or more favorite products into a dynamite eating sensation. Maybe a wild dream turns into a novel product. There are many different routes to new ideas.

Many new product ideas come in raw form from Marketing Departments. Marketers are free-thinking, creative people who are always thinking about new product concepts and how existing products can be different or more interesting, but such ideas are not necessarily practical. Marketing is about getting people to try new products. Ideas can also come from the Sales Department. Salespeople collect ideas from a variety of sources:

- Rumors of new products even before they hit the shelves
- Products that are currently available (including competitors)

- What is working and what is not (shelf stability)
- How good products could be made better
- New products consumers would like

Ideas from Sales tend to be less original and more practical than those coming from the Marketing Department because salespeople are on the front lines dealing with customers daily and must see their products from the customers' viewpoint.

Another source of product ideas is the consumer. As mentioned earlier, it is the consumer who makes or breaks a new product by either buying it or not buying it. Opening a conversation using social media is one way to start the process for obtaining consumer ideas. Marketing Departments spend much time and money using surveys and focus groups to systematically collect information. During a survey, consumers make known their likes and dislikes if asked about a new idea or given the opportunity to try a new product. Surveys may also be conducted through social media. Ultimately, a focus group may be used. A focus group consists of a few customers and a skilled moderator with a carefully scripted set of questions designed to get new ideas and test product concepts. Although some product ideas are generated from consumers, it is difficult to separate those that will appeal to the general market and those that are "unique" and will appeal to only a few.

Finally, ideas come from product developers themselves. They work with new ideas all the time. Sometimes, a failed product will give them an idea for a new product that may work. Other times, a product not previously envisioned happens quite by accident with the addition of the wrong ingredient or the right ingredient at the wrong level, which produces unexpected results. Product developers may be sent by their companies hundreds of miles to cities like Chicago, New York, or San Francisco to sample the latest local fare for new product ideas. Food scientists bring a systematic approach to the development process, but product development still includes art as well as science. A successful developer will be able to bring some of both to bear.

8.4 Improving Existing Products

We are all familiar with the phrase "new and improved." It may be just a more consumer-friendly package or a product that doesn't spoil as quickly. As times change, so do consumer tastes and preferences. A developer must diligently keep products current with changing times while simultaneously not making changes that will cause the loss of loyal customers. It can be a delicate balance.

Product line extensions are defined as changes in a product feature, such as flavor, content, size, name, or packaging. For example, a new papaya flavor for ice cream, milk, or juice mix adds a new product to an existing line. Adding cherry, lemon, or vanilla to colas or jalapeno peppers to cheeses represents a more dramatic line extension. Creating a line of vegetable yogurt was an even more revolutionary change that did not work in the American marketplace. To appeal to a different market such as children or seniors, products may be packaged in different sizes or under different names or labels. Any modification to product ingredients requires a corresponding change in the labeling.

Improvement of the flavor, color, or texture of a product generally happens because of consumer complaints. The sensory quality of a product may be fine when it leaves the manufacturing plant but is lost during distribution. The improvement needed here is to extend the shelf life by increasing the products' stability. This change can be accomplished with a new formulation (change in ingredients) or a modified process at a specific unit operation (change in temperature). Packaging can also be a source of product improvement simply by making it easier to open. Easier preparation, such as microwavable maple syrup containers, is a common type of product improvement.

Another reason to modify an existing product might be the need to substitute ingredients. Occasionally, an ingredient becomes unavailable. At other times, the ingredient is available but the quality is too variable, making it impossible to provide product consistency. Perhaps the ingredient is available but it has become too expensive. Then again, maybe the developer has found an ingredient that is simply better than the one presently being used.

Many products are now being formulated to produce low-calorie versions using fat and sugar substitutes such as Olestra or stevia. Substituting an ingredient is not as simple as it might seem. The product developer must conduct many experiments to find the right balance. It may take two or more ingredients to perform the same function as a single ingredient in the original formula, or one ingredient may substitute for two or more. Substitute ingredients may interact with other ingredients to provide quality or stability problems not encountered with the original formulation. The new ingredient(s) may induce slightly different sensory properties, but it is not clear whether these new properties are great enough to affect consumer acceptability. Another concern when ingredients are substituted is that the statement on the label must be changed. Companies want to be certain that the ingredient change is a definite improvement before changing their label and discarding a large stock of unused labels. Cost is always a concern when reformulating a product.

Product improvements could also result from process modifications. Production of truly new products (like 3-D corn chips) requires new equipment or at least major modifications to existing equipment. Major modifications in equipment or processes are rare because they are very expensive. Thus, new product sales projections must be high for management to make any changes. Sometimes, minor modifications are made to equipment in a food manufacturing plant, which results in a more consistent quality product, but in most cases, the developer will modify the product to fit the existing equipment rather than modify the equipment to fit the product.

8.5 Brand New Products

New products are developed for a variety of reasons, such as a new idea, a new trend, a problem confronting consumers, a new technology for food production, a new type of material for packaging, or the introduction of a foreign dish. Some new products represent major changes and are truly innovative. These products may change the way consumers eat or even think about eating.

Another source of truly innovative products is a new idea of what a food is or how to eat it. One of the more famous is the hot dog. There are many stories about how it was developed, but this one stuck. Apparently a vendor decided to put a German sausage into a French roll. The sausage, being long and round, prompted him to call it, dachshund. The name didn't work, but a modification—hot dog—did. The product had appeal because it could be eaten without utensils, a trait that is important in fast-food restaurants of today. This innovation led to the development of specific frankfurters for hot dogs, including the substitution of turkey for pork or beef. Buns were designed to fit the wieners, which then took on different lengths. More wieners and buns could be sold if there were different quantities of buns and wieners in their respective packages. Toppings like mustard, ketchup, coleslaw, sauerkraut, and chili have increased in sales and consumption thanks to the development of the hot dog.

The big trend these days is health foods. Developers like Alice and Malik have been trying to incorporate trendy ingredients into acceptable products. They have found that many of these ingredients have unpleasant flavors or odors. For example, garlic has been touted as being a healthy ingredient, proclaiming to help prevent cancer and heart disease, but garlic is also a major cause of halitosis (bad breath), a socially unacceptable condition. Some dispensers of garlic tablets provide the best of both worlds—odorless garlic. If, however, the physiologically active components are also the ones that provide its odor, any health benefits will be lost when the odor is lost.

As this edition is being written, consumers are cutting back on soft drinks for more flavored water, coffees, and teas. Exotic juices and protein drinks are also becoming popular. Many consumers want more veggies in their diets but don't find whole ones very convenient. New formulations incorporate vegetable pureés and other vegetable-based ingredients. Omega-3 oils, nuts, and ancient grains such as quinoa and chia are trendy ingredients, particularly in gluten-free products. Low-salt and low-sugar products that have full flavor with clean labels are being developed in many commercial laboratories. How long these trends will last is not clear.

New technologies become another source for truly innovative products. Extruders permit a whole range of new foods. By changing the die on the end of the extruder, new sizes and shapes can be created while still using the same piece of processing equipment. In the late 1960s, using extrusion technology, two companies collaborated to develop a new bite-size egg roll without the traditional fold. The companies decided it would be too expensive to retool the plant. A new company was started by some of the employees from each of the former two companies. The new manufacturing plant with new equipment produced a much better quality product. The two original companies sued the new one for breaking confidentiality rules that the ex-employees had signed with them, and the new company went out of business. Many years passed before the newer, better, bite-size egg rolls came back into the market.

A more recent development involving extrusion technology was undertaken at the University of Missouri by the research group led by Dr. Fu-Hung Hsieh. His team created a soy-based chicken substitute over a several-year period using the extruder to impart the precise layering and structure necessary to simulate the fibrous texture associated with real chicken meat. Seldom does the public see the dramatic impact of university research, but Dr. Hsieh's development was adopted by a commercial manufacturer and has been featured by the Institute of Food Technologists in one of their "Day in the Life of a Food Scientist" videos (http://www.ift.org/dayinthelife). A picture of the commercially manufactured strips is shown in Insert 8.2.

New technologies can also be introduced in the home. An important trend in the past 40 years has been to reduce meal preparation time. What used to take hours now takes minutes. In the 1950s, the TV dinner was a convenient item that took 45 minutes to prepare. The quality of the food was poor, but it was reasonably priced and required little effort. However, consumers wanted even more convenience, and they wanted it right away. In the 1970s, the microwave oven revolutionized the way Americans prepare meals and

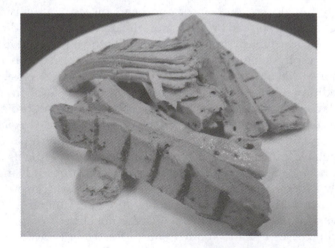

INSERT 8.2
A sample of the soy-based chicken substitute developed at the University of Missouri in its commercial form. (Photo courtesy of Andrew Clarke.)

how developers design new products. New packaging was needed and was designed to meet this requirement, and the food products were designed to meet the needs and wants of consumers. Initially, the quality of microwave products and packaging was as poor as their TV-dinner predecessors, but now, premium quality products can be produced by experienced preparers.

Innovation can also be inspired by a new type of packaging. An overlooked health food on the market, liquid milk, is not as popular as it once was. For consumers not getting enough calcium, more milk can be desirable. New products that contain reduced lactose, reduced fat, improved flavor, and richer texture of skim milk have helped it hang on despite competition from rice, soy, and other milk products. Traditional milk packages don't fit very well with today's lifestyle. They have been redesigned to open and pour more easily, which is particularly important to elderly consumers. Milk chugs are designed to fit into vehicle cup holders and are primarily marketed at one-stop gas stations as an option for students to replace colas and other sugared beverages.

Traditional foreign dishes provide new products in new environments. Good old American meals (meat, potatoes, two vegetables, and dessert) were eaten by almost all Americans in the 1950s and 1960s. Now, "pasta" and catchy-sounding foreign names are the primary products available in low-calorie, flavorful, microwavable entrées in the frozen food section of the supermarket. Pizza and yogurt entered the United States because American soldiers returning from the World Wars created a demand. Both products have become so Americanized in the intervening years that Americans in Europe are frequently disappointed with Italian pizza and French yogurt.

8.6 Reality Check

Not all new product ideas are practical, and not all product concepts are feasible. Marketing may come to Research and Development (R&D) indicating that they want a fresh broccoli, zucchini, bean, and pasta product with no preservatives, full flavor, and a shelf life of 75 days under refrigerated storage. By now, we know that this idea is not practical. It becomes the task of R&D to either design the product or let Marketing know the constraints and provide an alternative product that meets some, but not all, of the guidelines.

Food scientists must understand the capabilities and limitations of ingredients, processes, and distribution when designing new products. They rely on their technical training in chemistry, microbiology, processing, engineering, nutrition, sensory science, packaging, and quality control to modify an existing product or develop a new one. Usually, this effort, led by a food scientist, is conducted by a research team that contains members with a wide range of skills including marketing. Product developers must be particularly concerned about ingredient interactions and limitations, sensory quality, product safety, process constraints, shelf stability, and economics.

Sometimes, an idea sounds good, even to a food scientist, but it just doesn't work out. At other times, experienced food scientists can anticipate many of these problems and solve some of them through knowledge of the functionality of ingredients and processing techniques. They can also identify technical problems that are not likely to be solved and develop alternative solutions that meet some, if not all, of the desired characteristics. This approach was used in the development of the soy-based chicken substitute as overcoming the oxidation of soy lipids and replicating the meaty texture of chicken were significant hurdles in developing the product.

Ingredients have many limitations, but a developer with a good knowledge of different ingredients can usually find one that will perform the function needed. When substituting low-calorie sweeteners for sugar or replacing fats, sometimes a blend is needed to produce the desired effect. College students seem to be very sensitive to some low-calorie sweeteners, and many reject any product containing them. It is very difficult to develop a fat-free product that delivers both flavor and mouthfeel, but food scientists have become very good at producing high-quality products with much of the fat removed.

Many dieters would do well to find the low-fat, low-sugar alternatives that combine low calories with good sensory characteristics. Of course, there are some components that cannot be changed. For example, Jennifer's 1-calorie beer is technically impossible because ethanol (drinking alcohol) contains 7 calories per gram. To remove the calories, we must first remove the alcohol. Jennifer may be drinking beer for its flavor, but others may be looking for something else. No-alcohol malt beverages that taste like beer are available, but they are not very popular. Even these beverages have some calories, however, because they contain carbohydrates.

Product developers must be very sensitive to the quality of the product. Remember that quality doesn't have to be synonymous with perfection. It is more important that products meet or exceed consumer expectations. Developers would like to use the finest of ingredients for each product, but they must take into consideration the cost. As stated previously, they may develop the finest of products in the laboratory, but conventional processing, storage, and distribution can lead to loss of quality. Other factors must be considered. For example, with microwavable syrup, developers must consider how repeated heating and cooling will affect flavor, color and viscosity.

Product developers must always be concerned with safety. As we have learned, a properly canned product is about as safe a product as we can eat. Contrary to popular opinion, fresh foods are more likely to be unsafe than processed ones. Consumers demand foods with full, fresh flavor, and food scientists want to deliver. When a newer, fresher product is designed, the product developer must build safety measures into the process, package design, distribution and storage strategy, and preparation instructions to ensure that the product will be safe to eat under normal conditions. For

> When I was working for an egg-roll company mentioned previously in the chapter, my boss had a great idea that we would develop a ham-and-egg-roll, the same outside but ham and eggs on the inside. We worked on our formulation, using the freshest of ingredients, and these egg-rolls were great! I took one of our early versions around to the front office, and everybody loved them. Then my boss suggested that I do cost estimation based on the best price we could obtain for the ingredients. The cost of ingredients alone was greater than what we would be able to charge for the product. We started looking for less expensive ingredients, and we found them. We developed a formulation that was reasonable cost-wise. Then we produced our modified version. They were terrible! News of the disaster spread faster than I could move from office to office. No matter how hard we tried we couldn't get a decent flavored product for a reasonable cost. In the food industry many other great ideas meet a similar fate. —Rob Shewfelt

INSERT 8.3
Economic constraints associated with product development—a personal account.

perishable products, the food scientist also wants to make sure that the product will spoil before it becomes unsafe to eat.

Process constraints are another factor a developer must consider when designing new products. For example, any heat process, even mild heat treatments like blanching and pasteurization, can diminish flavor and nutritional quality. Trade-offs must be anticipated, and the developer or development team must consider all aspects from production to consumption in its design. The fewer changes needed to existing equipment, conditions, or operations, the greater the chance the company will adopt the product for production.

Distribution constraints also limit the development process. A product must reach the consumer at an acceptable level of quality or it will not last long in the marketplace.

Developers must test their new inventions under standard market conditions. Tests evaluating the quality changes of a refrigerated product at 35°F will not give the food scientist a clue as to how it will behave in supermarkets stored at 45°F–50°F. Shelf-life studies are critical in determining its likely success or failure in the marketplace. The Sales Department frequently wants a longer shelf life than is realistic or necessary. It is important to determine realistic shelf-life requirements and the necessary trade-offs to meet these requirements. Food scientists must also consider economic constraints as described in Insert 8.3.

8.7 Food Formulation

As we learned in Chapter 5, formulated foods involve mixtures of ingredients. Most of the food products many of us eat daily are formulated. Among the key responsibilities of product developers is to know and understand the function of each ingredient in a product and how the ingredients interact with each other. They also need to understand what ingredients are essential, what ingredients can be replaced, and what potential effects ingredient substitution will have on quality, nutrition, stability, and safety of that product. Some ingredients have their own identity and cannot be replaced without changing the product. Pistachios are critical components in pistachio ice cream just as strawberries are in strawberry jam. Others such as starches and gums vary widely in their functional properties. For a frozen custard pie, we might wish to use carrageenan for freeze–thaw stability. To maintain the thickness of a salad dressing at room and refrigerated temperatures, we could use carboxymethylcellulose.

Product matches are something that developers are asked to perform. The boss brings in a sample of a competitor's product her mother bought in the supermarket over the weekend and wonders why our company can't make as good a product. The ingredient statement on the label provides a place to start looking. Some ingredients, like citric acid, are easy to match, while others, like natural flavors, are obscure and part of trade secrets. Once we have a list of potential ingredients, we must start guessing at the levels of the ingredients. Most developers have a reasonable clue as to how much is needed from personal experience. An attempt at duplication may not produce a similar product if production details are unknown. Usually, the first new product on the market will be the market leader if it meets the expectations of consumers. Copycat products tend to be successful only if they come attached to a well-known brand that has loyal followers, have a noticeably lower price, or possess a clearly superior quality.

Knowledge of the functional properties of ingredients separates the good developers from the superior ones. Functional properties affect not only the flavor, color, and texture of a product but also its convenience, nutritional quality, safety, and stability. Formulations of some of our favorite products today started out as old family recipes. While some of these recipes remain intact, most require major changes in ingredients to become commercially viable. As we have seen, freshly prepared products are not likely to maintain their quality during conventional processing, distribution, and storage. A home recipe might not withstand freezing and thawing if it is produced as a frozen product. Fresh-squeezed juice blends will not retain their delicate flavors upon pasteurization to keep them safe. The cost of typical ingredients may be too high to produce a product that enough consumers are willing to purchase at a price necessary to generate a profit.

In developing a new formulation, the food scientist must determine which ingredients to use and how much. If it is a line extension or minor modification, the basic formulation is already determined and ingredients are substituted. It may be as simple as substituting papayas for strawberries in an ice cream product line, but most development projects are not as simple as they might seem. There may be ingredient interactions with the papayas we did not experience with the strawberries. An equivalent amount of papaya we used may be too overpowering or may be too weak. Papayas may give a strange color that would repel the consumer or the color may change from highly desirable to unacceptable during processing, handling, or storage. Papayas may become sticky and gooey in the product, resulting in a nauseating texture in the mouth. The nutritional level for selected nutrients may change greatly, resulting in a major modification of the product label. The microbial safety of papaya pureé may not be as good as that for strawberries requiring a more rigorous heat treatment. Changes in processing may lengthen the time of production, thus increasing the cost of the product and lowering nutritional and sensory properties. All of these factors and more must be considered by the developer for a seemingly simple change.

Another consideration that a product developer must make is the order of the addition of ingredients. It is not just as simple as adding them in the order as they appear on the ingredient statement. Anyone who has baked a cake knows that we can't dump all the flour into all the water and expect them to mix properly. In candy making, certain ingredients must be mixed in carefully to get them to distribute properly. Texture is the sensory property most often affected when ingredients are not added in the right order.

One factor that developers of low-fat and sugar-free products must consider is how to make up for the loss of fat or sugar. Assuming that a good sensory match can be made with the sugared, fat-filled product, the developer still has a problem. All sugar substitutes and many fat replacers are required at much lower levels than the ingredients they are replacing.

Consumers looking for low-calorie substitutes are not likely to be amused when given less product for the same price. Bulking agents must then be added to provide the same serving size at a lower-calorie level, and most of the time, these agents perform their function well. Sometimes, the consumer just eats a larger quantity, consuming as many calories as they would have had with the original product. Occasionally, overconsumption of bulking agents can lead to excess gas production and other evidence of gastric distress. In the case of reduced-fat almond butter, the fat replacer also has calories and the reduced-fat version actually has the same calories as the full-fat product (see Insert 8.4).

Initial product formulations are produced in a laboratory to achieve the desired sensory characteristics. The time it takes to develop a new formulation depends on the technical skill of the developer, differences in the new formulation from existing ones, and difficulties posed in modification. A successful formulation is called a **prototype**, which can then be evaluated for processing effects.

8.8 Process Operations

Even if the formulation is perfect, and the ingredients are added in the right order, the product still may encounter problems during processing.

Full Fat Almond Butter		
Nutrition		
Facts		
Serving Size		32g
Servings Per Container		16
Amount Per Serving		
Calories 190	Calories from fat 130	
		% Daily Value
Total fat 16g		25%
Saturated Fat 3g		16%
Trans Fat 0g		0%
Cholesterol 0mg		0%
Sodium 150mg		6%
Total Carbohydrate 7g		2%
Dietary Fiber 2g		9%
Sugars 3g		
Protein 8g		
Niacin 20%	● Riboflavin	2%
Vitamin E 10%	● Iron	4%

Reduced Fat Almond Butter		
Nutrition		
Facts		
Serving Size		36g
Servings Per Container		14
Amount Per Serving		
Calories 190	Calories from fat 110	
		% Daily Value
Total fat 12g		18%
Saturated Fat 2.5g		12%
Trans Fat 0g		0%
Cholesterol 0mg		0%
Sodium 250mg		10%
Total Carbohydrate 15g		5%
Dietary Fiber 2g		9%
Sugars 4g		
Protein 8g		
Vitamin B$_6$ 6%	● Folic acid	6%
Niacin 25%	● Iron	4%
Copper 10%	● Zinc	6%
Magnesium 15%	●	

INSERT 8.4
Nutritional labels for two types of almond butter.

The product developer must anticipate the potential effects of each step in the manufacturing process. Many of the processes that protect a food from spoilage rob it of its freshness and diminish its quality. Other preservation processes, such as fermentation and roasting, develop characteristics that enhance its acceptability. Heat can produce desirable browning, aromas, and textures, but it can also destroy delicate flavors and nutrients. Oxygen that is incorporated into the product speeds up reactions that generally decrease desirable characteristics, but air can provide light fluffy textures in bread and ice cream. Product developers work closely with process developers to make sure that the correct process is matched to the new product.

Process developers design new processes or modify existing ones, much like product developers. Process developers must have a strong understanding of engineering concepts. They must know the effects of each unit operation on microbial activity, ingredient functionality, ingredient interaction, and product quality. In completely new processes, the process developer or development team may design entirely new pieces of equipment to achieve the desired result. More frequently, they are interested in the order of operations and the specific conditions, such as time and temperature, for each operation using existing equipment. Process developers don't go straight to the manufacturing plant to test their ideas. The equipment in the manufacturing plant is too big, and the time it takes to run process development experiments is too valuable. A process developer uses a pilot plant, consisting of miniaturized pieces of equipment that mimic nonideal conditions that, unlike in the laboratory, occur in the manufacturing plant, to optimize process operations.

Products from a pilot plant are much more realistic than those made in the laboratory. The process developer can evaluate different orders and conditions of operations in a set of experiments. As in product formulation, the length of time to develop an optimal process for a new product depends on the technical skill of the process developer. Any modification in ingredients or time and temperature of the process can lead to unanticipated difficulties. The product and process developers must work closely together to ensure that the desired texture, color, and flavor are obtained. See Insert 8.5 for a schematic of the overall development of a new product.

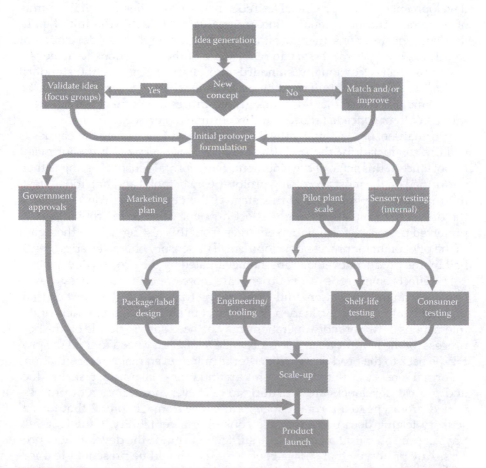

INSERT 8.5
Schematic of product and process development. (Diagram composed by Carlos Margaria.)

Even minor modifications in a process can have major implications in the microbiology and nutrition of a product. One result of a slight decrease in temperature in an operation could be inadequate killing of microbes, which then contributes to premature spoilage or, worse yet, a safety hazard. Heat and light also destroy vitamins, such that use of too much heat to ensure safety can lead to lower nutritional quality.

8.9 Quality Evaluation

Early in product and process development, a standard or specification for the product should be developed. Standards and specifications help guide the development of a new product. Desired sensory properties, acceptable limits of microbes, and nutritional value are evaluated. Usually, the initial standard and specifications are high and difficult to accomplish. As development continues, it may be necessary to relax some of the restrictions to achieve a viable product. Occasionally, standards are raised. Each time the standard is relaxed, a determination must be made as to whether to proceed with the new standard, reformulate or redesign the process to more closely achieve initial goals, or concede failure and discontinue the project.

Informal sensory testing by the developer and a few trusted colleagues is usually conducted for the initial formulations. Sensory quality is of major importance at this stage of development. More formal sensory testing is then performed on the most promising prototypes. Microbial and nutritional testing may also be performed at this stage if the developer is concerned that the differing formulations might affect nutrient value or microbial load. A preferred prototype formulation emerges from this testing, which then goes to the pilot plant for process development. The sensory characteristics identified by the product developer are then evaluated by the process developer.

The effects on microbes and nutrients are more important in process development than in formulation. Initial processing trials look at the effect on final product quality. Close evaluation of the effect of individual operations or the interactions of two or more operations may be necessary to decide on the best process for the new product. The process developer may need to send the prototype back to the product developer for minor or even major reformulation.

Formal sensory evaluation is a complex and time-consuming task. Product and process developers are unwilling to take every formulation or process-varied prototype to a formal panel. Remember from Chapter 7 that formal sensory testing does not guarantee consumer acceptability. Usually, a few physical and chemical measures are sufficient to guide the development process. Any prototype that shows good promise should be presented to a formal panel to make sure that it is in line with standards. In some tests such as product matching, the competitor's product may serve as a "gold standard" or the best possible product to be achieved. A gold standard can be very useful, but it can also eliminate formulations and process-tested prototypes that are superior. Storage stability is also a factor that must be considered when comparing our newly developed product to a gold standard.

8.10 Storage Stability

A superior formulation and process scheme does not guarantee success for our product. We must appreciate the effects of handling and storage on the quality of our best prototype. For example, the cookies on the end of a manufacturing line have much more fresh-cooked flavor than the same cookies in a vending machine. In a product match of a competitor's product, we should assume that a purchased item is not as good as it was when first manufactured. Shelf-life testing is necessary to determine if a new product meets minimum requirements, establish an expiration date, and assess the quality of the product under conditions likely to be seen by the consumer.

The same types of physical, chemical, sensory, microbial, and nutritional tests used to evaluate initial formulations and processing prototypes are also used in shelf-life testing. During shelf-life testing, it is necessary to understand which characteristics deteriorate most rapidly and thus limit product stability. Changes do not occur at the same rate. At least three temperatures are studied during shelf-life tests. One of those temperatures should be the most likely storage temperature. During testing, higher temperatures are used to accelerate quality losses testing to provide a quicker, but sometimes less accurate, estimate of shelf life.

8.11 Package Development

As a product is being developed, so is a compatible package. This task can be simple if it is a line extension or complex if it is a truly new product. In a large company, a packaging engineer will be on the development team, while in a smaller company, one person may serve as product developer, process developer, and packaging engineer. A packaging engineer from the company that supplies packaging materials to the company developing the product may also be involved in package development. Among other things, the package must contain the product, protect the product, provide important information to the consumer, and sell the product. The packaging engineer is responsible for choosing the right packaging materials, making sure the package and the product are compatible and that the package serves all of the technical requirements of the new product, as described in Chapters 4 through 6.

Before selecting the material and designing a new package, we should list the functions a package must serve. In addition to protecting the product from contamination, the package must also keep moisture, odors, and gases in and oxygen, odors, light, and water out. Permeability is the property of a package that selectively permits certain substances to cross the package barrier. Selection of the appropriate packaging material must also consider its effect on the environment as will be discussed in Chapter 9.

Graphics sell food products, and a great product will never be successful if it doesn't sell. A graphic artist may be part of the development team to design an appropriate label to merge the technical side of the product with the marketing campaign. Obviously, bright colors will help the product stand out but may not be appropriate for a staple product such as rice or beans. Package graphics must also be sensitive to the cultural impact of certain colors. In the United States, white stands for purity and black stands for death. Thus, we may see many white and few black food packages. In other countries, different meanings are attached to these colors; hence, package graphics may need modification for these markets.

In many cases, the package may serve in food preparation or consumption. Enclosed plastic utensils, easy-to-open caps, the ability to place a beverage container in a standard cup holder, and spill-proof containers for coffee all provide the convenience so attractive to students on the run. Innovations for microwave cooking include a metal sheet that helps brown our pizza or the syrup bottle that can provide hot syrup for waffles or pancakes. The packaging in use for the soy-based chicken substitute combines a deep plastic tray

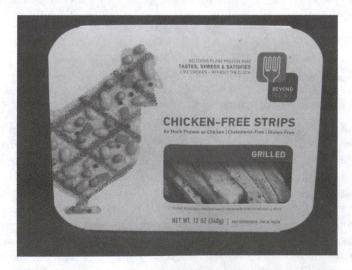

INSERT 8.6
Commercial packaging for a soy-based chicken substitute. (Photo courtesy of Andrew Clarke.)
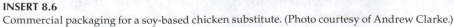

with flexible film to preserve a modified atmosphere around the product, which is then placed in a fiberboard sleeve with all the required labeling information (Insert 8.6).

8.12 Package Labels

Consumer information present on the label must include Nutritional Facts, product weight or size, and the ingredient statement. Contact information, such as the address of the manufacturer or distributor, a toll-free phone number, a website address, and marketing information (such as how to get a scary spider ring, T-shirt, or other valuable stuff) must also be included on the label. If a product requires special storage conditions or further preparation, there are generally specific instructions. For large products, package labels are not a problem; however, on small products, the label can easily become cluttered or the lettering can become so small that nobody over the age of 40 can read it.

Comprehensive nutritional analysis is needed for the Nutrition Facts. Larger companies have the facilities to routinely perform nutritional, formulation, and sensory tests on prototypes for the development team. Smaller companies may not have a good idea of the nutrient content of the product until late in the development process as such analyses can be very expensive. Strict rules govern which nutrients must be tested and what claims can be made for a particular product. Since the nutrients on the label are listed in relation to the serving size, it is important that the appropriate serving size be determined. Some serving sizes are tricky. Many beverage containers, usually consumed whole, may actually contain two or more servings.

Examples of nutritional labels for several foods are found in Chapter 3. As in other aspects of product development, it is not sufficient to perform nutrient analysis only on the freshly manufactured product. Rather, we must understand that the nutrients may change during handling, storage, and distribution. Generally speaking, the more rigorous the preservation technique (like canning), the more nutrients are lost during processing and the more stable they are during handling and storage. Over time, losses can also occur by interaction of nutrients with other components in the product or the package.

The ingredient statement is a very important, often ignored, part of the label. Much of this chapter emphasizes the importance of understanding the properties of ingredients in developing new products, processes, and packages. The statement warns allergic consumers about ingredients that may cause a reaction. It also alerts careful readers to unwanted preservatives or other chemical-sounding ingredients. Ingredient statements can provide useful clues to developers, making product matches as described earlier in the chapter. As stated in Chapter 2, the ingredients must be stated in order of quantity added with the first being present at the highest amount. Simple products may have few ingredients while others, like beef stew, may have many ingredients that have ingredients of their own (designated in parentheses). What can and cannot appear on a label and how it is displayed is under strict governmental regulation. See the labels shown in this and previous chapters for examples.

8.13 Scale-Up and Consumer Testing

Earlier in the chapter, we discussed how a promising formulation developed in a laboratory becomes a prototype. The prototype is then used to develop the processing technique in a pilot plant. After the process has been developed, some reformulation may be necessary to help match the product and the process. Consumer testing is then needed to assess consumer acceptability of the best prototype. If a competitor's product is in the market, our product may be tested against it. If it is a "new and improved" product, it may be tested against the existing product. If it is a completely new product, it may be tested on its own. At this point, marketing or brand information are kept secret to determine the reaction of consumers to the product's sensory characteristics rather than its image characteristics.

Some pilot plants are large enough to provide adequate material for a limited consumer test. Other tests may require more product than can be made in a small pilot plant, leading to a limited run in the regular processing plant. Scaling up a product from the pilot plant to the manufacturing plant is not as easy as it might seem. Mixing and heat-transfer operations are particularly difficult to scale up. While 2–10 pounds of a product might be produced at a laboratory bench and 50–200 pounds in a typical pilot plant, many manufacturing plants can produce tons of products in an hour. It may take hundreds of pounds of ingredients just to get a piece of equipment running effectively enough to produce useful samples and then hours to clean the equipment after the test run before resuming production of the regular product. See a pilot-scale retort for processing pouches in Insert 8.7.

What works easily in the pilot plant with careful controls may not work as well in the manufacturing plant. Thus, scaling-up runs must be carefully planned by the development team in conjunction with Plant Production. Frequently, these batches are done at the end of a normal production run before shutting down the operation for cleaning. Important lessons can be learned from running a test batch in a manufacturing plant. A complete microbiological, sensory, and nutritional analysis and shelf-life study should be conducted on the product from this batch. The results might suggest reformulation or modification of process conditions before a full market test.

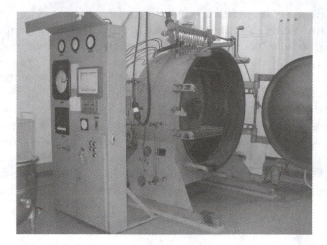

INSERT 8.7
Retort for sterilization of packaged foods used in producing canned foods in flexible pouches such as those used for Meals Ready to Eat for the military and disaster relief. (Photo courtesy of Katherine Herndon.)

8.14 Market Testing

At some point in the development process, a marketing plan for the new product is developed. A product name is selected and a target market is identified. Advertising themes and venues along with promotional materials are considered. Merchandising efforts and product placement are determined. Focus groups are employed to test these marketing concepts. If some of the prototype is available, it might even be presented at the end of the session to get consumer reaction. Collaboration between Marketing and Development is necessary to match the product to the marketing campaign (e.g., the sensory and image characteristics).

Market testing begins when the best formulation has been prepared using the best process and the best package has been matched to the best marketing scheme. Control of the new product then passes from the R&D Department to the Marketing Department. Consumer sessions, usually an intercept method at a shopping mall, are used to determine whether the marketing plan is reaching the right target market and if the product is acceptable. Image characteristics are more closely evaluated at this point than sensory characteristics. These tests are closely monitored. The results may suggest a need for modifications in the market campaign, package design, or product formulation. Major modifications may require backtracking to an earlier stage in development and repeating many steps. Complete rejection of the product or its marketing campaign by consumers may lead to its discontinuation. Minor modifications are feasible without further consumer testing.

Items from one or more full production run(s) are selected for a major market test. Many members of the development team will be present during the initial run(s) to help troubleshoot and be prepared for minor modifications. A certain region of the marketing territory is selected to present consumers with the new product in a typical setting. With full promotional effort, a fast-food chain will offer the new product for sale in small, medium, and large markets. A packaged food will be sold in a supermarket, possibly being promoted by someone offering free, prepared samples to passing shoppers. On the basis of market test results, an economic analysis is done to determine the probability of success. Full acceptance here sends the product to its launch. Problems with the economic analysis could lead to either further development or discontinuation. Many products disappear because of poor acceptance during market testing.

8.15 Product Launch

A new product faces many go, modify, or no-go steps along the way. To make it to the launch, a product must have passed the challenges of concept generation, formulation, process design, package design, scale-up, consumer testing, and market testing. Careful coordination is needed at this point to ensure that the product launch is successful. The news media is contacted to gain free publicity to enhance the marketing effort. All members of the development and marketing teams collectively hold their breath hoping that the launch is successful. Probably, at no other point in the product's life will it receive more attention and advertising. This time is make-or-break for the product. Some follow-up testing is done to track its performance. On rare occasions, modifications may be made after the launch.

8.16 Success or Failure

The first few weeks after launch are critical to the product's success. Marketers know that regardless of the marketing campaign, not everyone will try a new product. One consumer classification is the early adopter. These consumers, like Ignacio in Chapter 3, are usually the first in their neighborhood to try something new. Their opinion is influential as they pass on their judgment to friends. If the early adopter recommends it, then every time a friend is reminded of the product, the temptation to try it will increase. If the early adopter complains, the friend is unlikely to be tempted. As the second wave of friends make their personal judgments, the product will take off, build steadily, or die. Milestones are set up to see if the product is meeting company expectations.

The most important measure of product success is how much money it makes for the company. Investment costs of a nationally released product are such that it may take 1 to 1 1/2 years to break even. Sales projections are made as part of the economic analysis to see if the product is outperforming or underperforming expectations. Serious underperformance could result in withdrawal of the product. With this many chances to fail, it is not difficult to understand why so few products are successful.

Some products are very successful early, and it may be difficult to produce enough to meet market demand. Inability to meet market demand can do serious damage to the success of a product when frustrated consumers finally give up trying to find it on the shelves. Examples of dramatic increases in new product demand are when catfish was introduced into a fast-food chain in the southeastern United States and when colorless colas were introduced nationally. Possible reasons for unexpected early demand include that the new product represents an unfulfilled consumer want or need or that it is seen as a novelty that becomes a fad. Fast-food catfish apparently met an unfulfilled need in southern consumers, but the colorless colas represented a novelty that turned into a fad, which faded as quickly as it started.

The goal of every developer is for the product to have long-term success with worldwide recognition and be a money-maker for the company for several years. Such products exist, but for every one of these, there are many that appear in the market for a short time only to fade away and many more that never even enter the marketplace. Some of the successful products may cycle back to the original developer(s) or their successor(s) for consideration of a "new and improved" version or a line extension. Product and process development can be a very rewarding and challenging job for a creative person with strong technical training. Jobs always seem to be available for successful product developers.

8.17 Remember This!

- The most important measure of product success is how much money it makes for the company.
- The packaging engineer is responsible for choosing the right material(s), making sure that the package and product are compatible and ensuring that the package serves all of technical requirements of the new product.
- Shelf-life testing is necessary to determine if the new product meets minimum requirements, establish an expiration date, and assess

the quality of the product under conditions likely to be seen by the consumer.

- A process developer uses a pilot plant, consisting of miniaturized pieces of equipment that mimic nonideal conditions that, unlike in the laboratory, occur in the manufacturing plant, to optimize process operations.

- The ingredients must be stated in order of quantity added with the first being present at the highest amount.

- In developing a new formulation, the food scientist must determine which ingredients to use and how much.

- Food scientists must understand the capabilities and limitations of ingredients, processes, and distribution when designing new products.

- A developer must diligently keep products current with changing times while simultaneously not making changes that will cause the loss of loyal customers.

- Product line extensions are defined as changes in a product feature, such as flavor, content, size, name, or packaging.

- Creativity is important in designing a product or process that results in something many consumers will enjoy eating and come back for more.

8.18 Looking Ahead

This chapter introduced us to how food scientists develop new products and processes. Chapter 9 discusses sustainability of food products and packaging materials. In Chapter 10, we will learn about the role of food scientists in developing and enforcing regulations as well as in research. In the final five chapters, the fundamentals of food science will be presented from the chemistry to nutrition, microbiology, engineering, and sensory science.

Testing Comprehension

1. Develop a concept for a food product that is not currently available in the marketplace. Identify its most important quality characteristics. How would these characteristics be measured?

2. Outline the steps needed to develop the product selected in the previous question. Prepare a tentative ingredients statement. Does this

statement represent a clean label? Why or why not? What difficulties would we anticipate in trying to achieve a clean label for this product?

3. Describe the greatest opportunities and challenges associated with developing the product described in the previous questions. How could the challenges be overcome? How could the opportunities be exploited?

4. Diagram the unit operations necessary to produce the product selected in the first question. Identify any CCPs associated with this process. What is the primary preservation principle for this product? What would be the greatest safety concern for the product?

5. Compare and contrast the effort associated with line extensions and brand new products. Is the product selected in the previous questions a line extension or a brand new product? Outline a marketing plan for this product.

6. Describe the opportunities and challenges of developing a gluten-free product. List three products that would be relatively easy to develop as gluten-free and three that would be most difficult. Compare and contrast the sensory and hidden quality characteristics of these products. What are the primary reasons for the degree of difficulty in developing gluten-free products?

7. Select a line of beverages or flavor enhancers currently available in the market that feature at least five flavors. Identify five new flavors that could be extended to this line. Outline the steps a developer would need to take to extend this line to these new flavors. Anticipate any difficulties that could arise in developing these new flavors. Assume three of the new flavors make it through the development process and are ready to be launched. Which three current flavors should be discontinued to make way on the supermarket shelves for the new ones? What problems might occur if these flavors were replaced?

8. Identify three strategies developers of formulated foods for restaurants could take to lower the chances for the development of obesity in America. Rank in order the likelihood of success for these strategies from most likely to least likely and provide the rationale for the ranking. What contributions can restaurants make to lessen the obesity epidemic? What limitations do they have with respect to the epidemic?

9. Identify a package of a current food product that is not as good as it could be. Why is it not satisfactory? List all the functions that this package should have. Redesign this package. How is the redesigned package better than the current one? What problems could result from the redesigned package? What can be done to minimize these problems?

10. In substituting papaya for strawberry into an ice-cream line, a developer finds that there is a difference in sugar content and expense of the two fruit pureés. Papaya pureé has 60% more sugar than strawberry pureé, strawberry costs 20% less than papaya, and cane sugar is 15% of the cost of strawberry pureé. The pureé provides 4 g of the 14 g of sugar per half-cup serving of the strawberry ice cream. Calculate how many grams of sugar from the papaya pureé should be in each serving to maintain the same amount of sugar per serving and the same cost of ingredients. What other challenges could this ingredient substitution present to the developer?

Further Reading

Brody, A. L. and J. B. Lord, 2007. *Developing New Products for a Changing Marketplace*, 2nd ed., Boca Raton, FL: CRC Press, Taylor & Francis Group.

Carpenter, R. P., D. H. Lyon and T. A. Hasdell, 2013. *Guidelines for Sensory Analysis in Food Product Development and Quality Control*, New York: Springer.

D'Antonio, M., 2006. *Hershey: Milton Hershey's Extraordinary Life of Wealth, Empire and Utopian Dreams*, New York: Simon & Schuster.

Fuller, G. W., 2013. *New Food Product Development: From Concept to Marketplace*, 3rd ed., Boca Raton, FL: CRC Press, Taylor & Francis Group.

Nachay, K., 2014. Six ingredient trends shaping product development. *Food Technol.*, 68(9):16.

Sloan, A. E., 2014. What's bubbling up in beverages. *Food Technol.*, 68(9):17.

9

Sustainability and Distribution

Kyle does not buy all of this environmental activism. It sounds more like political correctness to him. He eats what he wants to eat and thinks all this talk about saving the world is a bunch of garbage. We'll always have what we want to eat available in the good old US of A.

Tiana is very concerned about the environment and the daily impact we are making on the healthiness of the globe. She bikes to school every day, has a hybrid car to get good fuel mileage, and eliminates unnecessary trips. She avoids as much food packaging as she possibly can by throwing fresh produce directly into her shopping cart, bringing her own clean containers to hold granola and nuts that are scooped out of bulk bins, and filling her own canvas bags to fill and carry out her groceries. She goes to farmer's markets when she can and prefers buying organic and local foods when available.

Nil has not been so concerned about the environment, but he learned in his biology classes that we are consuming the earth's resources at an alarming rate. They did an exercise in class that indicated we would run out of oil before he was his parent's current age! He has always been cautious with his money and thinks that maybe he should be more cautious about the resources he uses. He is learning about sustainability and that what looks environmentally responsible is not always as good as it appears. He wonders how food scientists can make foods more sustainable.

9.1 Looking Back

Previous chapters focused on food issues we deal with daily, the types of foods we eat, and the primary occupations of food scientists. Some key points that were covered in those chapters help prepare us for understanding the challenges that the food industry faces in sustainability and distribution:

- As food production becomes more mechanized and less personal, it is necessary to develop ways of making sure that each product is of good quality.
- Fresh fruits and vegetables deteriorate rapidly as they decay, die, and exude fluids.

- Expedited handling of fresh foods minimizes safety concerns and loss of quality.
- In selecting the ingredients for a formulation, the food scientist must consider the quality of the food, its safety, its stability, and its cost.
- A clean label is one that has only clearly recognizable ingredients, none of which sound like chemicals.
- The main function of a package is to preserve the physical and chemical integrity of a product including preventing microbial or chemical contamination.
- Food processing and preservation increase the shelf stability of a raw material usually at the cost of nutrition and quality.
- Although many of us try to eat healthy, there are many temptations and influences affecting our decisions that we do not consciously consider.
- Organic food production minimizes the input of fossil fuels and synthetic chemicals.
- Pests represent the greatest threat to availability of food, worldwide.

We are living in a world that is growing in population and using natural resources faster than we are able to sustain them. Throughout history, most people have assumed that these resources were limitless. Thomas Malthus, a clergyman in England, proclaimed in 1791 that the geometric growth of population would eventually outstrip the linear growth of food production, bringing on worldwide famine. Since then, pessimists have predicted global doom, and optimists have relied on technological innovation to head it off. Despite famines and plagues in places around the world brought on by both natural and man-made causes, advances of technology have been able to avoid the cataclysm Malthus forecast. Technology, however, has increased the appetites of an ever-growing population to consume a dwindling supply of natural resources. The ability to put us on the path to sustaining world resources may be the greatest challenge facing the generation of college students today.

9.2 Sustainability

Sustainability, like quality, is a term that is used widely and means many things to many people. We will use the definition of sustainability as "meeting the needs of the present" without compromising the ability of future generations to meet their needs" (http://lct.jrc.ec.europa.eu/glossary). For food, we must consider everything that happens from the time the field is tilled or an animal is born to the food and packaging waste is collected and recycled, treated, or buried. It is becoming more apparent that we should think beyond our personal desires to consider the needs of those who will inherit the earth after us. A sustainable food then is one "designed, manufactured, and sourced under process guidelines, based on the efficient use of natural resources, the minimization of all kinds of waste, and the reduction of negative impact in surrounding communities along their life cycle" (http://www .sustainabilityconsortium.org/glossary/). Animal welfare and social justice are also included in the sustainability philosophy.

The world population is currently more than 7 billion and is expected to grow to more than 9 billion by the year 2050. By that time, we will need to be able to produce at least 1.5 times the food we currently produce to adequately feed the additional population. At the same time, fertile land for food crops is being lost to competition with bioenergy crops, flooding, global climate change, topsoil depletion, urbanization, and other poor land-use practices. The quest for more land to produce more crops leads to deforestation and contributes to even greater concerns about global climate change.

Many solutions have been proposed, but critics of the "industrial food system" have branded advanced technology with its reliance on too much energy and destruction of our natural resource base as the problem. These critics appear to be advocating a major reduction of agricultural and food technology back to what was available 50–100 years ago. It is difficult to see how less technology will be able to produce the massive amounts of food that we will need to feed the rapidly growing world population. Continuation of current technological practices without modification to become much more sustainable is also unrealistic.

What appears to be best for sustainability is not always the best for the environment. For example, the concept of food miles was introduced to demonstrate how far a food had to travel from harvest to consumption. When studying the environmental footprint of a product, however, transportation rarely makes the most significant impact. For example, it is more energy efficient to raise sheep in New Zealand and ship the meat to England than to raise and process them in England. Thus, it is more important to study the life cycle of a food and where the most effective changes can be made.

There are 14 environmental impact categories that can be assessed in a life-cycle analysis as shown in Insert 9.1. Most life-cycle analyses focus on climate change, **eutrophication** (accumulation of nutrients in water to deplete oxygen or in soil to decrease plant fertility), resource depletion (including waste), and water depletion. Waste prevention is critical in sustaining our planet, and it becomes more critical the later the waste occurs in the life cycle as the inputs accumulate at each point in the cycle.

In ensuring a sustainable future, not only must we consider our impact on resources, energy use, water, soil, and air, we also need to pay attention to the welfare of humans and animals. We should be working to ensure that all humans have access to food and a living wage under safe working

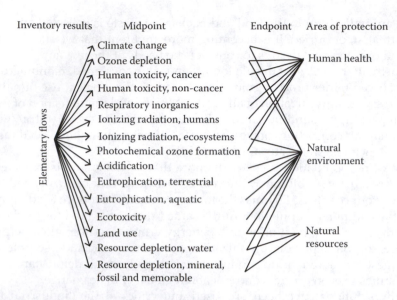

Inventory results   Midpoint   Endpoint   Area of protection

Climate change
Ozone depletion   Human health
Human toxicity, cancer
Human toxicity, non-cancer
Respiratory inorganics
Ionizing radiation, humans
Ionizing radiation, ecosystems
Photochemical ozone formation   Natural
Acidification   environment
Eutrophication, terrestrial
Eutrophication, aquatic
Ecotoxicity
Land use   Natural
Resource depletion, water   resources
Resource depletion, mineral,
fossil and memorable

Elementary flows

INSERT 9.1
Environmental impact categories that can be evaluated during a life-cycle analysis of a food product. (From Hauschild, M.Z. et al., *International Journal of Life Cycle Assessment* 18: 683, 2013. With permission.)

conditions. As resources become scarce, food becomes more expensive and more people will become hungry. The philosophy of sustainability also includes humane treatment of farm animals and protection of habitat for wild animals. Pollution of air and water should be minimized, and a virtuous cycle of recovery and regeneration of resources must be developed. All of these goals must be achieved economically as a business that fails to consistently generate a profit will eventually become a failed business.

The challenges are daunting, but the future of mankind depends on clear solutions. This book takes the position that it is only through effective use of technology and free-market capitalization that we can succeed. Before we look at sustainability from the farm or ocean to the consumer, we need to discuss the topics of distribution and the supply chain.

9.3 Distribution

Distribution involves everything that happens to a product from the time it is produced until it reaches the consumer. The goal of distribution is to deliver a product to the consumer in a reasonable time in acceptable quality with an adequate amount of shelf life remaining. Understanding the complete distribution system is critical in maintaining quality and reducing waste from the manufacturing plant to the consumer. To monitor potential problems, many producers use a **systems approach** to distribution—looking at how individual operations interact within the overall context of the system rather than focusing on specific steps. The shelf stability of the product determines the conditions of handling during distribution. Although perishable and shelf-stable products have similar distribution steps, refrigeration is of little consequence to stable products, but it is critical for maintaining the quality of perishable and semiperishable foods.

Chilled foods enter a cold chain in the processing plant, which is maintained through distribution until purchased by the consumer. These conditions can be met by backing a refrigerated truck up to enclosed bays in refrigerated warehouses and using electric forklifts to move pallet loads rapidly from truck to storage room. For example, fresh lettuce may be packed into pallet bins in the field, vacuum cooled, transported across the country in a refrigerated truck, unloaded, prewashed, treated with chlorine, washed, cut, spun dry, packaged, and palletized. It is then loaded on a truck, transported to a wholesale warehouse, unloaded, divided into smaller segments, loaded into a smaller truck, transported to a supermarket, unloaded, stored, and then moved to a display unit for consumer purchase. Cross-docking eliminates the need to warehouse products by taking them off the truck from the processor and immediately loading them onto the outbound truck headed to the retailer. During its trip from field to the consumer, lettuce should be held at 4°C or lower.

It is even more critical to maintain refrigerated temperatures in fresh meats as elevated temperatures can promote growth of pathogenic microbes. Other chilled items should be kept in a cold chain as well. Frozen foods are also perishable. They must be kept at temperatures below freezing as thawing will lead to major losses of quality and potential food safety problems. A large truck can be subdivided into zones that separate refrigerated, frozen, and shelf-stable foods. To maintain energy efficiency, trucks backhaul goods to the point of origin as an empty truck is wasting fuel. Whatever is backhauled, however, must not be a source of contamination for future loads of food.

Shelf-stable foods are generally those that can be stored at room temperature for more than a month. Many canned foods are stable for years because they are essentially sterile. Chips, other salted snacks, and some candies will develop off-flavors if not sold and consumed in time. Some companies package their products in nitrogen to reduce oxidation of the oils during handling and storage. Expiration or best-if-consumed-by dates are placed on items to help the consumer finish the product before noticeable quality changes are detected. Inventory management involves techniques to properly rotate stock. **FIFO** (First-In, First-Out) is the most common means to ensure that products don't lose their shelf life before they are sold. Fresh breads and other baked goods are susceptible to staling and development of mold. They are typically held at room temperature, but they must be transported to market and rotated on the shelves to allow sale before becoming spoiled. Breads with mold inhibitors have a longer shelf life but may become stale. A few minutes of heating can restore some of the lost flavor.

Careful monitoring of temperatures during distribution, sampling product at retail, and removing items at or near the expiration date to ensure that consumers get fresh products are ways that a company can maintain quality during distribution. Supermarkets must be careful that the amount of a specific item ordered closely matches the amount of that item sold. If sales exceed orders over a period, the supermarket will run out of it, angering its customers. If orders exceed sales, the storage rooms will fill up and the product on the shelves will become older over time. Donation of expired products or deteriorating fresh produce to food banks for distribution to consumers with low incomes is one way of preventing waste. Some processors sell damaged items that are still edible and safe at a company store at deep discounts to prevent waste.

Manufacturing plants also need to be concerned about treatment of the wastes that they produce. Some waste can be utilized in the manufacture of by-products, which may be produced at that plant or shipped to another location for further processing. For example, chicken feet, considered a delicacy in some Asian countries, are shipped from US poultry companies overseas. If waste cannot be converted to another usable product, it must be treated according to local, state, and federal regulations before being released to the environment.

9.4 Supply Chains

Not only must a food company be concerned about manufacturing and distribution, it must also be concerned about the resources it uses. Supply chains involve everything used in the plant from equipment to raw materials to ingredients to packaging materials to energy and water use and even to its workers. Suppliers are companies who provide goods or services to help produce a product. Sourcing is the act of finding suppliers and making sure that they are meeting company specifications. A congressman once asked our college dean how many companies it took to make a loaf of bread. A former student helped provide a realistic answer—at least 13 companies (see Insert 9.2).

Although processing and laboratory equipment are only purchased once, the supplier must be able to provide technical assistance when a piece is not working correctly, spare parts, timely upgrades, and anything else associated with its safe and effective operation. Raw materials are generally perishable and must be either shipped quickly to the manufacturing plant or

Baker—1

Flour—2

    Company that mills the flour

    Company that sells the flour company the enrichment

Water—1 (excluding the companies that sell the chemicals to treat the water)

Yeast—4

    Company that sells the yeast

    Farmer that produces the sugar cane

    Processor that converts the sugar cane to molasses

    Company that supplies the yeast nutrient

Salt—1 (miner)

Sugar—2

    Farmer that produces the sugar cane

    Processor that converts the sugar cane to sugar

Shortening—2 (soy)

    Farmer that grows the soybeans

    Processor that converts the soybeans to soy oil

That makes 13 companies for a very basic formulation and does not take into account any packaging companies, shipping companies, electrical companies, secondary water companies for the ingredients or any of the companies that the intermediate ingredient companies may need to use. The actual total of companies used to produce a loaf of bread would be much greater.

INSERT 9.2

How many companies does it take to make a loaf of bread?

kept under proper handling, storage, and transport conditions. Most companies that have fruits, vegetables, milk, or meat as raw materials have field departments that interact directly with the farmer and other companies or individuals within the supply chain.

Ingredients can be either perishable or stable and should be handled, stored, and transported appropriately. If they are coming from different suppliers, FIFO may not always be the best policy as an ingredient shipped from one company may come to the manufacturing plant last but may have been produced earlier. Fully formed packages such as cans and glass jars or bottles may come to the processing plant ready to be filled and capped. The materials for plastic jugs for milk and water are usually shipped to the plant where they are formed by special blow-mold machines shortly before filling.

Other suppliers that must be considered are sources of water and energy. County and municipal agencies are generally responsible for supplying water and electricity. Treatment of incoming water may be a necessary task if it does not meet product specifications. Generation of plant power may also be handled by the company if it can be produced more efficiently and economically. Anything that can be done within the processing plant to reduce water use or energy consumption without compromising product safety and quality can be beneficial to both the environment and the bottom line.

9.5 Sustainability Systems from Farm to Consumer

If food companies are able to meet the needs of the estimated 9 billion people on earth in 2050, they will need to implement changes through the supply chain, in the manufacturing plant, and during distribution. Earlier in the chapter, we mentioned pessimists who believe that we are doomed unless we break out of the industrial food system. Optimists tend to believe that every modern problem can be solved by innovative technology. The remainder of the chapter will follow food from the farm through the processing plant on into distribution and eventually to the consumer. Changes are being made by many companies at every stage of handling, processing, storage, and distribution, but many more changes will be needed to make the food system more sustainable.

Many companies rely on terms such as *eco-friendly, fair-trade, fresh, green, local, low energy, natural,* and *organic* to communicate sustainability in their products. It is becoming clear that some practices may improve sustainability in one way but impede it in another. For example, reducing fertilizer and pesticide inputs in the field prevents water pollution through runoff but may lead to lower yields in the field and increased waste during harvest and distribution. More advanced companies are moving away from these labels to basing decisions on outcomes—the most benefit for the least input—and working on developing a sustainability index. It will be a challenge to develop a useful index that accurately reflects the true environmental impact of a product, is easily understood, and will be accepted by the consumer. Concerted efforts are being made to turn the supply chain into a value chain such that all members are adding value and improving sustainability through the chain.

The remainder of the chapter will take a systems approach based on the idea that the whole is greater than the sum of its parts. It will follow items through the life cycle, to evaluate the sustainability of a product. Processors and retailers that are big enough are in the position to set specifications for raw materials, ingredients, and finished products, rewarding suppliers for meeting specific goals and penalizing those who do not. For example, Whole Foods Market favors organic products with clean labels. McDonald's has established standards for animal welfare and packaging materials. BASF has conducted more than 500 life-cycle analyses for food products and other consumer goods to maximize resource utilization and minimize waste.

9.5.1 Life-Cycle Analysis

A life-cycle analysis can identify hotspots or points in a system where improvements can be made in agricultural production, the supply chain, processing, distribution, retail operations, and with the ultimate consumer

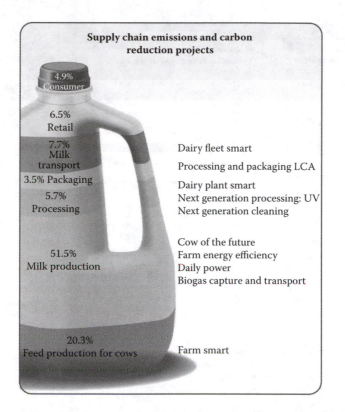

Supply chain emissions and carbon reduction projects

4.9% Consumer

6.5% Retail

7.7% Milk transport

3.5% Packaging

5.7% Processing

51.5% Milk production

20.3% Feed production for cows

Dairy fleet smart
Processing and packaging LCA

Dairy plant smart
Next generation processing: UV
Next generation cleaning

Cow of the future
Farm energy efficiency
Daily power
Biogas capture and transport

Farm smart

INSERT 9.3
Carbon footprint for a gallon of liquid milk produced in the United States as contributed to by the various stages in the supply chain, processing, and distribution. (From Miller, G.D. and Wang, Y., eds., *International Dairy Journal* 31(Supplement 1): S1, 2013. Provided by the Innovation Center for U.S. Dairy.)

to make a product more sustainable. Insert 9.3 shows the carbon footprint for liquid milk in the United States. With a life-cycle analysis, we can look at ways to reduce fertilizer and pesticide use without significant losses in crop yield and spoilage during handling and storage. Exploring ways to conserve water in the field and the processing plant must not compromise quality and safety of an item during distribution and in the home or at a restaurant. Life-cycle analysis is also used to determine how effective one type of process can be over another. For example, is it more energy efficient despite the high energy input to sterilize a canned vegetable than to keep its fresh counterpart in the cold chain, which requires refrigeration and is more likely to result in waste from field to consumer?

The life cycle of white wine is shown in Insert 9.4. The life-cycle analysis of carbonated beverages revealed that more than half of the environmental impact was attributed to packaging. The 2-liter plastic container provided the best solution for packaging over metal cans and glass bottles. Washing

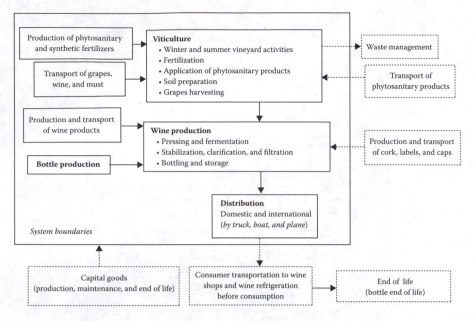

INSERT 9.4

A life-cycle diagram of Portuguese white wine. The dashed lines indicate that these steps were not analyzed in the study. (From Neto, B. et al., *International Journal of Life Cycle Assessment* 18: 590, 2013. With permission.)

and reusing glass bottles would reduce the carbon footprint, but greater recycling of plastic bottles would be even more beneficial than the reuse of glass.

9.5.2 Fieldprints

Since crop production for food and animal feed is a major factor in environmental impact, the field is a primary focus of attention and opportunity for improving sustainability. A major hotspot in many areas around the world for growing corn is the availability of water, particularly in southern Africa, the northeastern Mediterranean region of Europe, and southeastern South America.

A Fieldprint Calculator (http://www.fieldtomarket.org/) has been developed by The Keystone Center to help American farmers adopt more sustainable practices with respect to energy use, greenhouse gas emissions, irrigation water use, land use, soil carbon, and soil loss. By providing confidential information into the calculator, farmers can compare their performance to growers in their county, state, or nation. Competition between farmers can then lead to new ideas and overall benefit. An example of a fieldprint for a corn grower is shown in Insert 9.5. The field-to-market program lets environmental factors such as reducing carbon and water footprints

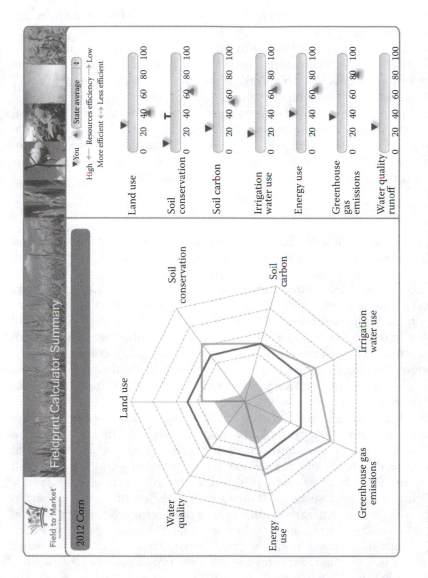

INSERT 9.5

Fieldprint of a corn field (shaded area) compared to state (gray line) and national (black line). (Prepared for use in this book by The Keystone Center, 1628 Sts. John Road, http://www.keystone.org. For additional information on fieldprint calculators, go to http://www.fieldtomarket.com.)

identify management changes rather than dictating specific practices that farmers must follow.

9.5.3 The Value Chain

Sourcing within a supply chain typically finds the least expensive raw material, ingredient, or service that results in minimally acceptable quality or safety. Value chains are developed to set higher standards for quality and safety with clear specifications that must be met by suppliers. Regional value chains are being developed for fresh items that combine the resources of many small farmers to compete with larger corporate farms. These value chains must be able to provide a consistent supply of an item within a local distribution system. Assessment of the life cycle for margarine indicates that the selection of the vegetable oils is the hotspot. If a regional chain can provide a more sustainable oil and be more responsive to the needs of the margarine processor, it will be selected over a national chain.

9.5.4 Processing Efficiency

In the processing plant, the focus has generally been directed at water and energy conservation. Any savings in water or energy use also provide savings in production costs. Reducing the amount of packaging used can also reduce costs. Selection of ingredients that are more sustainable may or may not lead to cost savings. Every change to processing or formulation of a finished product must be assessed for its effect on safety and quality. A slight decrease in quality may be acceptable for a significant increase in sustainability, but safety must not be compromised. Responsible companies must also view the effect of the process on sustainability during distribution. Higher energy use in a processing plant to increase shelf life of a product and thus reduce waste may be beneficial.

A very interesting study by Pardo and Zufia looked at the most energy-efficient way to process a precooked dish of fish and vegetables. They compared the sustainability of four processing techniques: two processes that required heat—steam and microwave pasteurization—and two that did not require heat—high-pressure pasteurization and modified atmosphere packaging. The most sustainable process for a shelf-life requirement of less than 30 days was modified atmosphere packaging even when packaging waste was considered. Both techniques that required heat contributed more to global warming than the processes without heat. Lower water requirements were also found for the nonheat processes over the heating processes. While there are ways to improve sustainability of processes requiring heat, it is likely that many of these processes will eventually be replaced by more sustainable techniques as new processing plants are built.

9.5.5 Sustainability of Packaging Materials

The most visible part of the waste stream for food products is the food package. Many food packages are disposable and end up in the landfill after use. Appropriate packaging materials for foods include glass, metal, fiberboard, paper, and plastics. Each material has its advantages and disadvantages. Glass containers hold a product nicely and prevent leakage of liquids and gases in or out of the product. Unfortunately, glass is heavy, which increases energy consumption and shipping costs, and makes a mess when broken. Metal provides a nice barrier for liquids and gases but will not break under normal conditions. Most metal containers, particularly those for traditionally canned foods, are heavy. Some product ingredients such as acids can interact with the metal. These containers require an enamel coating to protect the can. In-home carbonation such as the device shown in Insert 9.6 has been proposed as an alternative to the packaging for carbonated beverages.

Fiberboard is usually used for secondary containers. Fiberboard is strong, flexible, and, for the most part, recyclable, but it is susceptible to water damage and can collapse if placed under too great a load. Waxed fiberboard cartons provide protection from water damage, particularly with fresh fruits and vegetables, but waxed fiberboard is not recyclable. Paper and cardboard are relatively inexpensive and very good for displaying graphics, but they

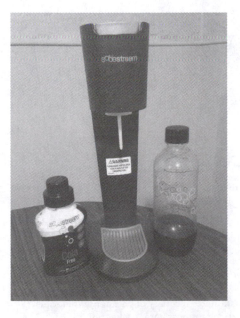

INSERT 9.6
SodaStream Source home carbonation machine. (Photo courtesy of Christine Gianella.)

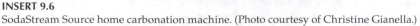

are not effective at keeping out gases or liquids and are easily penetrated by insects, pets, and vermin.

Plastics provide a wide variety of characteristics that can range from flexible to rigid, permeable to impermeable, clear to opaque, reactive with ingredients to inert, and graphic-friendly to graphic-hostile. Plastics have become the most widely used packaging material. A packaging engineer understands the properties of each type of plastic and selects the most appropriate material or blend of materials at the appropriate thickness to meet all packaging requirements. Plastic containers can be recycled, but many recycling

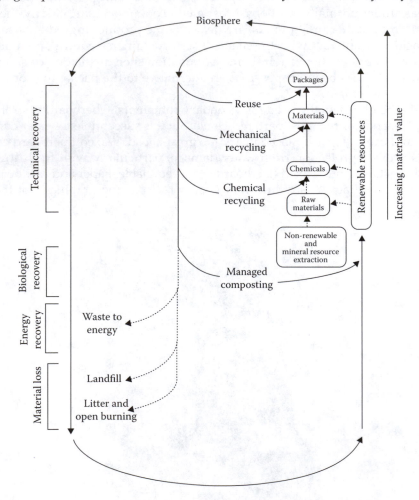

INSERT 9.7
Potential for a more sustainable recovery of packaging materials. (From Sand, C.K., Packaging sustainability for modified atmosphere packaging of fruits and vegetables. In *Modified Atmosphere Packaging for Fresh-cut Fruits and Vegetables,* Brody, A.L., Zhuang, H., and Han, J.H., eds. Hoboken NJ: Wiley-Blackwell, 2011, Chapter 15. Copyright Wiley-VCH Verlag GmbH & Co. KGaA. Reproduced with permission.)

stations are not set up to handle recycled plastic containers other than those for carbonated beverages, liquid milk, and water. More sophisticated containers frequently feature mixtures of plastics that are not readily recyclable.

Everyone understands that recycling is part of sustainability, but many of us forget that the three arrows in the familiar symbol represent REDUCE–REUSE–RECYCLE. Using recyclable packaging materials is one way to improve sustainability, but that is not always possible or desirable. **Source reduction**, using less total packaging material, is sometimes more important. The calculation must include the probability that a single item such as a glass jar or metal can be recycled by the ultimate user, how much the weight of the container will contribute to energy usage in transport, and how much the total amount of the packaging can be reduced. Any change in the selection of a package must consider safety, quality, and cost. It used to be that beverage cans were heavy and strong, but the industry went to a much thinner aluminum can requiring much less metal, which becomes susceptible to leaking if handled roughly.

The main benefit of food packaging with respect to sustainability is extending shelf life and thus reducing food waste. The primary problem with food packaging with respect to sustainability is the material that is discarded after use. Food companies are looking at ways to reduce packaging waste through biodegradable materials, composting, downcycling, recycling, and resource reduction as shown in Insert 9.7.

9.5.6 Distributor Sustainability

To improve sustainability during distribution, companies should transport fresh foods as directly as possible to minimize loading and unloading. Energy efficiency is needed during transportation and warehousing. **Cross-docking**, **backhauling**, and divided loads are all techniques that cut energy costs during transport, handling, and storage. Rapid turnover of stock, primarily using FIFO inventory management, helps ensure that a product gets to the consumer with sufficient shelf life to prevent waste. Truckers and other distributors need to make sure that products are stacked together properly and that proper storage conditions are maintained to prevent spoilage or damage that will result in more food waste.

9.5.7 Quality at Retail

When we think of retail outlets, we usually think of a supermarket, but we buy food at ballparks, co-ops, concert venues, gas stations, hospitals, restaurants, and numerous other sites. Retail outlets use large amounts of energy to store, display, and merchandise products. Generally, the more control the retail outlet is able to maintain, the more energy efficient it becomes and the less waste is generated. Supermarkets use the term *shrink* to describe the amount of product that is wasted from the time it enters the store to the time

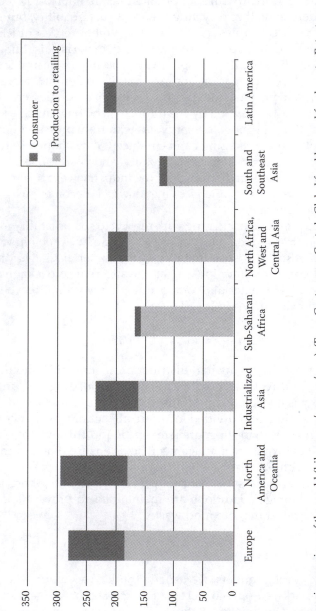

INSERT 9.8

Food losses in various regions of the world (kilograms/person/year). (From Gustavsson, C. et al., Global food loss and food waste: Extent, causes and prevention. Study conducted for International Congress SAVE FOOD! Interpack 2011, Dusseldorf, Germany. FAO, United Nations. With permission.)

it leaves as a purchased product. A life-cycle analysis of restaurants traced the greatest vulnerability to the raw materials and ingredients it buys, which suggests that sourcing and paying attention to the value chain are critical in maintaining sustainability for restaurant chains.

9.5.8 Consumer Responsibility

The end of the line for sustainability is not at the point of purchase. Note that, in Insert 9.3, almost 5% of the total carbon footprint for liquid milk is traced to the consumer. Factors that can affect the sustainability of the products we buy include

- The number of trips to a certain retail outlet
- The amount of food that was bought each trip
- Purchase of the proper size to minimize both excess packaging and food waste
- Proper transport, handling, and storage of the food from purchase to consumption to prevent waste
- Willingness to recycle or properly dispose of packages

Studies suggest that the greatest source of food waste in developing countries is immediately after harvest. Loss of perishable products after purchase by the consumer is the greatest source of food waste in affluent countries as shown in Insert 9.8. Note that, in North America, almost 300 kilograms (660 pounds) of food are wasted per person per year, with more than 250 pounds of that wasted directly by the consumer after purchase. We must remember that all resource, air, soil, water, energy, human, and animal inputs have gone into any product we purchase and that anything wasted by the consumer has a much greater environmental impact than waste incurred earlier in the value chain.

9.6 A Sustainability Index

Sustainability is in everyone's interest from us as ultimate consumers back to the producers of our foods. As consumers and other players in the value chain, we need *actionable information* to make intelligent decisions on what to purchase in order to improve sustainability. If terms like *organic, natural, low energy, local, green, fresh, fair-trade,* and *eco-friendly* are not sufficient in and of themselves to let us know what practices are and are not sustainable, what can we do?

Some major organizations including CARE, the Environmental Protection Agency, the Natural Resources Defense Council, the Nature Conservancy, and the World Wildlife Fund have teamed up with major companies including Coca Cola, Mars, MillerCoors, PepsiCo, Stonyfield Farm Organic, and Walmart to form the Sustainability Consortium (http://www.sustainability consortium.org/). This consortium is working on ways to encourage the use of life-cycle analyses and a systems approach to truly address problems in sustainability by valid measurement and reporting to have a direct, positive impact in our lives and on the environment. The consortium is also developing a sustainability index that will provide farmers, suppliers, processors, distributors, and consumers a tool to evaluate how well a product contributes to a better world.

Companies can be evaluated for their commitment to sustainability by the Dow Jones Sustainability Index. Such measures are difficult to develop and verify, but our future depends on our ability to evaluate the situation, support companies that strive to conserve resources and reduce their environmental footprint, and work toward constantly improving sustainability of life on earth. Food companies are more likely to adopt more sustainable practices if the sustainable practice

- Actually reduces overall costs of the product
- Increases overall costs but allows them to produce the product at a competitive selling price
- Entices enough loyal consumers because of their social responsibility

Sustainability goes beyond food products we consume to everything we do from the clothes we wear to the trips we take to the electronic devices we depend upon. As part of the global community, we all have a responsibility to the earth and its inhabitants. Numerous ideas have been floated from integrated cropping systems to high-rise vertical farms in cities. We all need to become part of the solution rather than contributing further to the problem.

9.7 Remember This!

- Sustainability goes beyond food products we consume to everything we do from the clothes we wear to the trips we take to the electronic devices we depend upon.
- To improve sustainability during distribution, companies should transport fresh foods as directly as possible to minimize loading and unloading.
- The most visible part of the waste stream for food product is the food package.

- The field-to-market program is to let environmental outcomes such as carbon and water footprints identify management changes rather than identifying standard practices to conserve resources or reduce waste.
- A life-cycle analysis can identify hotspots or points in the systems where improvements can be made in agricultural production, the supply chain, processing, distribution, retail operations, and with the ultimate consumer to make a product more sustainable.
- Supply chains involve everything used in the plant from equipment to raw materials to ingredients to packaging materials to energy and water outputs and even to its workers.
- Distribution is everything that happens to a product from the time it is produced to the consumer.
- Waste prevention is critical in sustaining our planet, and it becomes more critical the later the waste occurs in the life cycle as the inputs accumulate at each point in the cycle.
- The ability to put us on the path to sustaining world resources may be the greatest challenge facing the generation of college students today.
- We are living in a world that is growing in population and using natural resources faster than we are able to sustain them.

9.8 Looking Ahead

This chapter introduced the concepts of sustainability, the supply chain, and distribution. Chapter 10 will describe regulations that the food industry must follow and the future direction of research in food science. The final five chapters will go into the more fundamental aspects of food research.

Testing Comprehension

1. Outline the relationship between agriculture and the environment. List the steps that growers of crops, producers of animals for meat, and fish farmers can take to reduce their impact on the environment.
2. Compare and contrast the perspective of the authors of the book with those of the food industry, the federal government, the organic movement, and environmental organizations on sustainability. Rank these perspectives from most to least rational. Explain.

3. Describe the effect of storage temperature on spoilage of pasteurized milk. Why does milk spoil so quickly when held at room temperature? Identify ways that food scientists could extend the shelf life of milk. Organic milk generally has a much longer shelf life than other types of liquid milk. What are some possible reasons for the difference?

4. Analyze the strengths and weaknesses of a life-cycle analysis of a food product. Identify factors in the growth, harvest, processing, and distribution of foods that could lead to human toxicity. Describe any potential trade-offs between sustainability and food safety.

5. Describe and analyze the obligations of the farmer, supplier, processor, distributor, retailer, and the consumer in contributing to a more sustainable environment.

6. Select a food product and describe its primary, secondary, and tertiary packages. Enumerate the functions and analyze the sustainability of each of these packages. Which functions could be sacrificed to enhance the sustainability of its packages?

7. Compare and contrast the advantages and disadvantages of integrated cropping systems, vertical farms, and other ideas with respect to sustainability in the food system.

8. Diagram the life cycle of beer, identify potential hotspots, and construct a more sustainable value chain.

9. Calculate the number of tons of food waste that could be saved if consumers in the United States could practice sustainability as well as those in South and Southeast Asia. What are some reasons that Americans are not as environmentally responsible as those who live in these Asian countries?

10. Compare and contrast the effects of food packaging and food waste on sustainability. Which of these two things represents the greatest problem? What can be done to make food packaging more sustainable? How can we reduce food waste?

References

Gustavsson, J., C. Cederberg, U. Sonesson, R. Van Otterdijk and A. Meybeck, 2011. Global food loss and food waste: Extent, causes and prevention. Study conducted for International Congress SAVE FOOD! Interpack 2011, Dusseldorf, Germany: FAO, United Nations.

Hauschild, M. Z., M. Goedkoop, J. Guinee, R. Heijungs, M. Huijbregts, O. Jolliet, M. Margni et al., 2013. Identifying best existing practice for characterization modeling in life cycle impact assessment. *Int. J. Life Cycle Ass.*, 18:683.

Miller, G. D. and Y. Wang, Eds., 2013. Carbon and water footprint of U.S. milk, from farm to table, Special Issue. *Int. Dairy J.*, 31(Suppl. 1):S1.

Neto, B., A. C. Dias and M. Machado, 2013. Life cycle assessment of the supply chain of a Portuguese wine: From viticulture to distribution. *Int. J. Life Cycle Ass.*, 18:590.

Pardo, G. and J. Zufia, 2012. Life cycle assessment of food-preservation technologies. *J. Clean. Prod.*, 28:198.

Sand, C. K., 2011. Packaging sustainability for modified atmosphere packaging of fruits and vegetables, in *Modified Atmosphere Packaging for Fresh-Cut Fruits and Vegetables*, A. L. Brody, H. Zhuang, and J. H. Han, Eds., Hoboken, NJ: Wiley-Blackwell.

Further Reading

Amienyo, D., H. Gujba, H. Stichnothe and A. Azapagic, 2013. Life cycle environmental impacts of carbonated soft drinks. *Int. J. Life Cycle Ass.*, 18:77.

Baldwin, C., N. Wilberforce and A. Kapur, 2011. Restaurant and food service life cycle assessment and development of a sustainability standard. *Int. J. Life Cycle Ass.*, 16:40.

Boye, J. I. and Y. Arcand, 2012. *Green Technologies in Food Production and Processing*, New York: Springer.

Despommier, D., 2010. *The Vertical Farm: Feeding the World in the 21st Century*, New York: Thomas Dunne Books.

Florkowski, W. J., R. L. Shewfelt, B. Brueckner and S. E. Prussia, Eds., 2014. *Postharvest Handling: A Systems Approach*, 3rd ed., New York: Academic Press, Elsevier.

Fraser, E. D. G., E. Simelton, M. Termansen, S. N. Gosling and A. South, 2013. "Vulnerability hotspots": Integrating socio-economic and hydrological models to identify where cereal production may decline in the future due to climate change induced drought. *Agric. Forest Meteorol.*, 170:195.

Gonzalez-Garcia, S., E. G. Castanheira, A. C. Dias and A. Arroja, 2013. Using life cycle assessment methodology to assess UHT milk production in Portugal. *Sci. Total Environ.*, 442:225.

Mackey, J. and R. Sisodia, 2013. *Conscious Capitalism: Liberating the Heroic Spirit of Business*. Boston: Harvard Business Review Press.

McWilliams, J. E., 2009. *Just Food: Where Locavores Get It Wrong and How We Can Truly Eat Responsibly*, New York: Little Brown and Company.

Milài Canals, L., G. Rigarlsford and S. Sim, 2013. Land use impact assessment of margarine. *Int. J. Life Cycle Ass.*, 18:1265.

Parfitt, J., M. Barthel and S. Macnaughton, 2010. Food waste within supply chains: Quantification and potential for change to 2050. *Philos. Trans. R. Soc. B*, 365:3065.

Population Reference Bureau, 2014. World Population Data Sheet. Available at http://www.prb.org/Publications/Datasheets/2014/2014-world-population-data-sheet/data-sheet.aspx.

Saunders, C., A. Barber and G. Taylor, 2006. Food miles—Comparative energy/emissions performance of New Zealand's agriculture industry. Lincoln University Research Report No. 285.

Sonesson, U., J. Berlin and F. Ziegler, Eds., 2010. *Environmental Assessment and Management in the Food Industry: Life Cycle Assessment and Related Approaches*, Philadelphia, PA: Woodhead Publishing.
Stuart, T., 2009. *Waste: Uncovering the Global Food Scandal*, New York: W.W. Norton & Co.

10

Government Regulation and Scientific Research

Angela E. Edge, Mark A. Harrison, and Robert L. Shewfelt

Selina is fortunate enough to have landed a summer internship with the Food Safety and Inspection Service (FSIS) of the United States Department of Agriculture (USDA). Every morning, she receives a shipment of raw chicken products, kept cool in sealed containers with dry ice, purchased from supermarkets in many parts of the country. Her job is to carefully record the purchase information and company names, perform routine sampling of the surface of the bird, and conduct testing for *Salmonella*. If *Salmonella* is detected and the frequency of positive samples from a particular company is out of tolerance, more sampling is done on products from that brand and source. Evidence of a continuing problem will result in a visit to the offending plant and a possible recall of product.

Malik's graduate research project focuses on folate deficiencies in women of child-bearing age. Folic acid, a B vitamin, is of vital importance in the proper development of the fetus in the womb. Since critical events in this development process can occur before a woman even knows that she is pregnant, folate supplements administered to deficient mothers during pregnancy may not be sufficient to prevent defects in the baby. He plans to use the new field of **nutrigenomics** to help understand genetic factors that affect differences in intestinal absorption of this vitamin by women consuming diets containing similar levels of folate.

Selina and Malik are food scientists in training who are learning some of the aspects of the profession. Although most food scientists work in the food industry, many are employed by regulatory agencies of the government or by universities conducting research. In this chapter, we will explore food science opportunities outside the food industry.

10.1 Looking Back

Previous chapters focused on food issues we deal with in our daily lives and with food products we encounter in the marketplace. The following are some key points that were covered in those chapters to help prepare us for understanding governmental regulation and research:

- Supply chains involve everything used in the plant from equipment to raw materials to ingredients to packaging materials to energy and water outputs and even to its workers.

- Waste prevention is critical in sustaining our planet, and it becomes more critical the later the waste occurs in the life cycle as the inputs accumulate at each point in the cycle.

- Food processors must be careful to prevent contamination, beginning with the raw materials and on through every unit operation, using sanitation as the key to preventing contamination.

- The Hazard Analysis and Critical Control Point (HACCP) system is a means of ensuring microbial safety of a product.

- Molecular gastronomy has been developed in Europe to merge food science with the culinary arts to better understand the chemical and physical changes that food materials undergo during cooking processes.

- Maintaining adequate refrigeration of perishable products like deli meats is necessary, and expiration dates should be strictly observed.

- A clean label is one that has only clearly recognizable ingredients that do not sound like chemicals.

- Food is preserved to make it safer by reducing or eliminating harmful microbes and to extend its shelf life by reducing or eliminating spoilage microorganisms.

- The Nutrition Facts part of the label indicates the serving size, how many servings per container, calories per serving, and the fat calories per serving.

- Many governmental agencies are responsible for monitoring the safety and quality of our food supply.

Most food scientists work in the food industry. They primarily work in quality management, product development, or process development, but there are many other functions they can perform. They may be involved in marketing, technical sales, manufacturing, regulatory issues, and packaging. Many food scientists work directly for manufacturers of food products, but others work for ingredient, packaging, and equipment suppliers. Other food scientists work for government agencies and universities. Many government agencies develop and enforce regulations to keep the food supply safe and prevent fraud. Both applied and basic research projects are conducted by food scientists in government, universities, the food industry, and trade organizations.

10.2 Governmental Regulation

Food laws and regulations vary widely from country to country around the world, as the ruling authorities operate under different principles to protect their citizens. This chapter will describe the regulatory environment in the United States because we are familiar with it and US regulatory practices have served as a basis for systems used in many countries around the world.

When a bill is passed by Congress and signed by the President, it becomes a law. Once a law is official, it is put into practice. Laws often do not include all the details needed to explain how an individual, business, state or local government, or others might follow the law. To make the laws work on a day-to-day level, Congress authorizes certain government agencies including the Food and Drug Administration (FDA), the USDA, and the Environmental Protection Agency (EPA) to create appropriate regulations.

Regulations carry the authority of a law and set specific requirements about what is legal and what is not. For example, a regulation issued by the FDA to implement the Federal Food, Drug, and Cosmetic Act (FFDCA) could explain what levels of a contaminant might pose a human health concern. It tells food manufacturers what specific level of a defined substance could be legally present in food and what the penalty will be if an excessive level is found. Once the regulations are in effect, regulatory agencies then work to help the industry and others comply with the law and to enforce it. A list of most of the acronyms used in this chapter is provided in Insert 10.1.

AMS	FSIS	HACCP
DSHEA	FSMA	HARPC
EPA	GAP	NLEA
FDA	GHP	SOP
FFDCA	GMP	SSOP
FQPA	GRAS	USDA

INSERT 10.1
Alphabet soup. Identify the acronyms with the regulatory agencies, governing laws, and programs established through regulation.

10.2.1 Food Safety

In the United States, FFDCA is the main law influencing the food industry. The law grants power to the FDA, to ensure the safety of our food supply. This agency carries out this task by implementing inspections of food manufacture operations, examining products within the marketplace, microbial testing, issuing licenses, and other controls. The FDA regulates a large spectrum of food products in interstate commerce excluding meat, poultry, and processed egg products, which belong under the jurisdiction of the USDA in most cases. The FDA has developed Good Manufacturing Practices (GMPs) that cover the proper operation of food manufacturing plants. GMPs target sanitary procedures, minimizing safety risks, maintaining microbiological standards, design of facilities, production controls, and proper handling of ingredients and raw materials.

During a plant inspection of a candy factory, for example, FDA inspectors look at the cleanliness and safety of the raw materials, the cleanliness and condition of molding trays, the condition of scrap candy, the proper use and levels of food additives, and appropriateness of food labels. These inspectors would collect samples of molding starch, scrap candy, and the finished product. They also would sample the finished products for misbranding, deceptive packaging, or filth and possibly dangerous items (glass, stones, or pins) that could find their way into the candy.

USDA's FSIS, under other food safety laws, is responsible for regulation of all meat and poultry products that are distributed in interstate commerce. Every carcass of poultry, pork, beef, and other edible animals is visually examined by a USDA-trained and certified inspector. No diseased animals are allowed to be processed or distributed for human food. All meat or poultry processing operations must have at least one certified inspector present any time product is handled and processed. While the inspectors are employed by the government, the meat processor must pay the USDA for the service. USDA/FSIS is also responsible for approving mandatory HACCP plans.

The intention of the FFDCA is to control aspects of food that could adversely affect the health of the consumer and prevent fraud by food companies. It has been amended and updated throughout its lifetime. The newest changes come from the implementation of the Food Safety Modernization Act (FSMA), the most sweeping reform of food safety laws in more than 70 years. FSMA aims to ensure that the US food supply is safe by shifting the focus from only responding to contamination to preventing it. FSMA allows the FDA to respond to and contain food safety problems when they arise. The law also directs the agency to ensure that imported foods follow the same standards as foods domestically produced. Most importantly for states, it directs the FDA to build an integrated national food safety system in partnership with state and local authorities.

Through its regulatory authority and extensive contracts with state and local food and health officials, the FDA is responsible for food safety in the country, with the exception of meat, poultry, and processed egg safety requirements, which are handled by USDA/FSIS. Thus, food under the jurisdiction of the

FDA should be an unadulterated product and should not be misbranded. The term **misbranding** under the FFDCA applies to false or misleading information, lack of required information, conspicuousness and readability of required information, misleading packaging, and improper packaging and labeling of color additives. Also, according to the FFDCA, a determination that labeling is "misleading" includes considering both what the label says and what it fails to reveal. Simply put, adulteration implies that the product is somehow corrupted and should not be offered for sale in the market.

Food additives are also a largely monitored aspect of food safety. Only additives that are approved by the FDA or are accepted through GRAS (Generally Recognized as Safe) approval are allowed in food. GRAS substances are shown through conducted studies to be safe and have also been reviewed by a panel of experts for acceptability and safety. Any substance that is not GRAS and is intentionally added to food is an approved food additive that has been subjected to a premarket review and approval by the FDA.

The USDA is governed under many laws including the Meat Inspection Act, Poultry Products Inspection Act, Egg Products Inspection Act, and US Grain Standards Act. It has regulatory control over different aspects of the food system such as meat, poultry, processed egg products, and raw agricultural commodities. The power of inspection has been given to USDA inspectors so that they can work to prevent adulterated or misbranded meat and poultry products from being sold as food. It also ensures that meat and poultry products are slaughtered and processed under sanitary conditions. These requirements also apply to imported meat products, which must be inspected under equivalent foreign standards.

The EPA is also a regulatory agency that plays a major role of ensuring food safety. The EPA regulates pesticide application and sets the limits for pesticide residues on foods through the Food Quality Protection Act and the Federal Insecticide, Fungicide, and Rodenticide Act. The EPA registers all pesticides that are used in the United States and determines the label requirements for each registered pesticide including application conditions on specific crops. Pesticides cannot be applied legally to unauthorized crops or under conditions other than those specified on the label without written consent from the EPA. A list of useful websites for regulatory agencies is shown in Insert 10.2.

Food and Drug Administration: http://www.fda.gov

United States Department of Agriculture: http://www.usda.gov

USDA Food Safety and Inspection Service: http://www.usda.gov/fsis

USDA Agricultural Marketing Service: http://www.usda.gov/ams

Environmental Protection Agency: http://www.epa.gov

Codex Alimentarius Commission: http://www.codexalimentarius.org/

INSERT 10.2
Useful websites for information on food regulatory agencies.

10.2.2 Preventive Control Programs

Preventive controls are put in place in order to anticipate food safety problems before they happen. They are risk based, which means they identify and address areas where the probability of an issue is the highest. Preventive control programs include reasonably appropriate procedures, practices, and processes to significantly minimize or prevent the hazards identified in hazard analysis.

To assist growers and food processors, regulatory bodies such as the FDA and USDA have created programs and procedures that are useful in attempting to prevent food safety problems. On farms and in fresh produce packing houses, preventive control programs such as Good Agricultural Practices (GAPs) and Good Handling Practices (GHPs) are commonplace. GAPs refer to farming methods that reduce the likelihood of contaminating produce, by implementation of practices that address water quality, manure and compost use, worker health and hygiene, and contamination from wildlife, domestic animals, and livestock. GHPs refer to postharvest handling of produce to minimize contamination. Practices include water quality, sanitation of the packing house, pest control programs, and sanitation of containers. Fruit and vegetable producers implement GAPs and GHPs to reduce the risk of microbial contamination that can cause consumer illness from consumption of contaminated fresh fruits and vegetables.

In food manufacturing plants, preventive control programs are used as well. Common ones include GMPs, Sanitation Standard Operating Procedures (SSOP), Standard Operating Procedures (SOP), HACCP, and Hazard Analysis and Risk-based Preventive Controls (HARPC). Current GMPs provide for systems that assure proper design, monitoring, and control of manufacturing processes and facilities.

GMP, SOP, and SSOP are prerequisite programs for HACCP. In order to have an HACCP program, a company must first complete those programs before an HACCP program may evolve. HACCP is a tool to assess hazards and establish control systems that focus on prevention rather than relying on end-product testing. HACCP programs are required in all meat, poultry, juice, and seafood processing operations in the United States. HARPC is a new term developed by the integration of FSMA. It requires facilities to maintain a written food safety plan and to keep records of preventive controls, monitoring, corrective actions, and verification. Only an individual qualified through either training or experience should develop the plan. All Preventive Control Programs are used to combat food-borne illness before occurrence.

10.2.3 Recalls

When preventive control programs fail and harmful microbes or other substances are introduced to the food system, recalls are issued. Recalls are typically voluntary actions by a company to send out a notice to consumers and distributors that a product they have manufactured and introduced into the market may be contaminated or mislabeled and should not be consumed. The FDA anticipates that its mandatory recall authority allowed under the FSMA will be used in rare instances, since companies will be provided with an opportunity for an informal hearing before an order to require recall is made and may opt to take the corrective action themselves.

For FDA-regulated foods, recalls are always a concerted effort between the agency, other regulatory bodies, and companies that are closely involved with the problem. Outside the FDA, the recall network includes the Centers for Disease Control and Prevention, the USDA, and food safety, agricultural, regulatory, public health, and laboratory professionals at state and local government agencies. State and local governments, in conjunction with public health, are often the first investigators of a complaint from a consumer.

When a problem has been identified as legitimate, then the FDA is contacted. The FDA is then charged with the responsibility of judging if an official recall is needed or if another action is required. A Class I recall is one where a clear danger to the public has been identified. For meat, poultry, and processed eggs, similar actions occur with the USDA being the lead federal agency. A Class II recall involves less serious health hazards, in which people may get sick but are expected to recover. Class III recalls involve a violation of agency rules, but the public is not endangered. Recalls frequently involve the presence of dangerous levels of pathogenic microorganisms, the presence of a toxin such as a cleaning fluid in a product, or the presence of a potent allergen like peanuts in a product not properly labeled. A picture of a product involved in a Class I recall is shown in Insert 10.3.

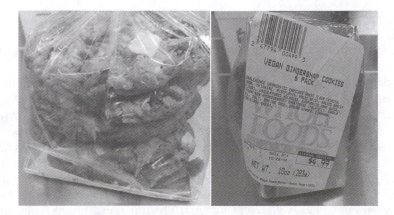

INSERT 10.3
Vegan gingersnap cookies involved in a voluntary Class I recall by the company from the only store in the chain because of failure to declare potential allergens such as egg, milk, soy, and tree nuts (almond and walnut).

10.2.4 Quality

Quality of a food has little to do with safety. Quality parameters are established to increase the value of the product. The USDA offers grading services through the Agricultural Marketing Service. Grading is not mandatory, but rather it serves as a marketing tool for manufacturers. USDA quality grade marks are usually seen on beef, lamb, chicken, turkey, butter, and eggs. For many other products, such as fresh and processed fruits and vegetables, the grade mark is not always visible on the retail product. In these commodities, the grading service is used by wholesalers, and the final retail packaging may not include the grade mark. Grade standards make business transactions easier whether they are local or made over long distances. Consumers, as well as those involved in the marketing of agricultural products, benefit from the greater efficiency permitted by the availability and application of standardized grade standards.

The grading branch of the USDA uses standards that have been researched at universities, developed within the USDA, and recognized by industry. For example, meat grading determines the quality and yield of carcasses. Quality grades vary depending on the animal species. USDA quality standards are based on measurable attributes that describe the value and utility of the product. For example, beef quality standards are based on attributes such as marbling (the amount of fat interspersed with lean meat), color, firmness, texture, and age of the animal, for each grade. Standards for each product describe the entire range of quality for a product, and the number of grades varies by commodity. There are eight grades for beef, and three each for chickens, eggs, and turkeys. On the other hand, there are 38 grades for cotton, and more than 312 fruit, vegetable, and specialty product standards.

10.2.5 Labeling

The information available on our FDA-regulated product label is regulated under the Nutrition Labeling and Education Act. Each label must have an ingredient statement; a net weight; an address of the processor, distributor, or importer; and the name of the product that can be clearly understood by the consumer. The address must be provided so that the FDA or the consumer can contact the company about a complaint or problem with the product. Ingredients are listed in descending order of the level in the product's formulation. They must be identified using a common name. When an ingredient in the product is composed of other ingredients, the other ingredients are enclosed in parentheses. Many products also have a processing date or expiration date. However, except for infant formula, expiration dates are not mandatory.

Most products require a statement of Nutrition Facts. There are very specific guidelines for the Nutrition Facts in a standardized format including permissible font sizes for different aspects. All nutritional information on the label is presented in the amount per serving. As this book is being written, changes in labeling regulations are being considered, which means that by the time this chapter is read, food labels may look different. USDA products are similarly labeled with some additional information such as cooking instructions and warning labels on the dangers of under-cooked meat and poultry, as well as the USDA inspection symbol that is mandatory.

Dietary supplements are regulated by the FDA under the Dietary Supplement Health and Education Act. Although producers of food additives must demonstrate the safety and **efficacy** (i.e., ability to perform the specific purpose for which it was added) of the additive, dietary supplements can be added without meeting safety and efficacy requirements. The FDA regulates claims of nutrient content and health benefits based on strict guidelines they have developed. The USDA is the agency that certifies meat, poultry, fruits, vegetables, and other items as organic using clearly developed standards as to what items are and what items are not organic. As stated previously, the USDA has developed quality standards for many raw items such as corn, oil, soybeans, and wheat. These designations may appear on the label.

10.2.6 Imports/Exports

The FDA and USDA share duties of monitoring food that is imported into the United States, but they differ in the ways they carry out this duty. The FDA relies solely on point-of-entry inspection. The FDA's inspection requirements are company specific, meaning companies must register with the FDA before importing food products. The USDA/FSIS, on the other hand, works collaboratively with the importing establishments' government to verify that the other countries' regulatory systems for meat, poultry, and egg products are equivalent to those of the United States. The USDA coordinates with the government of the country before accepting meat, poultry, or egg products for sale into US commerce.

With recent changes to the import process attributed to the implementation of FSMA, for the first time, importers will be specifically required to have a program to verify that the food products they are shipping to this country are safe. Among other things, importers will need to verify that their suppliers are in compliance with reasonably appropriate risk-based preventive controls that provide the same level of public health protection as those required under FSMA. The Foreign Supplier Verification Program requires importers to conduct risk-based foreign supplier verification activities to verify that imported food is not adulterated. They must also show that the product was produced in compliance with FDA's preventive controls requirements and produce safety standards, where applicable.

10.2.7 Other Agency Involvement

The FDA and USDA work with many different agencies on a regular basis. Some of the most frequent contact is with those at the state level, such as those that are involved in agriculture and public health. The names of these state agencies can vary from state to state, but the responsibilities are typically divided between departments. These agencies work to promote and protect consumer safety actively on a daily basis. State inspectors help bridge the gap in food safety where the FDA or USDA may not be able to reach. State-level inspectors have oversight of grocery stores, like convenience stores and discount dollar stores, and other retail food and foodservice establishments.

Typically, the state department charged with agricultural responsibilities regulates processors and distributors of food in intrastate commerce, as well as that in interstate commerce. Interstate regulations are done in agreement with the designated federal agency to ensure that the process is done at equivalent levels. Dairy farms, poultry processing facilities, and meat processing facilities are also some other facets where a state-level inspector would be conducting regular inspections.

On an international basis, the FDA and USDA work with different countries. US agencies depend on the food safety standards and enforcement bodies within these foreign countries to monitor the food supply. Regulatory bodies within the United States also work closely with an international organization that promotes food regulations known as the Codex Alimentarius Commission. Codex offers a collection of internationally recognized standards, codes of practice, guidelines, and other recommendations relating to foods, food production, and food safety. Codex states that its mission is to

---

Labeling and Nutrition Guidance Documents and Regulatory Information:
http://www.fda.gov/Food/GuidanceRegulation/GuidanceDocumentsRegulatory Information/LabelingNutrition/default.htm

Food Facts for Consumers:
http://www.fda.gov/Food/ResourcesForYou/Consumers/ucm077286.htm

Guides for People at Risk of Foodborne Illness:
http://www.fda.gov/Food/ResourcesForYou/Consumers/ucm2006968.htm

FDA's Education Resource Library:
http://www.fda.gov/Food/ResourcesForYou/Consumers/ucm239035.htm

USDA/FSIS Fact Sheets for Consumers:
http://www.fsis.usda.gov/wps/portal/fsis/topics/food-safety-education/get -answers/food-safety-fact-sheets

USDA/FSIS Ask Karen, Karen provides information for consumers:
http://www.fsis.usda.gov/wps/portal/informational/askkaren

Food Safety Information: http://www.foodsafety.gov/

Partnership for Food Safety Education: http://www.fightbac.org/

INSERT 10.4
Websites that supply important information for consumers.

harmonize international food standards, guidelines, and codes of practice to protect the health of the consumers and ensure fair practices in the food trade.

Codex Alimentarius and the FDA often do not agree on some major issues affecting our food supply, for example, genetically modified organism (GMO) labeling. One thing they do agree on is that cohesion between all organizations that are concerned with food is essential to making our food as safe as possible and their policies stronger so that the consumer is always first. Useful information for consumers can be found at the websites listed in Insert 10.4.

10.3 Scientific Research and Technology Development

Another function of a food scientist is research. The terms **basic research** and **applied research** are relative. A fundamental chemist or microbiologist might consider basic food science to be applied chemistry or microbiology. In the pure sciences, basic research is generally regarded as work that has no immediate direct application to practical problems, whereas applied research focuses on solving specific problems. In food science, applied research is directed at specific problems associated with food; basic research focuses on a deeper understanding of the properties of food materials.

Both basic and applied research are conducted at universities, in governmental laboratories, and in large food companies. University and government researchers have an obligation to publish scientific journals. Industry scientists, however, may keep their results secret to provide long-term economic advantage to their company.

As the problems facing the world become more complex, scientists are working together to approach problems from different disciplinary perspectives. For example, food microbiologists work with food engineers to develop more effective ways of killing microbes to better preserve foods. Food chemists and sensory specialists may also be needed to assess the effects of such processes on the quality of a functional food product. Food scientists work with nutritionists, molecular gastronomists, biochemists, molecular biologists, physicists, and many other types of scientists to help better understand the science behind our food.

10.3.1 Processing and Engineering

Most material in the universe is neither a gas, a liquid, nor a solid. It is plasma, a highly charged substance that is very hot and the component of our sun and all of the stars. Cold plasma is partially charged and can be produced on earth. The primary use of cold plasma in the food industry is in sterilizing plastic packaging. Treating a plastic polymer with inductively coupled plasma kills microbes on contact without leaving a residue on the package and no toxic liquids that require disposal. Thus, plasma technology is more environmentally friendly than other sterilizing technologies.

The idea of processing food products at home for personal consumption may become possible with three-dimensional (3D) printing. This technology has the potential for individuals to tailor their products based on personal health concerns, sensory preferences, and amount needed for a specific meal without the problems associated with leftovers or food waste. 3D printing of foods uses a template for a specific food item and prints it out one layer at a time from an inventory of available ingredients. See some printed items in Insert 10.5. If the food is to be consumed immediately after printing, the use of preservatives and many other additives might not be required. Research in this area will require studies to overcome potential problems with regard to quality, safety, and stability concerns.

Some of the innovative new processes to preserve foods that are being studied by food engineers were described in Chapter 4. New techniques are being evaluated that are as effective as heat on microorganisms and enzymes but not as damaging to vitamins and flavor. One such preservation technology uses high pressure. High-pressure techniques are being used to extract health-promoting chemicals from plants and improve homogenization of dairy, alternative-milk, and juice products. Whole foods are a source for numerous beneficial compounds, but they are not always convenient to prepare and consume. These molecules can be extracted from different sources and added as ingredients in functional foods. Ultrahigh pressure can be applied to fluids that break up particles and improve shelf life with little increase in temperature. This process can also provide greater stability in food emulsions.

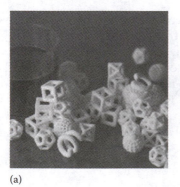
(a)

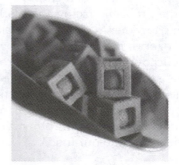
(b)

INSERT 10.5
Printed food objects using the ChefJet 3D printer: (a) 3D printed sugar cubes and (b) 3D printed chocolate sugar. (Images provided by 3D Systems.)

10.3.2 Microtechnology and Nanotechnology

Microtechnology cuts across all areas of food science. Analytical devices are now being produced that can detect very small levels of nutrients, oxidation products, toxins, and microorganisms using miniature electrodes. These probes can be inserted into a single cell and monitor physiological activity. Liquid crystals can be used to encapsulate nutrients or other functional compounds to more effectively deliver them to the needed site in the body. Microstructure of starch is being modified to slow its glycemic response and thus even out the release of glucose into our bloodstream.

Miniaturization is now moving from microtechnology to nanotechnology. It promises advances in food packaging, targeted delivery and improved bioavailability of nutrients and bioactive compounds, and improved sensory quality of foods. Among the many applications in food packaging are better control over permeability of the package. These changes can also make a package more biodegradable, bind antimicrobial and antioxidant compounds to prevent them from entering the food directly, and improve the functional properties of edible coatings. New techniques such as **electrospinning** and **electrospraying** can add coatings layer by layer, allowing more effective customization for different products produced on the same processing line with lower material requirements.

Nutrients such as β-carotene and pro-vitamin A can be encapsulated in nanoparticle ingredients and targeted to specific sites in the body. Antioxidants, omega-3-fatty acids, phytosterols, and other beneficial compounds can be incorporated into nanoparticles to increase their bioavailability. Nanoparticles with antimicrobials can be added to foods to improve their functionality as ingredients by more effective distribution of the additive than current systems. Nanotechnology can also improve delivery of flavor compounds to improve sensory perception and customize the texture of specific products. The form of a nanoparticle affects its ability to function as an ingredient. Thus, research is active on how to best prepare them to be most effective.

10.3.3 Chemistry

The physical state of a food product plays a critical role in whether a chemical reaction can take place and how fast it can occur. For molecules to react, they must be able to touch each other. Molecules within most foods are not stationary; they vibrate and move around in what we term a *phase*. They can also be transported from one phase to another. Examples of phases are the states of matter (gas, liquid, and solid), as well as water-based and oil-based phases. In living organisms, membranes separate compartments within a cell, providing limited transfer of molecules from one compartment to another. As the temperature increases within a food product, molecular motion speeds up, more molecules bump into each other, and chemical reactions are more likely to occur. When a product cools, molecular motion slows and so do molecular interactions and chemical reactions.

As the demand for new sensory sensations at fine-dining establishments is growing, food scientists are collaborating with research chefs to satisfy this market. Molecular gastronomy is driving this exploration with particular attention to the chemical and physical properties of specific chemical compounds as they contribute to the functional properties of ingredients. Flavor release is of particular importance in these investigations and how they relate to consumer acceptability. Scientific study of the complex reactions in the food resulting in a favorable or unfavorable experience by the diner require an understanding of the

- Chemical composition of the food and compound-to-compound interaction within the food
- Changes at the molecular level resulting from cooking and other preparation techniques
- Sensory perception of the released flavor compounds

Chemical analyses in industry and academic laboratories are energy and resource intensive. As we try to become greener in food production, manufacture, and distribution, it is imperative that we introduce green technologies in the laboratory. The first place to look is waste reduction as shown in Insert 10.6. Ways to reduce waste include the following:

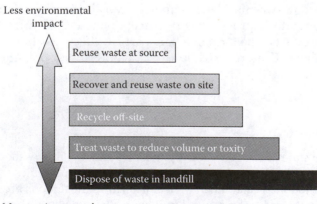

INSERT 10.6

Environmental impact of laboratory wastes. (From Boye, J.I. et al., Greening of research and development. In *Green Technologies in Food Production and Processing*, Boye, J.I. and Arcand, Y., eds., New York: Springer, 2012.)

- Microtechniques, which use very small levels of solvents and reactants to determine a solution
- Purchasing small amounts of chemicals at a time to reduce the inventory of those items that might need to be discarded after the expiration date
- Careful planning of experiments to minimize the use of toxic substances and failed tests

Other possible ways to improve the laboratory environment include reducing the need for printed material, decreasing the amount of disposable plastic materials used, and automatic shutoff of unnecessary electrical power when the laboratory is not in use. Although regulations to protect laboratory worker safety tend to increase energy demands, construction of new laboratories can take advantage of many innovative technologies to decrease the environmental footprint of a laboratory.

10.3.4 Nutritional Properties

New functional foods hit the supermarket weekly, targeting a wide range of diseases: obesity, diabetes, cancer, heart disease, and other diseases of civilization. Research is being conducted to determine how molecules that act as antioxidants and anticarcinogens work to slow or prevent diseases. For example, phenolic compounds, like anthocyanin pigments and tannins, are of particular interest. Overall, food scientists are studying

- The molecular mechanisms of these diseases and compounds
- The doses needed to produce a positive outcome
- Whether higher levels can lead to toxicity or harmful interactions with other beneficial compounds such as vitamins
- How food processing affects the amount and potency of these compounds

As the interest in health and wellness grows in the general population, consumers are demanding healthier foods. Media reports, blogging sites, and marketing campaigns tend to be the primary sources consumers use to determine which foods are or are not healthy. Frequently, the guidance provided by these sources is not based on carefully planned scientific studies. Research is being conducted on the actual health benefits of specific ingredients in functional foods, how much of the active compound needs to be consumed to be effective, its bioavailability, and how much can be counterproductive. For example, α-tocopherol (vitamin E) is the most effective antioxidant in the body at certain levels, but it can increase oxidation at higher levels.

Nutrigenomics refers to the interaction of nutrients with body metabolic processes. This field combines a knowledge in chemistry with that of molecular biology to better understand how ingredients in foods contribute to human health. From this type of research, scientists like Malik can explore areas of nutrition that might have effects on certain subpopulations of humans that are unrecognized in the general population. The field of nutrigenomics points to an ultimate goal of discovering a combination of nutrients required to promote health for an individual consumer. Nutritionally correct foods and diets can then be designed for each person on the basis of their body chemistry. Understanding what is best for a specific consumer, however, doesn't guarantee that the person will consume the proper combination.

10.3.5 Microbiology and Toxicology

Food microbiology involves the isolation, identification, and sometimes classification of microorganisms in foods, which we will explore further in Chapter 13. Basic food microbiology, however, explores the molecular mechanisms of pathogenesis, which include questions such as the following:

- Why are some microorganisms pathogenic, but most are not?
- Why are some microorganisms pathogenic to some animal species like humans and not to other species?
- What is the molecular basis of pathogenicity?
- How can we rapidly determine the presence or absence of food-borne pathogens in a food product?

One example of a contaminant that is not a microorganism is a **prion**. Prions are proteins found in contaminated food that can infect the brain. At present, we have no way of treating or curing people who are infected with a prion, but we prevent transmission by keeping prions out of the food supply. The greatest concern is contaminated feed infecting animals, which then can infect those consumers of meat from these animals. Prions are resistant to processing methods we use to kill microorganisms. Thus, infected animals are normally killed and burned to prevent them from infecting other animals and entry into the food supply. Promising research is being conducted on prion infection of yeasts where the biology, structure, and methods of replication can be studied. As if prions are not scary enough in themselves, microbiologists are finding other infectious agents from animals that can be transmitted to humans though food, water, and even pets who can be asymptomatic carriers.

Toxicology studies the toxins in the environment and how they affect health of humans and other organisms. In addition to prions, toxicologists are studying the formation of polycyclic aromatic hydrocarbons (PAHs) that are formed when food is heated above 120°C. Concerns were first raised about acrylamide, a PAH found in French fries, but it is now apparent that any heating in a fryer or oven can produce this class of compounds. The amount of acrylamide precursors can be reduced in potatoes through genetic modification, but consumer fears about GMOs make it unlikely that genetic techniques offer a solution.

Concerns have also been raised about the safety of new compounds produced by advanced technological methods such as nanoparticles that could enter our bodies from foods and packages modified by this technology. Many particles in the whole and formulated foods we consume now contain nanoparticles that form in animal and plant tissue and during accepted processing operations without any safety concerns. Some protein nanostructures found in nature have been found to be toxic, however. Research is needed to determine whether nontoxic compounds, when incorporated into a novel nanoparticle, are safe for human consumption.

10.3.6 Sensory Quality and Other Frontiers

Advances in these fields tend to focus on economics, efficiency, and safety. Traditionally, once the details have been worked out, sensory testing begins. Unacceptable quality may mean slight tweaking of previous research or extensive reevaluation of newly developed techniques. Efforts are now being made to integrate sensory studies earlier in the evaluation process. Although it would seem to be a simple task, greater treatment and sample sizes challenge the logistical capabilities of traditional sensory research. Predictive models, advanced statistical techniques, and **chemometrics** are being used to decrease the demand for extensive panel testing. Sensory scientists are continually studying basic psychology research to find new ways to measure consumer response to food stimuli. Brain scans using an instrument called functional magnetic resonance imaging (fMRI) can provide insight into consumer likes and dislikes as described in Chapter 15.

The social aspects of food are receiving increased attention. Questions on the acceptance of new food technologies, agricultural practices, and governmental policies are being raised and studied. The role of specific foods in the development of obesity and the promotion or deterioration of human health is also being explored. Frequently, single studies do not offer enough information to draw broad conclusions or serve as the basis for policy decisions. Statistical investigation of numerous studies, a process known as **meta-analysis**, can tease out more information. Such research requires

- Selection of appropriate search terms
- A search for all potential articles in relevant databases

- Criteria for appropriateness of the identified articles
- Screening out all articles identified that fail to meet the criteria
- Rescaling all relative quantitative measures so that appropriate comparisons can be made
- Conducting the final analysis

10.4 Remember This!

- Questions on the acceptance of new food technologies, agricultural practices, and governmental policies are being raised and studied.
- Nutrigenomics combines a knowledge in chemistry with that of molecular biology to better understand how ingredients in foods contribute to human health.
- Nutrients such as β-carotene and pro-vitamin A can be encapsulated in nanoparticle ingredients and targeted to specific sites in the body.
- Basic research is generally regarded as work that has no immediate direct application to practical problems, whereas applied research focuses on solving specific problems.
- Cohesion between all organizations that are concerned with food is essential to making our food as safe as possible and our policies stronger so that the consumer is always first.
- Each food label must have an ingredient statement; a net weight; an address of the processor, distributor, or importer; and the name of the product that can be clearly understood by the consumer.
- Recalls are typically voluntary actions by a company to send out a notice to consumers and distributors that a product they have manufactured and introduced into the market may be contaminated or mislabeled and should not be consumed.
- Preventive controls are put in place in order to anticipate food safety problems before they happen.
- The intention of the FFDCA is to control aspects of food that could adversely affect the health of the consumer and prevent fraud by food companies.
- To make the laws work on a day-to-day level, Congress authorizes certain government agencies including the FDA, USDA, and EPA to create appropriate regulations.

10.5 Looking Ahead

This chapter focused on the roles of food scientists as governmental regulators and researchers. The final five chapters of the book will provide more depth in the primary subdisciplines of food science, which form the basis for further advances in the field.

Testing Comprehension

1. A poultry processing company has two separate facilities on the outskirts of a city—one that receives live birds and packs refrigerated and frozen chicken parts and the other that manufactures frozen products such as pot pies and entrées. Both plants ship product in interstate commerce. Describe the regulatory oversight needed for these facilities by state and federal agencies and the governing authority for each.

2. Explain the differences in safety and quality as perceived by food scientists and journalists. What are the main reasons for these differences?

3. Outline all the steps and actions an FDA inspector would need to take to evaluate a plant that produces ramen noodles. List all of the advantages and disadvantages of such an inspection from the perspective of the FDA, the company being inspected, and the consumer of ramen noodles.

4. Diagram all the steps needed in a voluntary recall of contaminated dog food. Identify at least three possible reasons for this recall. For each reason listed, describe an action that could have been taken by the company to have prevented the problem. What agency would be in charge of the recall? Why?

5. Identify three specific vulnerabilities to the food supply that could be taken advantage of by terrorists. Describe the responsibility of the government, the food industry, the distribution chain, and the ultimate consumer in maintaining a safe food supply.

6. Compare and contrast the goals and benefits of basic research, applied research, and technology. How do basic and applied research in food science differ from each other? How does food science differ from food technology? How does basic research in food science differ from basic research in biochemistry? How does applied research in food science differ from applied research in microbiology?

7. Select one of the areas of scientific research described in the chapter. Describe several potential changes in the food supply resulting from advances in this type of research. Are there any potential problems that could result? Why or why not?

8. Identify at least five "potential problems with regard to quality, safety, and stability concerns" with respect to 3D printing of food based on what has been learned in this book so far. Rank these potential problems in order from most difficult to least difficult in development of specific solutions to overcome each one. What food product would be most interesting to print in 3D form? Why?

9. Kiwifruit slices lose approximately 1 milligram of ascorbic acid (vitamin C) per 100 grams of fresh weight every 12 hours when left in refrigerated storage at 7°C. Calculate the loss of vitamin C during 3 days of storage in a refrigerator of slices from a 70-grams kiwifruit containing 80 milligrams of ascorbic acid at the time of slicing. If the RDA for ascorbic acid is 90 milligrams, what percent daily value of vitamin C was in the kiwifruit before slicing and in the slices after 3 days in the refrigerator?

10. Carefully study Insert 10.6. Analyze the accuracy and usefulness of the diagram. Describe how this concept could be applied to other wastes in our lives.

Reference

Boye, J. I., A. Maltais, S. Bittner and Y. Arcand, 2012. Greening of research and development, in *Green Technologies in Food Production and Processing*, Boye, J. I. and Arcand, Y., Eds., New York: Springer.

Further Reading

Akrititis, N., 2011. Parasitic, fungal and prion zoonoses: An expanding universe of candidates for human disease. *Clin. Microbiol. Infect.*, 17:331.

Barham, P., L. H. Skibsted, W. L. P. Bredie, M. B. Frost, P. Moller, J. Risbo, P. Snitkjaer and L. M. Mortensen, 2010. Molecular gastronomy: A new emerging scientific discipline. *Chem. Rev.*, 110:2313.

Crowe, K. M. and C. Francis, 2013. Position of the academy of nutrition and dietetics: Functional foods. *J. Acad. Nutr. Diet.*, 113:1096.

Dumay, E., D. Chevalier-Lucia, L. Picart-Palmade, A. Benzaria, A. Gracia-Julia and C. Blayo, 2013. Technological aspects and potential applications of (ultra) high pressure homogenization. *Trends Food Sci. Technol.*, 31:13.

Fabra, M. J., M. A. Busalo, A. Lopez-Rubio and J. M. Lagaron, 2013. Nanostructured biolayers in food packaging. *Trends Food Sci. Technol.*, 31:79.

FAO/WHO Scientific Basis for Codex, 2014. *CODEX Alimentarius: Home.* World Health Organization and Food and Agriculture Organization of the United Nations, January 1. Web: September 1, 2014. Available at http://www.codex alimentarius.org/.

Food Safety Modernization Act; Effect on States, 2014. *Food Safety Modernization Act.* National Conference of State Legislators, January 1. Web: September 1, 2014. Available at http://www.ncsl.org/research/agriculture-and-rural-development /food-safety-modernization-act.aspx.

Frewer, L. J., I. A. van der Lans, A. R. H. Fischer, M. J. Reinders, D. Menozzi, X. Zhang, I. van den Berg and K. L. Zimmermann, 2013. Public perceptions of agri-food applications of genetic modification—A systematic review and meta-analysis. *Trends Food Sci. Technol.*, 30:142.

Huang, H.-W., C.-P. Hsu, B. B. Yang and C.-Y. Wang, 2013. Advances in the extraction of natural ingredients by high-pressure extraction technology. *Trends Food Sci. Technol.*, 32:73.

Joye, I. J. and D. J. McClements, 2013. Production of nanoparticles by antisolvent precipitation for use in food systems. *Trends Food Sci. Technol.*, 34:109.

Lagerwall, J. P. F. and G. Scalia, 2012. Review: A new era for liquid crystal research: Application for liquid crystals in soft matter nano-, bio- and microtechnology. *Curr. Appl. Phys.*, 12:1387.

Liebman, S. W. and Y. O. Chernoff, 2012. Prions in yeast. *Genetics*, 191:1041.

Lipson, H., and M. Kurman, 2013. *Fabricated: The New World of 3D Printing.* Indianapolis, IN: John Wiley & Sons.

Pankaj, S. K., C. Bueno-Ferrer, N. N. Misra, V. Milosavljevic, C. P. O'Donnell, P. Bourke, K. M. Keener and P. J. Cullen, 2014. Applications of cold plasma technology in food packaging. *Trends Food Sci. Technol.*, 35:5.

Raynes, J. K., J. A. Carver, S. L. Gras and J. A. Gerrard, 2014. Protein nanostructures in food—Should we be worried? *Trends Food Sci. Technol.*, 37:42.

U.S. Food and Drug Administration, 2014. *Frequently Asked Questions.* Food and Drug Administration. Web: September 1, 2014. Available at http://www.fda.gov /Food/GuidanceRegulation/FSMA/ucm247559.htm.

Vergeres, G., 2013. Nutrigenomics—Linking food to human metabolism. *Trends Food Sci. Technol.*, 31:6–12.

Section IV

Scientific Principles

11

Food Chemistry

As a Chemistry major, Ignacio was more interested in what toxic chemicals the microbes made than in the microbes themselves. He was also interested in all the chemicals that were added to foods, like preservatives, but he wasn't so sure that he wanted all those chemicals in his mouth. While he was looking for an elective course online during open registration, he came across one called Food Chemistry. It sounded interesting, like it might be a course where he could apply his basic knowledge in chemistry to the real world. He took the course, loved it, and found out that he had much more to learn about the chemicals in his food. Much of what he learned changed his understanding of and appreciation for chemistry in everyday life.

Jennifer, by now a committed vegan, decided to major in Nutrition because she wanted to learn how to eat healthier. We can imagine her shock when she learned that nutrition is mainly about chemicals and how they act in the body. It really doesn't have much to do with food at all. There was in-depth study of digestion and all the metabolic pathways that occur to food components once they are broken down, but healthy eating wasn't exactly the main topic of discussion. When her professors talked about a vegetarian diet, they had some good things to say but also a lot of negative things. Mostly, they talked about chemicals. They talked about large chemical compounds like carbs (only they called them carbohydrates), fats (lipids), and proteins. She learned that vitamins are actually organic chemicals and that minerals are elements straight from the periodic table she had memorized (and quickly forgotten) in first-year chemistry. She wanted to know more about nutrients, but she wanted to know about the nutrients in the types of foods she ate regularly.

Kyle is a Food Science major and is learning more about all the chemicals in his foods. He learned about the toxins and preservatives Ignacio was into, as well as about the nutrients that Jennifer was studying. He was fascinated by the many other chemicals in foods and how they all work together to produce the quality of a food. He found out that foods are made of ingredients and ingredients are made of chemicals. Each ingredient has a function in the food, but it is actually the chemical components that give an ingredient its function. The more he learned about pigments and stabilizers, the more he wanted to learn about texturizers and humectants. He thought that the taste of a food was simple, but now he knows that flavor combines taste and aroma. He learned that tens and even hundreds of chemical compounds could be contributing to the aroma of foods. Upon completion of his degree,

Kyle plans to go to graduate school to learn more about food chemistry and then to work in the food industry to develop new food products.

11.1 Looking Back

In previous chapters, we looked at general food issues, the types of food products we encounter in the marketplace, and the activities that food scientists perform. In this chapter, we focus on the most basic science we need to know as it relates to foods: chemistry.

The key points that follow were covered in previous chapters and will help prepare us for a basic understanding of the chemical aspects of foods:

- Waste prevention is critical in sustaining our planet, and it becomes more critical the later the waste occurs in the life cycle as the inputs accumulate at each point in the cycle.

- Molecular gastronomy has been developed in Europe to merge food science with the culinary arts to better understand the chemical and physical changes that food materials undergo during cooking processes.

- Stabilizers are added to formulated foods to keep them from breaking down.

- Individual fat replacers cannot perform all functions of lipids.

- A clean label is one that has only clearly recognizable ingredients, none of which sound like chemicals.

- The main function of a package is to preserve the physical and chemical integrity of a product including preventing microbial or chemical contamination.

- The Nutrition Facts part of the label indicates the serving size, how many servings per container, calories per serving, and the fat calories per serving.

- Nutraceuticals are foods specifically designed to act as drugs.

- Although not a true allergic reaction, celiac disease is an autoimmune disorder in which microvilli in the intestinal tract react with gliadin, a component of gluten found in wheat and other grains.

- Preservatives are food ingredients that slow spoilage and help prevent food-associated illnesses.

By now, it should be apparent that all foods are composed of chemicals—edible chemicals, but chemicals nonetheless. All food components, macro- and micronutrients, and any processing additives and preservatives, colors, and flavors are of chemical nature. Proteins, carbohydrates, and fats are chemicals that provide calories. Vitamins and minerals are chemicals that are needed for proper body metabolism. Dietary fiber is a complex mix of chemicals that aids digestion and binds toxins. Even the most important nutrients of all, water and oxygen, are chemicals. People who do not have a background in nutrition, physiology, or food science may not understand or even want to believe that our bodies are complex organisms composed of chemicals and will need chemical replacements to maintain health. Food scientists believe that chemicals are not to be feared but rather to be understood.

11.2 Chemistry of Our Foods

11.2.1 Water

Water, with its simple chemical formula (H_2O), is the most abundant compound in the majority of fresh foods although it is not listed on most nutritional labels. Fruits and vegetables are made of as much as 90%–95% water, while full fat cheeses and bread may contain 35%–40% water, and nuts and chocolate, between 0.5% and 1%. Vegetable oils are among the few foods that contain no water.

Water is the only chemical commonly found as a solid, liquid, and gas under normal conditions, and it is both an amazingly simple compound to understand and a deceptively complex component of almost all food systems. Water is also known as the universal solvent as it will dissolve many solids and liquids, but some compounds such as fats, oils, and organic solvents like hexane are not soluble in water. The solubility of organic compounds in water is a function of hydrogen bonding. Hydrogen bonding is primarily a function of the presence of hydroxyl (–OH) groups with the H in the hydroxyl group forming a hydrogen bond with the O in water and the O in the hydroxyl group forming a hydrogen bond with an H in water. The longer the chain of a hydrocarbon, the less soluble it will be.

Water is important in foods as it provides a medium to support microbial growth (which can have a positive or negative effect as we will see in Chapter 12) and for chemical reactions to occur. Generally speaking, the more water present, the greater the opportunity for microorganisms to grow. More important than the amount of water is the amount of water available to the microbe. **Water activity** (A_W) is the term that relates to the ability of a microbe to grow in a particular environment.

Manipulation of water content and availability in a food product by drying or concentrating or by addition of salt or sugar will reduce its susceptibility to microbial attack. Water also has a profound effect on the product's texture as well as its color and flavor. Food scientists use **moisture sorption isotherm** figures to determine the relationship between water content and water activity. Such plots help predict the behavior of a food during drying and rehydration. A large difference in the plots of the drying and rehydration isotherms (known as **syneresis**) of a breakfast cereal means that it will not become soggy in a bowl of milk.

Water is also the medium for many chemical reactions in food. Molecules must be able to move within a food product to react with each other. During food storage, many of these reactions can be detrimental to food quality (although aging of wine and beef as well as ripening of fruits are notable exceptions). **Molecular mobility** is the term used to describe this movement of molecules within a food product. During freezing, the molecular mobility decreases as the water freezes. With decreased molecular mobility, the chemical reactions can be slowed down and the quality can be prolonged. Not all water freezes at the same rate, however; hence, the water in a food does not go immediately from a liquid to a solid state.

Water content also affects the sensory quality of foods. The presence of water in a food product can be perceived as both juicy and succulent or watery and soggy, depending on the product. Likewise, the absence of water can be perceived as dry or crunchy. **Water-holding capacity** (WHC) results from physical entrapment of the water within the food matrix that restricts flow but no other physical properties of the water molecules. In packaged meats, lack of WHC leads to drip loss or unsightly microbe-laden water in the bottom of the package and a tougher cooked product.

11.2.2 Carbohydrates

We derive energy from macronutrients—proteins, lipids, and carbohydrates. Most people around the world obtain more than half of their calories from carbohydrates. **Monosaccharides**, known as simple sugars, are the basic unit of carbohydrates and consist of carbon, hydrogen, and oxygen. The most common monosaccharides are glucose (blood sugar) and fructose (the primary sweetener in honey). Monosaccharides combine to form **disaccharides**, **oligosaccharides**, and **polysaccharides** (see Insert 11.1).

Common disaccharides include sucrose (table sugar) and lactose (milk sugar). Sucrose is composed of a molecule of glucose linked to a molecule of fructose, and lactose is a molecule of glucose linked to a molecule of galactose (another monosaccharide). Oligosaccharides are short chains (between 3 and 10) of monosaccharides. Among them, inulin and oligofructose are gaining popularity in food applications as well as for their potential health benefits as prebiotics.

Examples of polysaccharides are starch, cellulose and dietary fiber (in plants), and glycogen (in animals). Starches are complex carbohydrates that consist of long chains of monosaccharides (primarily glucose). Cellulose is

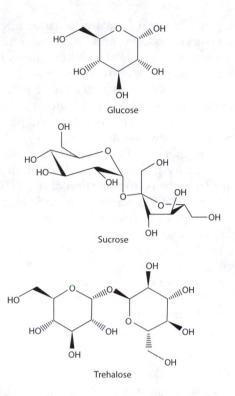

Glucose

Sucrose

Trehalose

INSERT 11.1

Chemical structures of three naturally occurring sugars—a monosaccharide (glucose), a disaccharide (sucrose), and a trisaccharide (trehalose).

another long molecule consisting of glucose molecules linked together. The molecular linkage in starch is different from that of cellulose. Our digestive systems have enzymes that can break down the bonds in starch into single glucose units, which, in turn, can be used by our bodies, but we do not have the enzymes that can break the cellulose linkages. Cattle and other ruminants do have the enzymes that can break down the bonds in cellulose, allowing them to eat grass and derive energy from it. Dietary fiber, found in fruits, vegetables, whole grains, and their products, is also composed of complex carbohydrates. These compounds (hemicellulose, pectin, and lignin) are more complex in structure than starch and cellulose and are not broken down during digestion. Glycogen is the energy storage of glucose in animals and humans.

Food scientists are interested in carbohydrates for more than their nutritional value. Sugars are sweet and add to the flavor of many food products, and complex carbohydrates contribute to food texture. Starches can be chemically modified to improve ingredient functionality. Modified starches have desirable properties that make it possible to produce instant foods (instant puddings or quick grits), maintain creamy textures upon thawing (frozen custard pies or other frozen desserts), and cause thickening (gravies). Pectin, cellulose, and gums are also effective at providing desirable textural properties. Food scientists must be aware of the properties of the carbohydrate, the properties of the food, and how both will change with typical processing operations. For example, the usefulness of a gum as a thickener depends on its solubility, stability to changes in temperature and pH, compatibility with other gums, and its freeze–thaw stability.

Starch is the major component of bread and other bakery products. One of the most common quality problems associated with bakery products is staling, which results from the **retrogradation** of starch. This retrogradation involves the crystallization of the starch molecules such that they begin to separate from the other molecules present in the product, which leads to loss of acceptable color, flavor, and texture of the product. Anyone who has used starch to prepare a food product knows that starch can't just be dumped in water, because it will not dissolve. The hydroxyl (–OH) groups on the starch molecule interact with the water. Using just a small amount of water with the starch permits hydration of these hydroxyl groups by hydrogen bonding. Once these groups are hydrated, the starch will more easily dissolve in the water.

11.2.3 Lipids

The chemical category that includes fats and oils is lipids. Fats are solid at room temperature while oils are liquid. Lipids are defined as chemical compounds that are soluble in organic solvents but not soluble in water. The three primary groups of lipids found in foods are **triacylglycerols**, **phospholipids**, and **sterols** (see Insert 11.2).

Triacylglycerols contain three fatty acids and are found in bulk lipids such as the visible fats we cut off of a steak, lard used in baking, and vegetable oils that come in bottles. Phospholipids contain two fatty acids with a polar head group and are found in cellular membranes of plants and animals. Since phospholipids are soluble in both water and lipid, they can be used as emulsifiers. Lecithin, the most common phospholipid emulsifier found in many food products' ingredient lists, can be extracted from egg yolks and soybeans.

Cholesterol is the most well-known sterol, but there are many other sterols in plants and animals. Sterols are multiringed structures without fatty acids that help stabilize cellular membranes in living tissue. They are also precursors of hormones in our bodies. Other lipids may act as antioxidants and pro-vitamins. Thus, although many of us consume too many lipids, it is important to remember that small amounts of lipids in our diet are necessary to maintain our health.

In earlier chapters, we learned about saturated, unsaturated, polyunsaturated, and *trans* fats. It is the fatty acid part of a lipid molecule that varies by

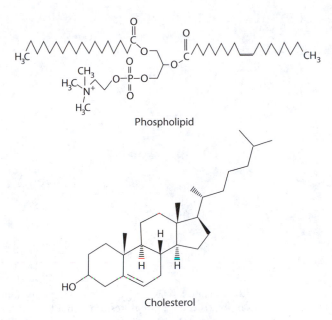

Phospholipid

Cholesterol

INSERT 11.2
Chemical structures of a phospholipid and a sterol.

degree of saturation. Fatty acids consist of chains of hydrocarbons (a carbon backbone with hydrogen atoms attached). A fatty acid is classified by the number of carbon atoms and the degree of saturation and is completely saturated when it has the maximum number of hydrogen atoms attached and no double bonds. A monounsaturated fatty acid contains a double bond and two fewer hydrogen atoms than a saturated fatty acid. A polyunsaturated fatty acid contains at least two double bonds. As the number of double bonds increases, the melting temperature decreases and the more likely the lipid is to become an oil. Saturated lipids are solid fats and spreads and are often associated with heart disease.

Polyunsaturated lipids tend to be oils, but these oils can be hydrogenated by adding hydrogen atoms across a double bond to make the fatty acid more saturated. While this process results in a better spread, *trans* fatty acids become an unwanted by-product. *Cis* fatty acids, which occur in fats and oils that have not been modified, have the hydrogen atoms on the same side of the double bond, while *trans* fatty acids have the hydrogen atoms on opposite sides (see Insert 11.3). Our bodies cannot use *trans* fatty acids, and there is growing scientific evidence that *trans* fatty acids provide more serious threats to our health. Partially dehydrogenated oils represent a major source of *trans* fatty acids in foods, and these oils are being phased out in food products.

Lipids are considered unhealthy by many consumers. The health risks associated with lipids include a doubling of calorie content for the same weight of carbohydrates or proteins and the accumulation of lipids in our

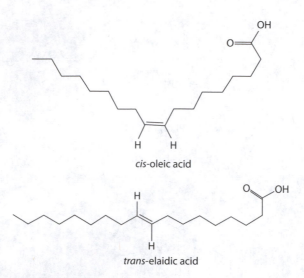

cis-oleic acid

trans-elaidic acid

INSERT 11.3
Chemical structures of a *cis* fatty acid and a *trans* fatty acid. The hydrogen atoms are on the same side of the double bond in the *cis* configuration, resulting in a kink in the chain. The hydrogen atoms are on the opposite side of the *trans* conformation.

arteries leading to atherosclerosis and heart disease. Contrary to popular belief, however, we do need some fat in the diet. Linoleic (18:2, 18 carbon atoms and 2 double bonds) and linolenic (18:3) are essential fatty acids that we must get in our foods as we cannot produce them in our bodies. The fat-soluble vitamins require some amount of lipid in order to be absorbed by our body in the intestines. In addition, lipids contribute to satiety as well as many of the pleasant aromas and provide lubrication of foods in the mouth. If we cut out too many lipids, our food becomes tasteless, we may not get enough intake of fat-soluble vitamins, and we might not eat enough to keep us healthy. Low-fat foods may be popular, but if we overconsume them, we will still gain weight.

Chemical reactions in foods involve breaking down of lipids by hydrolysis and oxidation. **Lipid hydrolysis** involves the separation of a fatty acid from the glycerol backbone of a triacylglycerol or phospholipid. If these fatty acids are short chain (four carbons or less), the aromas can be objectionable, but longer-chain fatty acids usually do not cause quality problems. **Lipid oxidation** is a reaction of lipids with molecular oxygen that proceeds through a free-radical mechanism. Lipid oxidation can result in severe off-odors and -flavors (known as oxidative rancidity). Too many of these oxidative products can be toxic to humans. The free radical consists of a carbon atom with an extra electron, resulting from the removal of a hydrogen atom. Oxygen can attach to the free electron, resulting in a lipid hydroperoxide. Through a very complex series of chemical reactions, these compounds leading to oxidative rancidity are formed.

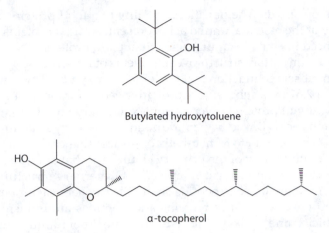

Butylated hydroxytoluene

α-tocopherol

INSERT 11.4

Chemical structures of two potent antioxidants. Butylated hydroxytoluene (BHT) is an artificial antioxidant found in many formulated foods. The α-tocopherol molecule is vitamin E and the most effective antioxidant in cellular membranes.

Antioxidants either inhibit or retard oxidation through one or more mechanisms. Antioxidants such as β-carotene (pro-vitamin A), α-tocopherol (vitamin E), lycopene (red pigment in tomatoes), or ascorbic acid (vitamin C) may occur in the food tissue itself and help slow or prevent oxidation. Other compounds such as butylated hydroxyanisole (BHA) and butylated hydroxytoluene (BHT) are artificial antioxidants that are added to foods to prevent rancidity. The naturally occurring antioxidants tend to be more effective in tissue foods to prevent oxidation of phospholipids in cellular membranes, while the artificial antioxidants tend to be more effective in the triacylglycerols in formulated foods (see Insert 11.4).

11.2.4 Proteins

Proteins are another class of macronutrients in our foods. Although they can be used for energy in the body, they are much more important as a source of essential amino acids. Proteins are large molecules composed of long, folded chains of amino acids that are linked together by peptide bonds. Amino acids can act both as acids and as bases with the carboxyl (–COOH) end acting as the acid and the amino (–NH$_2$) group acting as a base. The peptide bond forms as the carboxyl group from one amino acid binds with the amino group from the next one with the net loss of a water (H$_2$O) molecule. There are 21 amino acids that are typically found in food products, but only 9 are essential to human health (phenylalanine, methionine, tryptophan, isoleucine, threonine, histidine, leucine, lysine, and valine). The remaining 12 amino acids can be synthesized by our bodies and thus do not need to be ingested in our foods. The nutritional quality of a food protein is based on the balance of the essential amino acids present. Animal proteins tend to be more balanced in essential amino acids than plant proteins.

Proteins are important structural components of muscle tissue and are also involved in muscle contraction and movement. Enzymes (as we will discuss in Section 11.2.5) are a subgroup of proteins needed for metabolic processes.

The structure of proteins is very complex. Primary structure refers to the chain of amino acids linked by peptide bonds. Secondary structure relates to whether the chains tend to form α-helix or β-sheet shapes. Tertiary structure involves the interfolding of the primary chain such that amino acid number 42 may be close to amino acid number 16. Quaternary structure refers to the linkage of more than one peptide chain. Physiochemical properties (how they act in living systems) of proteins and peptides are influenced by the **hydrophobicity** and **hydrophilicity** of the constituent amino acids. Some amino acids are soluble in lipids and not in water (hydrophobic) while others are soluble in water and not in lipids (hydrophilic). In the tertiary structure of a protein, regions can form that are primarily composed of hydrophobic or hydrophilic amino acids. These regions then associate with like environments within a cell resulting in the folding of the chain. Other factors that affect physiochemical properties of proteins include ionic charge, hydrogen bonding, and van der Waals forces.

Food scientists are also very interested in the functional properties of proteins in foods. The texture of omelets, meringues, yogurt, and many other products is attributed to the presence of denatured proteins. Denaturation of proteins affects the secondary, tertiary, and quaternary structure of the protein by inactivating the physiochemical properties while changing the physicochemical properties (physical and chemical properties that, in turn, affect the functional properties) of the protein. Chemical modification of amino acid side chains alters functional properties of the proteins, which, in turn, alters the physicochemical properties of the food. During denaturation or chemical alteration of the proteins, some of the essential amino acids lose their nutritional value. Lysine is particularly susceptible to these changes.

While proteins are an essential part of the diet, problems can develop when too much protein is consumed. During digestion, the proteins are broken down into individual amino acids in the intestines and absorbed across the intestinal mucosa into the bloodstream where they are then transported to the tissues and cells where they are needed. Athletes who want to build muscle mistakenly think that an increase of protein consumption and a decrease of carbohydrates will help build muscle. Actually, carbohydrates are needed to build muscle. Increased protein consumption relative to carbohydrates increases hunger and causes the body to use the amino acids (both essential and nonessential) for energy rather than to build proteins. The brain needs glucose to function properly, but the body cannot produce enough glucose for the brain if there is insufficient carbohydrate present.

11.2.5 Enzymes

Enzymes are specialized proteins that catalyze specific reactions converting substrates to products. Living systems need enzymes to speed up reactions in the cell. Enzymes like pepsin and trypsin break down foods in the stomach and intestine into small components that can be absorbed across the intestinal walls into the bloodstream. Enzymes are also needed to synthesize new proteins and pigments, build and repair membranes and cell walls, replace worn-out DNA, and perform many other functions in cellular metabolism. Without enzymes, life as we know it would not be possible. Many compounds in the cell are stereospecific (the structure represents one side of a mirror image). The enzyme will recognize one side of the mirror image and not the other (e.g., L-amino acids and not D-amino acids). Enzyme reactions thus are stereospecific while normal chemical reactions produce equal amounts of the two mirror images.

Cellular compartmentation is an important factor in controlling enzyme reactions in plant and animal tissues. The plasma membrane, composed primarily of phospholipids and proteins, surrounds each cell. Within the cell are smaller structures called organelles that are also surrounded by or composed of membranes. Substrates can be protected from enzymes by cell membranes or they can be directly attached to a membrane. When these membranes are broken by a physical blow, bruising develops as evidenced in a muscle or in a fresh peach. In the peach, the enzyme polygalacturonase causes the flesh to become mushy, while another enzyme, polyphenoloxidase, is responsible for brown color development. During cutting, slicing, and other processing operations, these membranes can become damaged, and quality of the product suffers because of the effects on the enzymes.

Many enzymes are inactivated during processing, handling, and storage. Heat can denature an enzyme. Once an enzyme unfolds from its secondary and tertiary structure, it cannot operate as an enzyme, but it can still contribute functional properties that affect the structure of the food product. Enzyme activity (the rate at which it acts) is also affected by the pH and moisture content of the food, the storage temperature, the presence of oxygen and carbon dioxide in the food environment, and light.

Genetic engineering alters genetic composition to modify a specific trait of a raw food product. Genetic engineering works on modifying the DNA in the cell's nucleus (transformation), which affects RNA synthesis (transcription) and placement of amino acids in sequence in the proteins (translation). Many of the proteins affected are enzymes, which results in the increased or decreased formation of specific compounds in the cell.

11.2.6 Vitamins and Minerals

Vitamins are organic chemicals essential to health. Fat-soluble vitamins are more difficult to incorporate into formulated foods than water-soluble vitamins and are also susceptible to oxidation. Vitamins A, C, and E are anti-oxidant vitamins (see Insert 11.5) because they help protect fats from becoming oxidized. Processing, particularly heat processing, can be very damaging to vitamins. Canning or home cooking can destroy more than 50% of the vitamins, but further losses during subsequent storage are minimal. Most consumers don't realize that vitamins in fresh foods degrade during storage, either through normal metabolic processes or in response to external stress. Thus, major losses in vitamins, particularly water-soluble vitamins, can occur in whole foods stored in the refrigerator. Unlike vitamins, minerals are inorganic elements and at least 25 are essential for life (see Insert 11.6).

Next time we see a weird chemical-sounding name like ferric orthophosphate or pyridoxine hydrochloride, we can rest easier knowing that these are simply iron and vitamin B_6.

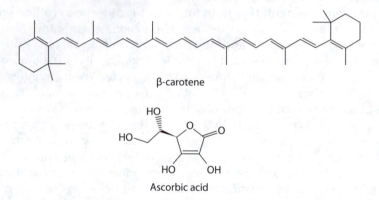

β-carotene

Ascorbic acid

INSERT 11.5
Chemical structures of a lipid-soluble vitamin (β-carotene or pro-vitamin A) and a water-soluble vitamin (ascorbic acid or vitamin C).

Calcium	Ca	Nickel	Ni
Chlorine	Cl	Phosphorous	P
Chromium	Cr	Potassium	K
Copper	Cu	Selenium	Se
Fluorine	F	Silicon	Si
Iodine	I	Sodium	Na
Iron	Fe	Sulfur	S
Magnesium	Mg	Tin	Sn
Manganese	Mn	Vanadium	V
Molybdenum	Mo	Zinc	Zn

INSERT 11.6
List of essential minerals and their chemical symbols.

11.2.7 Preservatives and Other Food Additives

In addition to the physical and chemical properties of compounds, food chemists are interested in functional properties of chemicals that translate into the **functionality** of ingredients. The functionality of ingredients is defined as the physicochemical properties that affect their performance in a food product during processing, storage, and preparation. Product developers must know about the functionality of ingredients when designing a new food product or modifying an existing one.

Our first thought about chemicals in our food usually is about preservatives and additives. Chemical preservatives provide one of the oldest and most effective defenses against microbial activity in foods, and the two most widely used chemical preservatives, sugar (sucrose) and salt (sodium chloride), are not usually considered chemicals, but *they are*. Preservatives will slow down or stop the growth of a microorganism, or even kill it. One way that preservatives work is by binding water and making it unavailable to microorganisms. Sugar and salt are very effective at decreasing water activity and thus impeding microbial growth.

Other preservatives like organic acids such as acetic acid (vinegar) and benzoic acid (a primary component of cranberry juice) lower the pH in the food, which results in an unfavorable environment for most microorganisms. Still others, like potassium sorbate, prevent microorganisms from growing. Acidulants like citric acid (found naturally in orange juice and many other fruits and their products) are added to citrus-flavored soft drinks to impart a tart flavor sensation as well as to act as a preservative (see Insert 11.7).

Additives are incorporated into food products for many reasons other than as preservatives. Antibiotics show up in milk as residues of treatments given to prevent diseases in dairy cows. Anticaking agents are added to powders to prevent clumping, such as the addition of calcium

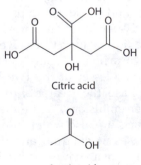

Citric acid

Acetic acid

INSERT 11.7
Chemical structures of acids found in natural and formulated foods. Citric acid is the primary acid in citrus fruits and carbonated beverages. We most commonly consume acetic acid in vinegar.

silicate to sodium chloride so that it will flow smoothly when the relative humidity (RH) is high. Antioxidants prevent fats from becoming rancid because rancid fats smell bad and can become toxic. **Sequestrants** or chelating agents like sodium tripolyphosphate bind metal ions, preventing them from oxidizing fats that would cause flavor problems. Gums are a class of chemicals that serve as texturizers helping to make ice creams and yogurts smooth.

Many foods and beverages that we consume are **dispersions** (a discontinuous phase dispersed in a continuous phase). For example, milk is a dispersion of lipid in water. A milk fat globule is composed of triacylglycerols layered by proteins and encapsulated by a plasma membrane. Milk, as it comes out of the gland, is not a stable dispersion. Left out, the milk fat globules (the discontinuous phase), which are less dense than the water (the continuous phase), float to the top of the milk. This fat can be skimmed of the top of the milk with the fatty portion called the cream and the remaining watery product the serum (or skimmed milk). To prevent this separation, milk processors **homogenize** the milk by disintegrating the fat globules into tiny fat particles that are too small to **coalesce** (come together) and rise to the top.

Dispersions can consist of a phase of one state (gas, liquid, or solid) dispersed in the phase of another. For example, a solid dispersed in a liquid is called either a solution or a suspension. True solutions are homogeneous mixtures with the individual molecules of the solute (solid discontinuous phase) dissolved in the solvent (liquid continuous phase). **Suspensions** are less stable than solutions. Colloidal suspensions are formed when bigger particles are dispersed in a liquid, but the particles are still not visible to the naked eye. Liquid spreads are colloidal suspensions called sols with fat globules dispersed in liquid oil. Jelly is also a colloidal suspension of pectin in a sugar solution with water as the solvent. A semisolid colloidal suspension like jelly is called a gel. Other interesting dispersions are foams like whipped cream (air dispersed in liquid fat), aerosols like breath spray (liquid flavorants dispersed in air), and smoke (solid particles dispersed in air).

The most common food dispersion is an emulsion, which consists of a dispersion of two **immiscible** liquids (don't dissolve in each other). Emulsions can be subdivided into two primary types—oil-in-water and water-in-oil. The discontinuous phase (the lesser of the two liquids by volume) is dispersed in the continuous phase (the greater of the two liquids). Salad dressings tend to be oil-in-water emulsions, while mayonnaise is a water-in-oil emulsion. Chocolate products are also water-in-oil emulsions formed when both the oil and water phases were liquid and then cooled to form a solid product. Since the two liquids of an emulsion are immiscible, help is needed to form the emulsion. Physical methods can be used to form this emulsion, such as vigorous shaking of oil and vinegar to form a salad dressing. Unfortunately, these two liquid phases separate quickly.

Food additives known as stabilizers are used to form and maintain a dispersion. Emulsifiers are specific stabilizers used to form and maintain an

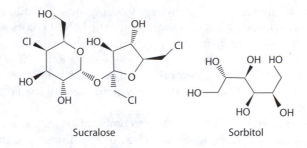

Sucralose   Sorbitol

INSERT 11.8
Chemical structures of artificial sweeteners in foods.

emulsion. Emulsifiers are classified according to their hydrophile/lipophile balance (HLB) index. A high HLB indicates that the emulsifier is more soluble in water than in oil and would be more suitable for use in an oil-in-water emulsion while one with a low HLB would be more effective in water-in-oil emulsions. Phospholipids like lecithin are particularly effective emulsifiers as there are both hydrophilic and lipophilic ends in the molecule.

As consumers become more health conscious, they want less sugar and fat in their products, but they still want full flavor. Food scientists use many classes of additives to help achieve these objectives. Bulking agents like starches and maltodextrin are added to compensate for the fats that are removed during the making of low-fat foods. Fat replacers like sucrose polyesters (e.g., Olestra in the fat-free potato chips) must be able to substitute many functions of fats, including flavor, mouthfeel, and cooking properties. Few compounds can perform all of these functions. Thickeners are added to foods to provide a pleasant mouthfeel. They have been particularly effective in making skim milk products more appealing. Artificial sweeteners like aspartame (NutraSweet) and sucralose (Splenda) replace sugars, permitting dieters and diabetics the opportunity to eat sweet foods without guilt (see Insert 11.8).

11.2.8 Colors and Flavors

Natural and artificial colorants differ in structure and stability. Nature provides a wide range of colors including the reds of lycopene in watermelons and heme in uncooked steaks to the oranges of β-carotene in carrots and astaxanthin in salmon. Plant pigments include the yellows of xanthophylls in summer squash, the greens of chlorophyll in broccoli, and the blues of anthocyanins in blue corn and blueberries. Brown pigments are formed enzymatically in a cut apple or nonenzymatically in golden brown pancakes. Unfortunately, many of these compounds are unstable under most processing conditions and even during storage of fresh, whole foods. Many times, the color is lost when the flavor, texture, safety, and nutrition are still fine. Consumers may throw away perfectly good food because it does not look "right."

Because of the instability of many natural pigments, food scientists frequently rely on artificial colorants to produce the bright colors so important in beverages, candies, and breakfast cereals. These artificial colorants are listed in the ingredient statement (e.g., Yellow #6 and Red #40). They provide a bright color at very low concentrations. These artificial dyes are derived from petroleum products and are carefully regulated by the Food and Drug Administration (see Insert 11.9).

Flavor can be narrowly defined as the combination of the senses of taste and smell or broadly defined to encompass all sensations encountered in the eating experience. Taste occurs when specific compounds come in contact with receptors on the tongue. Sugars and artificial sweeteners interact with sweet receptors, whereas acids interact with sour receptors. Bitter perception is stimulated by many compounds, including caffeine, theobromine (responsible for bitterness in chocolate), quinine, and humulone (a component of hops that contributes to bitterness in beer). Sodium chloride is the most common chemical affecting saltiness perception.

Aromatic compounds contribute to a full-flavor sensation. Character-impact compounds are chemicals associated with a particular product such as benzaldehyde in cherries and almonds, isoamyl acetate in bananas, and methyl anthranilate in grapes. Many foods are complex mixtures of many aromatic compounds, none of which qualify as character-impact compounds.

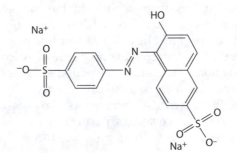

Yellow #6

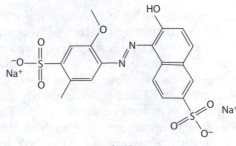

Red #40

INSERT 11.9
Chemical structures of two artificial food colors found in many formulated foods.

Limonene is a compound that contributes to the flavor of many fruit products, but it is not distinctive for any fruit. Most meat flavors develop during the cooking process. Among these heat-generated compounds are the pyrazine compounds associated with **Maillard browning**, which contributes to the golden to brown colors of beer, bread crust, chocolate, coffee, French fries, maple syrup, pastries, and toast.

Although most flavors are colorless and most colors are flavorless, the browning-reaction products also contribute to flavor. In addition to taste and aroma compounds, other components are responsible for the sensations we experience as spicy heat, coolness, pungency, and astringency. The heat of hot peppers is attributed to capsaicin, and menthol provides the cooling sensation of mints. Onion pungency is attributed to sulfur compounds, and tannins are responsible for the astringency of tea and unripe persimmons (see Insert 11.10).

Numerous chemical compounds contribute to the flavor of fresh and cooked whole foods. Extracted natural flavors or added artificial flavors are present in formulated foods. Thus, individual compounds serve as flavor additives in these foods. Vanillin is a synthetic compound that is added to foods to provide vanilla flavor. Many fruit-flavored beverages, soft drinks, and frozen desserts use extracted or synthesized chemicals to convey a particular flavor. Character-impact compounds can be used for these applications. The

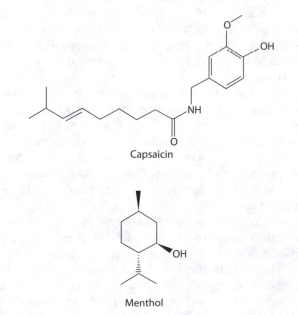

Capsaicin

Menthol

INSERT 11.10
Chemical structures of natural compounds responsible for chemical feeling factors. Capsaicin provides the heat in hot peppers and menthol gives us the cooling sensation in mints, candies, and cough drops.

addition of specific compounds that are not normally found together can produce unique flavor sensations.

Other compounds, like monosodium glutamate (MSG) and maltol are flavor enhancers. At high concentrations, MSG has a unique taste (called umami), but at lower concentrations, it brings out flavors, particularly meaty/brothy flavors. Maltol, a component of sweet potatoes and the character-impact compound for cotton candy, is a product of nonenzymatic browning and can enhance flavors in sweet products. Flavor compounds are delicate and can be easily inactivated by enzymes during storage of fresh items or by heat processing. Interaction with oxygen or light can also change flavor compounds.

11.3 Sources of Food Chemicals

11.3.1 Plants

The chemicals in some foods we derive from plants go far beyond the pesticides that normally come to mind. Solanine in green potatoes and amygdalin (a compound that releases cyanide) in apricot and peach pits are among the many naturally occurring toxins. Organic acids like citric acid in citrus fruits and benzoic acid in cranberry products are effective natural preservatives. Caffeine is a bitter chemical extracted from the coffee bean and cola nut to stimulate our senses. Plant pigments are chemicals. Pigments like chlorophyll make lettuce green, lycopene makes tomatoes red, and anthocyanins make grapes purple.

More than 200 chemical compounds contribute to the flavor of fresh-squeezed orange juice and even more may be found in a glass of wine or a slice of ripened cheese. Vitamins A and C are important nutrients found in fruits and vegetables. Grains provide carbohydrates; soybeans and peanuts are good sources of protein and oil. Papain is an enzyme that can be extracted from papayas and used as a natural meat tenderizer. The most abundant chemical in plants, however, is water, which can be as high as 96% in lettuce and cucumber.

We don't eat whole plants, but we do eat raw plant parts, processed plant parts, or ingredients derived from plant parts. Harvested plant products like fruits, vegetables, grains, and oilseeds are living tissues. As a result, these tissues are undergoing chemical and biochemical changes owing to the metabolic activities driven primarily by enzymes. The genetic differences between species (wheat vs. rye) or variety (Red Delicious vs. Gala apples) will also affect these changes. Chemical reactions can also be affected by the plant part (organ) like a broccoli head (flower), celery stalk (stem), corn (seed), and carrot (root). Microbes on the plant can lead to decay by breaking down the chemical components of cell walls and membranes.

Physiological changes in metabolic activities occur in a fruit or vegetable from initial development to refrigerated storage. During growth and development of plants, rapid changes are occurring as those parts of the plant change from inedible to edible. One of the most dramatic changes occurs during fruit ripening. After pollination of the flower, a tiny fruit forms. This fruit grows in size as cells divide rapidly and minerals are taken in through the roots and stems. Then, a series of complex metabolic reactions occur to produce

- The pigments that provide its color
- Volatile compounds for the aromatic component of flavor
- Conversion of starch to sugar to provide sweetness
- Breakdown of cell walls to induce softening
- Synthesis of vitamins
- Numerous other compounds that affect its quality

Another dramatic physiological event is the separation of the organ from the parent plant. Chemical signals from the detached plant organ, particularly from the simple gas ethylene, cause major changes in enzymatic activity, leading to a cascade of chemical reactions. The mechanical damage caused by cutting, impact, and vibration increases these signals as well as breaks apart the delicate membranes around and inside each cell that maintain the normal metabolic reactions. Too much mechanical damage can cause visible bruising and lower the quality of the produce.

Physiological and microbial changes in the plant organ are affected by environmental conditions like temperature and RH. Generally speaking, the lower the temperature, the slower the chemical reactions in the cell and the longer the shelf life. Most fruits and vegetables have a range of RH that is best for that item. If the RH is too low, it will wilt or shrivel; if the RH is too high, microbes can grow more rapidly, and the item will deteriorate more quickly. Each day that a fresh fruit or vegetable is stored, there will be a loss in sensory and nutritional quality.

During the processing of plant organs, there are several unit operations that cause changes in the chemical composition of that fruit or vegetable. Washing or soaking operations remove microbes; however, the water can remove (called leaching) soluble minerals and vitamins, reducing the nutritional value of the product. Cutting and slicing operations can increase enzymatic activity, causing unacceptable texture, off-flavors, product discoloration, and a loss of nutrients.

Heating bleaches pigments, softens cell walls, and changes flavor compounds. If we compare a raw green bean with a canned green bean in our minds, we can see the difference between the two. Heating is also very destructive to vitamins and minerals. On the other hand, heating inactivates

Introducing Food Science

the enzymes in the product that cause it to deteriorate, and therefore canned products are more stable than fresh products.

Drying is usually a more gentle process than heating, although some heating may be involved. Some of the same chemical reactions may occur in drying as in heating, but the biggest change is in the loss of water. As water is lost, other chemicals become more concentrated. Water loss causes an increase in some reactions like browning of sugars and oxidation of lipids but a decrease in others (such as enzymatic reactions) because these reactions require water to function effectively. Freezing is a more gentle food process than heating and drying, leading to much slower chemical reactions during frozen storage. If a frozen food is held for a long time, however, even small changes can add up to quality losses.

11.3.2 Animals

Food from animals is also composed of chemicals. Most of the meat and fish we consume is muscle tissue. Muscle tissue contains fat, protein, vitamins, minerals, and hormones but very little carbohydrate. Meat flavor is produced by the chemical reactions that are induced by heating. Heat changes chemicals already present (called precursors) into volatile compounds that we associate with the flavor of cooked meat. The type of cooking (roasting, frying, and baking) affects the temperature and the types of reactions and reaction products that occur, thus affecting the flavor. As with plants, the most abundant chemical in muscle is water (70%–80%). The chemical composition of muscle tissue is similar to the chemical composition of our bodies, making them much more complete sources of essential nutrients than plant products. Other foods from animal origin include milk, eggs, and organs (liver, kidney, etc.). These foods are very good sources of protein, vitamins, and minerals.

Unlike fresh plant tissues, animal products are not living. Physiological changes in muscle tissue are associated with the physiology of death. After harvest, two major proteins in muscle tissue, actin and myosin, react with each other to form a thick, tough complex called actomyosin during the development of rigor mortis. The presence of actomyosin causes toughness in meat, particularly beef and pork. The larger the animal, the longer and more severe the toughening effect. Rigor is resolved by conditioning the meat at low temperatures to allow natural enzymes called proteases to break down the actomyosin at sites away from the main point of attachment of the actin and myosin.

Meats, milk, and eggs are very rich sources of nutrients for consumers and for microbes. Meats are perishable because the microbes use their enzymes to convert the nutritious chemicals (known as substrates) in the meat to slime, off-colors, off-odors, off-flavors, and other reaction products that make the meat less desirable. Some metabolic disorders in the meat itself can result in poor quality meat. One example is pale, soft, exudative (PSE) pork. The pork is soft and mushy because of a rapid decrease in the pH of the meat right after slaughter.

Processing is very important in meat products because it prevents the growth of spoilage and harmful microbes. Processing also causes changes in flavor, color, and texture. Since we typically eat most of our meats cooked, we associate many of these changes with improvements in quality. The red color of wieners and bologna is produced by addition of nitrates and nitrites, which are added to inhibit the growth of microbes as well as to stabilize meat color. Drying removes water and provides unique flavor sensations by encouraging specific chemical reactions in intermediate-moisture products such as pepperoni and moist pet foods. Freezing of meats slows the growth of microbes and preserves the flavor, color, and texture of fresh meats. Many meat products, like chicken nuggets and surimi (ground fish), use ground muscle tissue and rely on proteins to form gels to help in holding the muscle fibers together.

As indicated earlier, pasteurization of milk and eggs kills harmful microbes but does not kill all the spoilage microbes. This process changes the flavor of the milk or egg and may decrease the nutritional quality. In most processes, particularly those involving heat, food scientists are willing to trade off some loss in nutritional quality to keep the food safe and extend its shelf life. Although processed meats, milk, and eggs are much more stable than their fresh counterparts, the fats in these products can become oxidized and cause off-flavors and toxic compounds.

11.4 Toxic Compounds in Foods

As we learned in Chapter 1, some foods can make us sick because toxic compounds in foods come in many forms. The most likely chemicals in foods that can make us sick are the toxins produced by bacteria and molds (see Insert 11.11). Pesticides in foods are also toxic. Fortunately, pesticides permitted in foods are chosen for their ability to break down rapidly into nontoxic reaction products before purchase and consumption. Most pesticides are very toxic to pests in the field, but, if handled properly, they are not toxic to consumers.

The toxicity of a chemical is related to its dose. Most of us consume minute amounts of toxic compounds daily without feeling their effects because the dose is less than what was needed to make us sick. Some compounds, like the botulinum toxin, are so powerful that very small doses can make us ill and even cause death. On the other hand, micronutrients, like vitamin A and many minerals, which are necessary for life, can be toxic when consumed at

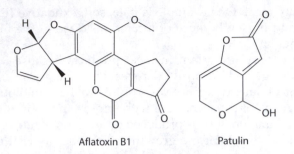

Aflatoxin B1   Patulin

INSERT 11.11
Chemical structures of mycotoxins in foods. Mycotoxins are produced by molds.

high concentrations. Thus, food scientists must not only know which compounds are toxic, but they must also determine the toxic dosage level. Toxic compounds are carefully monitored, and any compound that is a known carcinogen cannot be used in foods.

11.5 An Integrated Approach to Food Chemistry

One thing that makes food chemistry so interesting is that foods are complex mixtures of many chemical compounds. As a result, there are many chemical reactions that can occur in foods—some of them are desirable, and many are undesirable. It is not sufficient to know about individual chemical compounds in a food, but rather we must know how chemical compounds react with each other in the environment within a food product and as influenced by environmental factors. Such reactions could lead to compromised safety, loss of nutritional quality, or loss of sensory quality.

Safety hazards develop from the production of a toxic compound usually produced by a microbe, but the presence of a natural toxin or development of a toxin during storage is also hazardous to our health. Solanine is a toxic alkaloid that can develop in potatoes exposed to light. Fortunately, toxic potatoes tend to turn green (production of chlorophyll) under the same conditions, providing a warning to observant consumers. Another protection for the consumer is that solanine is readily inactivated by heat such as baking, boiling, or frying. Toxic compounds can enter a food from package materials or the interaction of the food with the primary package. Food scientists carefully screen package materials and study food/package interactions to make sure that the products are safe.

Loss of sensory quality of a food is the result of an increase in an undesirable characteristic or a decrease in a desirable characteristic. Development of slime on wieners, yellowing of lettuce and broccoli, and objectionable aromas in milk are all undesirable characteristics that signal poor quality. More subtle changes such as softening of bananas, loss of bright red color in strawberry jam, or decreased flavor of fresh tomatoes are all examples of losses of desirable characteristics. Frequently, an undesirable characteristic develops as a desirable characteristic is lost. All of these characteristics can be traced back to specific chemical reactions.

Food chemists can measure the loss of a reactant or the accumulation of a product in a chemical reaction to predict the loss of quality. Food engineers use these data to calculate the rate of deterioration using chemical kinetics. Many reactions in foods can be classified as zero-order (linear degradation such as nonenzymatic browning) or first-order (semilogarithmic such as loss of vitamins or lipid oxidation) reactions. Food engineers can then use equations to estimate the shelf life of a product under typical handling and storage conditions and develop an expiration date for the product.

11.6 Remember This!

- The toxicity of a chemical compound is related to its dose.
- Flavor can be narrowly defined as the combination of the senses of taste and smell or broadly defined to encompass all sensations encountered in the eating experience.
- Natural and artificial colorants differ in structure and stability.
- The most common food dispersion is an emulsion, which consists of a dispersion of two immiscible liquids.
- Functionality of ingredients is defined as the physicochemical properties that affect its performance in a food product during processing, storage, and preparation.
- Chemical preservatives provide one of the oldest and most effective defenses against microbial activity in foods.
- Chemical modification of amino acid side chains alters functional properties of the proteins, which, in turn, alters the physicochemical properties of the food.
- Lipid oxidation is a reaction of lipids with molecular oxygen that proceeds through a free-radical mechanism.
- Starches can be chemically modified to improve ingredient functionality.
- All foods are composed of chemicals—edible chemicals, but chemicals nonetheless.

11.7 Looking Ahead

This chapter introduced us to food chemistry. Chapter 12 will introduce nutrition, Chapter 13 will discuss food microbiology, and Chapter 14 will cover food engineering, including the design of processes to protect us from disease and foods from spoilage caused by unwanted microorganisms. Chapter 15 will describe the science associated with the use of human subjects to evaluate the quality of food products.

Testing Comprehension

1. Identify five food products that represent a wide range of water concentrations. How does water level in a food affect its quality and how it is processed? What is the preservation principle for each of these products?

2. Describe the benefits and detriments of high-carbohydrate foods. What foods are likely to be high in carbohydrates? Which ones are likely to be low in carbohydrates? Which is healthier, a high-carbohydrate diet or a low-carbohydrate diet? Why?

3. List all of the effects of lipids on our health. What determines whether a lipid is beneficial or detrimental? What foods should we incorporate into and eliminate from our diets to improve our lipid profile?

4. Compare and contrast the chemical nature of proteins and vitamins. How are they digested? How are they used by the body?

5. Outline the functions of enzymes in our foods, our digestive tract, our blood, and our cells. Identify the beneficial and detrimental aspects of enzymes. What would happen if all enzyme activity ceased?

6. Select four preservatives and four additional food additives from ingredient statements of a favorite food product. Identify at least one function of each of these ingredients. How many of these additives are chemical in nature? How could the label of these products be cleaned up without losing the function of each additive?

7. Differentiate between the terms *chemical*, *compound*, and *molecule* with respect to their use in the popular and scientific literature. Rank these three from most dangerous to least dangerous. Explain the rationale for this ranking.

8. Analyze the rationale for using artificial flavors and colors instead of natural flavors and colors. What types of products are more likely to contain artificial ingredients? What types of products are more likely to contain natural ingredients?

9. Calculate the number of ounces of creamed potatoes Jennifer who weighs 110 pounds and Kyle at 183 pounds would need to eat to become sick if the potatoes had been stored in the light accumulating 18 milligrams of solanine per 100 grams of potato. The recipe they used for their home-made potatoes included 4 pounds of potatoes, 1/4 cup of margarine, 1 ounce of soft soy cheese, and 1/2 cup almond milk. A dose of 2 milligrams per kilogram body weight could produce severe gastroenteritis and a dose of 5 milligrams per kilogram body weight can be lethal. How likely would it be that either Jennifer or Kyle could become sick or die? What could they do to minimize their risk of solanine poisoning? Are there any warning signs that could have helped them realize the danger?

10. Critique the popular idea that we should avoid any food product with an ingredient with an unpronounceable name or more than five ingredients. Also critique the premise of this chapter that "chemicals are not to be feared but rather to be understood." Which of these two concepts makes the most sense? Why?

Further Reading

Brady, J. W., 2013. *Introductory Food Chemistry*, Ithaca, NY: Cornell University Press.

Coultate, T., 2008. *Food: The Chemistry of Its Components*, 5th ed., Cambridge: Royal Society of Chemistry.

Damodaran, S., K. L. Parkin and O. R. Fennema, 2007. *Fennema's Food Chemistry*, 4th ed., Boca Raton, FL: CRC Press.

deMan, J. M., 1999. *Principles of Food Chemistry*, 3rd ed., Gaithersburg, MD: Aspen Publishers, Inc.

Hui, Y. H., 2007. *Food Chemistry: Principles and Applications*, 2nd ed., West Sacramento, CA: Science Technology System.

Pollan, M., 2009. *Food Rules*, New York: Penguin Books.

Singh, R. P., 2000. Scientific principles of shelf-life evaluation, in *Shelf-Life Evaluation of Foods*, 2nd ed., Editors C.M.D. Man and A.A. Jones. Gaithersburg, MD: Aspen Publishers, Inc.

USDA-ARS, 2014. National Nutrient Database for Standard Reference. Release 26. The National Agricultural Library. Available at http://ndb.nal.usda.gov/.

12

Nutrition

Leah is very interested in the contribution of specific foods to the growing obesity problem in America. She has read many diet books, and they seem to contradict one another. She wants to get a better perspective, based on true scientific data and not on propaganda. For her senior thesis project, she decided to research the physiological mechanisms that lead to obesity. As she got into her library research, she found that nutrition was only one part of the obesity problem.

Jennifer is now interested in the health benefits of whole grains, fruits, and vegetables. When they changed the food pyramid to MyPlate, she noticed that plant products took on an added importance. She was also beginning to realize that, as a vegan, she had to be careful or she might miss out on some essential nutrients. She was still a vegan and needed to be careful that she was eating a balanced diet and that she was getting enough calories to maintain her weight.

Kyle learned about food ingredients when he worked as part of a team that designed an edible soup bowl. One of the most interesting things they studied was nutrient loss during formulation and processing. He wanted to learn more about how nutrients are lost during manufacturing and storage and what could be done to prevent these losses from happening. Upon completion of his degree, Kyle plans to go to graduate school to learn more about the interrelationship between nutrition and food chemistry and then to work in the food industry to prevent the loss of nutrients during the processing of foods.

Leah, Jennifer, and Kyle are learning more about nutrition and how it interfaces with food science. Although food scientists aren't nutritionists, they must understand basic nutrition to properly evaluate food products and processes because many of the activities food scientists perform affect the nutritional quality of a product. Many times, these activities require trade-offs between nutrition and some other factor like sensory quality or shelf stability.

12.1 Looking Back

Chapter 11 focused on the function of chemicals in foods. This chapter expands that idea to the function of food chemicals when they are consumed. The following key points were covered in previous chapters and will help prepare us to understand the nutritional aspects of foods:

- Functionality of ingredients is defined as the physicochemical properties that affect its performance in a food product during processing, storage, and preparation.

- Chemical modification of amino acid side chains alters the functional properties of the proteins that, in turn, alter the physicochemical properties of the food.

- Each food label must have an ingredient statement; a net weight; an address of the processor, distributor, or importer; and the name of the product that can be clearly understood by the consumer.

- The unlimited supply of food in college dining halls and other facilities on campus is frequently cited as a major cause of the Freshman Fifteen.

- Diets containing gluten are more likely to provide the nutrients we need than gluten-free diets.

- The conditions that affect nutritional value also affect sensory quality.

- The higher the temperature of a heat process with the shorter time needed to kill the intended microbes, the less the loss of nutrients.

- Food processing and preservation increase the shelf stability of a raw material usually at the cost of nutrition and quality.

- Although many of us try to eat healthy, there are many temptations and influences affecting our food choices that we do not consciously consider.

- Good nutrition involves adequate consumption of required nutrients in the context of moderate energy intake.

12.2 Nutrients in Foods

As we learned in Chapter 2, the main function of food is to provide us with the energy we need. The energy in food comes in the form of calories (technically speaking, kilocalories). We can obtain kilocalories from four sources—carbohydrates, lipids, proteins, and ethanol. Dieticians recommend that our kilocalories come from a balance of foods and not a single source. Too many or too few kilocalories can cause severe health problems and can even lead to death. Likewise, too much reliance on any one of the four sources of energy can cause disease, either from consuming too much of something or from not consuming enough of certain nutrients. The most serious nutritional problem affecting Americans and Western Europeans is related to the consumption of too many kilocalories.

In many parts of the world, the most serious nutritional problem is consuming too few kilocalories. When we consume too few kilocalories, we are unlikely to consume adequate amounts of vitamins and minerals. Vitamins and minerals do not provide kilocalories, but, rather, they are key components of the metabolic processes needed to perform daily functions. Without them, we would be unable to stretch and contract our muscles so that we can breathe, eat, walk, talk, perform other movements, and conduct numerous other life activities that we take for granted. Without sufficient levels of mineral cofactors and vitamin coenzymes, our bodies would develop deficiency diseases such as anemia and pellagra.

Other substances have nutritional implications in our bodies. Dietary fiber does not provide energy, nor does it function as an enzyme cofactor, but it helps prevent constipation and has been associated with the prevention of or decrease in the incidence of a number of diseases, from varicose veins to colon cancer. Oxygen and water are essential to the maintenance of life. Many other components, such as antioxidants and dietary supplements, are also thought to contribute to health, but their role is not as clearly defined.

12.2.1 Proteins

As we learned in Chapter 11, proteins are composed of amino acids. Our bodies are constantly turning over proteins (breaking down old proteins and building new ones). We can synthesize many, but not all, of these amino acids. Those protein components that the body can't synthesize are called essential amino acids (shown in Insert 12.1). If an essential amino acid is not available, either from the recycling of the ones from old proteins or from dietary sources, protein synthesis cannot continue. Animal proteins are much more likely to have a balance of essential amino acids than plant proteins. Protein is also more abundant in muscle foods than in fruits, vegetables, and grains. Thus, vegans must get their proteins from different sources to ensure that they have an appropriate mix of essential amino acids. Fortunately, with a little study, this balance is not difficult to achieve.

During digestion, the proteins are broken down into individual amino acids in the intestines and absorbed across the intestinal mucosa into the bloodstream. Then, the individual amino acids are then transported to the tissues and cells where they are assembled back into proteins. Among the many important roles that proteins play in our bodies are as structural

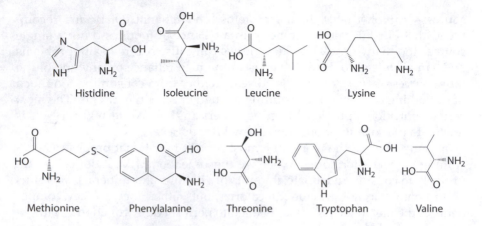

INSERT 12.1
Chemical structures of the essential amino acids.

components of muscles and as metabolic enzymes. Although proteins are an essential part of the diet, problems can develop when too much protein is consumed. The use of proteins as an energy source results in the production of ketone bodies leading to bad breath associated with ketoacidosis and the excretion of urea in the urine. The presence of excess ketones in the body and urea in the urine is unhealthy as it is an indication of insufficient glucose for the brain and can lead to a coma or even death.

12.2.2 Lipids

As described in Chapter 11, fats and oils are lipids. In the diet, we generally refer to all lipids as fats. Fats are critical components of our bodies; we could not function without them. As described in Chapter 2, fats provide twice the energy per gram as carbohydrates and proteins. They are compact sources of kilocalories, which can be quite convenient on long hikes where weight and volume are a concern. Fats contribute to the overconsumption of energy, however, particularly among sedentary consumers. Fats are also associated with the accumulation of undesirable lipids in the arteries, contributing to heart disease.

Lipids are found in every cell of our bodies. The plasma membrane surrounding each cell and the membranes within each cell contain phospholipids, cholesterol, and specialized proteins. When we consume excess food, our bodies can convert that food to lipids. This reserve lipid is stored for times when we do not have enough food, is burned to keep us warm (thermogenesis), and is used as a padding to protect vital organs. Prolonged overconsumption of kilocalories leads to excess padding. This excess padding is additional weight that stresses the heart, skeletal muscles, and other organs. These additional burdens can make exercise difficult, which, in turn, makes the problem worse.

We need to consume lipids for the essential fatty acids they provide and because lipid-soluble vitamins cannot be absorbed unless there is sufficient lipid in the intestinal tract to permit absorption. Vitamins A, D, E, and K are the lipid-soluble vitamins. Our bodies cannot synthesize essential fatty acids, so they must be consumed in the diet. These fatty acids are needed to synthesize phospholipids, the major component of cell membranes (see Insert 12.2).

Sterols are also very important in our bodies. Cholesterol, which is found only in animal products, and other sterols help stabilize cell membranes. Consumption of plant sterols is associated with lowering blood cholesterol, particularly low-density lipoproteins as the plant sterols are more readily absorbed across the intestine than cholesterol. Sterols are also needed for proper brain function and to produce key hormones such as progesterone and testosterone. In an effort to reduce kilocalories by cutting our lipid consumption drastically (e.g., less than 10% of total kilocalories), we may be trading one problem (too many kilocalories) for a more serious one (a vitamin deficiency).

Too much lipid in the diet can be a problem. In addition to contributing to an overconsumption of kilocalories, cholesterol can also accumulate in our arteries and cause heart disease. Heart attacks are caused by either thrombosis (blood flow is blocked because of clotting of platelets) or atherosclerosis (a buildup of plaque thickens arterial walls). A blood test can check the level of lipoproteins in the blood and indicate a consumer's risk of heart disease. The presence of a higher proportion of high-density lipoproteins (HDLs) is

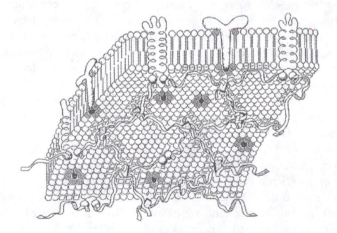

INSERT 12.2
Schematic of a cellular membrane. A membrane is composed of a phospholipid (lollipop-like structures with a water-soluble head group on both surfaces of the membrane and two fatty acids in its interior) bilayer spanned by proteins (structures that cross from one side of the membrane to the other) and sugars (the ribbon-like structures coming out of the bottom of the membrane). (From Tuszynski, J.A. and Kurzynski, M., *Introduction to Molecular Biophysics*, Boca Raton, FL: CRC Press Taylor & Francis Group, 2003. With permission.)

an indicator of a reduced risk of heart disease. A higher proportion of low-density lipoproteins (LDLs) and total cholesterol are indicators of a greater risk of the disease.

Evidence is growing that the presence of oxidized lipids in the arteries increases the risk of heart disease, suggesting that the consumption of anti-oxidant vitamins will help lower the risk of heart disease. Unfortunately, experiments relating increased consumption of antioxidant vitamins to heart disease have not been conclusive. Some of the most common contributors to heart disease are body weight, diabetes, gender, genetics, high blood pressure, and smoking (including secondhand smoke). In general, we have more control over the lipids we put into our mouths than any of the other risk factors.

As we have learned earlier, fats and oils contribute to the flavor and enjoyment of our foods. For those who enjoy eating but don't want to consume too many kilocalories, food scientists have developed fat replacers. If fat replacers are used as part of an overall plan to cut kilocalories, they can be useful. Too often, however, the consumption of food made with fat replacers provides us with an excuse to eat more food and not reduce kilocalories at all. Fat replacers may lead to other problems: sucrose esters can cause loose stools and other digestive difficulties when consumed in excess.

12.2.3 Carbohydrates

Carbohydrates should be our primary source of kilocalories. Carbohydrates include sugars, starches, and nondigestible cell-wall materials. Starches are broken down into simple sugars before absorption. Our bloodstream circulates glucose, a simple sugar, which is essential to proper brain function. Any excess glucose is converted to glycogen, which is an "animal starch." Glycogen is stored in the muscles as a source of immediate energy reserves. Since our muscles have limited capacity to store glycogen, additional excess glucose is converted to body fat or muscle protein.

Nondigestible cell-wall materials are the components of dietary fiber. Although fiber is not absorbed into the bloodstream, it has an important dietary function. Dietary fiber helps maintain peristalsis (keeping the material moving in our bowels). The slowing or stopping of peristalsis leads to constipation. Constipation, in addition to the discomfort it can bring, has been associated with a range of diseases and disorders, including varicose veins. Fiber is also an excellent binder of toxins, as well as some nutrients in our foods. Although the binding of toxins can protect our bodies, excess fiber consumption limits the absorption of essential vitamins and minerals. Few Americans, however, are guilty of consuming excess amounts of dietary fiber.

Unlike proteins and lipids, there are no essential carbohydrates that we need to consume, but we must have glucose circulating in our bodies. Insulin and glucagon are the hormones responsible for regulating sugar metabolism. Our bodies must properly regulate the levels of glucose in our bloodstream. Diabetes is a disease that results from an inability to maintain normal blood-sugar levels. Too much glucose in the blood over long periods can lead to blindness, or it can damage nerves and blood vessels, requiring amputation of the hands and feet. Too little glucose in the blood, or hypoglycemia, when untreated can lead to fainting, seizures, brain damage, and even death. Amino acids can be converted to energy sources, but they cannot provide enough glucose to adequately maintain brain function. Since too much protein and too much lipid can cause dietary problems, that leaves carbohydrates as our best energy source.

The consumption of too much carbohydrate is also a problem. Products high in sugar, such as pies, cakes, and candies, are quick sources of energy that are very appealing. We can consume them rapidly without feeling full. There is strong evidence to suggest that the level of glucose in our blood helps regulate our feeling of fullness. We can consume large amounts of sugar or starchy treats, however, before we receive the signal to stop consumption, which, over time, can lead to weight gain. Sugar replacers present the same advantages and disadvantages as fat replacers described in Section 12.2.2. Diabetics must be particularly careful of consumption of excess carbohydrates to prevent elevated blood-sugar levels soon after a meal followed by a sugar crash when the glucose is eventually broken down. Additionally, excess sugar on the teeth can cause dental caries (cavities).

12.2.4 Vitamins and Minerals

In our bodies, vitamins are cofactors to enzymes. Without these cofactors, enzymes can't catalyze reactions, and our metabolism is affected. Prolonged deficiency of these vitamins leads to the diseases discussed in earlier chapters. Many vitamins, including the B vitamins and vitamin C, are soluble in water. These vitamins are added to most foods but are susceptible to leaching during processing operations. Like vitamins, minerals also serve as cofactors in enzyme-catalyzed reactions in our bodies. Minerals also become parts of important molecules, such as the calcium in our bones, phosphorus in our cell membranes, and iron in our blood. Usually, they enter our bodies as parts of other chemicals (both organic and inorganic) in our foods. The difference between a vitamin and a mineral is that vitamins are compounds containing carbon while minerals are elements.

The usefulness of a vitamin or a mineral depends on its bioavailability. Bioavailability refers to how much of a vitamin or mineral can actually be used by the body. First, the vitamin or mineral must be absorbed in our intestinal tract. A food enters our body through our mouths, but, with the exception of dietary fiber, its nutrients don't function in the body unless they are absorbed. Some chemicals, like oxalic acid in spinach and rhubarb, inhibit absorption of nutrients; other chemicals, like ascorbic acid (vitamin C), enhance absorption of minerals, particularly iron. As indicated above, some lipids are necessary for the absorption of lipid-soluble vitamins. The chemical form of a nutrient also affects its absorption. Even when a nutrient is absorbed, there is no guarantee that it will be used by the body, and certain forms of nutrients are more likely to be used than others.

Although vitamins and minerals are essential to health, overconsumption can be dangerous. Lipid-soluble vitamins like A, D, and E can be toxic at levels not that much higher than those required. For example, too much vitamin D can cause hypercalcemia, which is an irreversible accumulation of calcium in the kidneys, heart, and lungs. Excess lipid-soluble vitamins are not excreted but are deposited in body fat. Most water-soluble vitamins are excreted in the urine when consumed in excess and do not pose a health threat. Likewise, we can overconsume minerals. For example, too much iron can cause increased oxidation of lipids in the body and can interfere with the absorption of zinc, and too much magnesium interferes with the absorption of calcium and iron.

12.2.5 Water and Electrolytes

Water neither contributes to calories nor serves as a cofactor in enzyme reactions, but it is a necessary chemical in our bodies. Too little water and we become dehydrated, but too much water dilutes our electrolytes resulting in water toxicity and potentially death. Water is a major component of most foods except vegetable oils. It is even present in dried foods such as flour and dried fruits.

Electrolytes are ionic forms of minerals, generally found in beverages like sports drinks. The electrolyte that we need in our cells is potassium (K^+), whereas the one found in our bloodstream is sodium (Na^+). Chloride (Cl^-) is also a common electrolyte found in conjunction with both K^+ and Na^+. For every positive charge in the body, there must be a corresponding negative charge. When table salt (NaCl), the most abundant source of sodium in our diets, is dissolved in water, it dissociates into Na^+ and Cl^-. As the primary electrolyte in intracellular fluids, potassium is a critical nutrient in our diets. Fortunately, we can find a ready source in fruits and their juices, vegetables, sports drinks, and milk.

Low levels of K^+ or high levels of Na^+ lead to high blood pressure since it is the balance of K^+ and Na^+ that determines the blood pressure. K^+ is particularly important in helping the body burn kilocalories, in ensuring a proper acid–base balance, and in helping the muscles relax after contraction. Na^+ is also an essential nutrient in the body, maintaining the **osmotic pressure** of the blood and other fluids located outside the cell. For most of us, getting enough Na^+ is not a problem; rather, we tend to consume too much sodium, which can cause high blood pressure. Light salts have an equal ratio of NaCl and KCl to help prevent an electrolyte imbalance.

When we work out or perform any strenuous exercise, we lose electrolytes through perspiration. Sports drinks and energy bars help replenish these electrolytes. The consumption of other fluids is also recommended since perspiration leads to a loss of water as well. In environments of low relative humidity, we need even more fluids since the perspiration evaporates quickly, and we don't always realize that we are losing water. Dehydration initially causes reduced urination and thirst; if not corrected, it can cause rapid respiration, pulse elevation, muscle spasms, nausea, and an inability to perform physically.

12.3 Alcohol

The fourth source of kilocalories in the human diet is alcohol. Ethanol provides 7 kilocalories per gram (190 kilocalories per ounce), intermediate between the other sources. A moderate amount of alcohol each day—a 4-ounce glass of wine, 12 ounces of beer, or a single mixed drink—is recommended by many physicians for good health. Originally, it was thought that the antioxidants in red wine provided the health benefits, but more recent evidence suggests that the ethanol itself is the beneficial component. One of the more highly regarded popular guides to healthy eating (*Eat, Drink and be Healthy*) suggests a daily alcoholic drink. All too often, however, we don't limit ourselves to a single drink. Excess alcohol puts the kilocalories on quickly (see Insert 12.3). An evening of binge drinking (five drinks for a male at a sitting and four drinks for

Product	Calories/serving	Calories/5 servings
Amaretto sour, 4.5 ounces	295	1475
Beer, 12-ounce bottle	155	775
Beer, 32-ounce small pitcher	413	2065
Bowl of ice cream, 2 scoops	285	1425
Cola, 12-ounce can	136	680
Dark chocolate, miniature bar	42	210
Diet cola, 12-ounce can	4	20
Light beer, 12-ounce bottle	104	520
Margarita on the rocks, 12 ounces	250	1250
Popcorn, buttered, 1 cup	83	415
Salted peanuts, 1 ounce, 32 peanuts	170	850
Frappuccino, 20 ounces	366	1830
Red wine, 4-ounce glass	85	425
Sex on the beach, 6.5 ounces	274	1370
Whiskey sour, 8 ounces	155	775
Whiskey and cola, 8 ounces	145	725
Wine cooler, 12 ounces	204	1020
White wine, 5-ounce glass	121	605

INSERT 12.3
Kilocalories associated with popular items on college campuses. (Calculated from http://www.choosemyplate.gov and http://www.myfitnesspal.com/food/calorie-chart-nutrition-facts.)

a female) can result in an increase in kilocalories with little or no vitamin or mineral intake.

Heavy drinkers tend to either gain weight (the infamous beer gut) or, to keep from gaining weight, cut back on their food intake, thus depriving themselves of needed nutrients. Of the total kilocalories an average American consumes, approximately 6% comes from alcohol, 10% by social drinkers, and more than half of total calories by alcoholics. In addition, excess ethanol impairs motor skills and judgment. As a drug and a weak toxin, ethanol probably causes more emotional problems, injury, and death than any other single chemical consumed. Responsible consumption of the chemical can be enjoyable and even health promoting, but too often it is misused and abused.

12.4 Nutrient Composition of Foods

Although we can buy and consume multivitamin tablets, most of which also contain minerals, it is usually better if we consume our nutrients in the foods we eat. Once nutrients enter the body, they are broken down into forms that we can use. It is easier to design diets around foods than around nutrients. Thus, it is important to understand the composition of various food groups.

12.4.1 Grains

Grains such as corn, oats, and wheat are cereal crops that are grown for their seeds, which are then further processed into foods or feeds. Grains are the most prominent source of carbohydrates in the world, and most people around the world get more than half of their kilocalories from carbohydrates. The primary carbohydrate in grains is starch. Starch molecules have one of two structures: linear or branching. The body has enzymes to break down both linear and branched starches.

Whole grains also have indigestible carbohydrates: cellulose, hemicellulose, lignin, and pectin, which are found in dietary fiber. Milling removes the coarser fractions of the grain resulting in more desirable, more functional, and whiter flour, but it also removes dietary fiber. The website ChooseMyPlate.gov recommends that at least half of the grain products we consume be whole grains. It is generally agreed that the average American does not get enough dietary fiber. Generally, fiber containing more pectin and less cellulose is better at achieving desired results. Oat fiber is considered to be one of the best food fibers.

12.4.2 Vegetables

Vegetables are defined as vegetative plant tissues that do not contain the reproductive parts of the plant. They can include leaves (lettuce, turnip greens), flowers (broccoli, cauliflower), stems (celery, asparagus), roots (carrots, parsnips), and tubers (potatoes, sweet potatoes). Tomatoes, squash, and cucumbers are classified as fruits botanically but are commonly considered vegetables by most consumers and at ChooseMyPlate.gov. By choosing vegetables of different colors, we are getting a wider range of nutrients than sticking with just one color.

Although vegetables have minerals and vitamins, particularly water-soluble vitamins, the most important nutrient in vegetables may be its fiber. Vegetable fiber tends to be higher in pectin and lower in cellulose than most whole grains. Another nutritional benefit of most vegetables is that they have high moisture content. Foods high in moisture and fiber and low in lipids and protein are more filling and less loaded with calories than their alternatives. The carbohydrates in vegetables tend to be indigestible fiber and starch, not sugars. Canned and frozen vegetables tend to be lower in vitamins than fresh vegetables, but the dietary fiber is frequently more beneficial to the body in processed products than in fresh products.

12.4.3 Fruits

A fruit is defined as a ripened ovary. Like vegetables, fruits contribute vitamins, minerals, and fiber to our diets. The nutritional benefits of fruits are similar to those of vegetables. In addition to the benefits listed above, fruits and vegetables are excellent sources of potassium. Fruits tend to have less starch and more sugars than vegetables. Bananas are an example of a fruit that is starchy when unripe, but the starch turns rapidly into sugar at the later stages of ripening.

The fruit group at ChooseMyPlate.gov also includes processed fruit products, including juices. Juices tend to have much less dietary fiber than whole fruits. With the exception of avocado, olive, and coconut (yes it is a fruit not a nut), most fruits and vegetables are low in lipids. Once again, it is good to vary the colors of the fruits we consume. Americans tend to eat less fruits and vegetables than consumers in other countries.

12.4.4 Dairy

Milk, cheese, and yogurt are considered part of the dairy group. Dairy products are high in calcium, protein, potassium, and vitamin D. The protein in milk has an excellent balance of essential amino acids. Low-fat alternatives are available for most dairy products and are highly recommended. Many cheeses are high in fats, particularly saturated fats; thus, caution should be exercised in choosing cheese products. Ice cream is high in fat and sugar with much less calcium than other dairy products and thus not considered part of this food group and should be eaten only occasionally. Reduced fat and sugar dairy desserts are available.

The calcium and vitamin D present in dairy products are important in maintaining bone health and preventing osteoporosis. Most dairy products

are fortified with vitamin D. As a fat-soluble vitamin, vitamin D is susceptible to oxidation. Oxidized vitamin D is toxic. Since milk is highly perishable,
the product is likely to spoil before vitamin D is oxidized, making it an excellent fortification vehicle. It is difficult to get sufficient calcium and vitamin D
in American diets without consuming adequate amounts of dairy products
or the use of mineral and vitamin supplements. Lactose-intolerant consumers tend to be deficient in calcium and vitamin D because they avoid dairy
products. Fortunately, yogurt is low in lactose and is an excellent source of
both nutrients. Low-lactose milks are also available in supermarkets.

12.4.5 Protein Foods

The protein foods group contains dry beans and peas, eggs, seafood, poultry,
nuts, processed soy products, and red meats. In addition to protein, many of
these items are also rich in the B vitamins, iron, magnesium, vitamin E, and
zinc. The animal products in this group tend to be higher in fat, saturated
fat, minerals, vitamins, and balanced proteins than the dry bean and pea
products. Lacto-ovo vegetarians who consume milk and egg products will
have no trouble balancing proteins. As noted above, vegans must ensure that
their protein comes from diverse sources. By careful mixing of amino acids
in plant sources such as grains and legumes, even vegans like Jennifer can
balance their proteins.

Although many beans and peas contain iron, the iron in them is not as
bioavailable; rather, it is more likely to be bound by indigestible carbohydrates and excreted in the stool. Consumption of an iron supplement such as
iron-fortified yeast can help overcome this deficiency. Vitamin B_{12} (cyanoco-
balamin) is readily available in animal, but not plant, products. As we age, it
becomes harder to absorb sufficient B_{12} and supplementation may be necessary for older adults. Strict vegetarians can get their vitamin B_{12} from fortified breakfast cereals, soy beverages, veggie burgers, yeast, a supplement, a
transdermal pouch, nasal spray, or injection.

12.4.6 Oils

Fats are solid at room temperature and have higher levels of saturated fats
than oils, which are liquid at room temperature. Oilseeds are crops whose
seeds are high in lipids. Primary examples of oilseeds are peanuts, soybeans, and sunflowers. For examples of the saturation of fatty acids present
in selected oilseeds and meats, see Insert 12.4. Oils pressed from seeds are
used for cooking and frying. They are also necessary ingredients in many
formulated foods such as salad dressings. It is important to have some oil in
our diet because they are sources of essential fatty acids and omega-three
and omega-six fatty acids, which are associated with maintaining proper
HDL/LDL ratios. It is recommended that any oil product containing *trans*
fats be avoided. The Food and Drug Administration requires manufacturers

Food	Percent daily value	
	Total fat	Saturated fat
Fried, breaded chicken breast	57	50
French fries, 8 ounces	46	25
Grilled chicken, 4 ounces	9	10
Ground beef, quarter pound	31	45
Macaroni and cheese, 1 cup	34	20
Oatmeal, 1 cup	3	3
Pinto beans, 1 cup	0	0
Pork chop	18	23
Quarter-pound hamburger with cheese	45	65
Salter, oil-roasted peanuts, 1 handful	37	18
T-bone steak, 12 ounces	120	175
Taco salad	86	80

INSERT 12.4

Lipids from selected animal and plant sources. (Calculated from http://www.choosemyplate .gov.)

of formulated foods to remove partially hydrogenated vegetable oils from their products, the primary source of *trans* fats in foods.

12.4.7 Processed, Formulated, Chilled, and Prepared Foods

The effect of food processing on the nutritional quality of food is described in Chapter 4. Many vitamins and minerals are lost during processing. To compensate for these losses, products are enriched with lost nutrients during processing operations. Products such as breakfast cereals may also be forti-fied by increasing the amount of vitamins and minerals above those found in the original grain. Some consumers mistakenly believe that vitamins that occur naturally are better than added ones. If the natural chemical form and the synthetic form of a nutrient are the same, the body cannot distinguish the difference between the two compounds. Processing can change the form of a nutrient to increase or decrease its bioavailability. Processing can also remove components that help in the absorption of key nutrients. For exam-ple, if vitamin C is removed, calcium and iron absorption will be restricted. Generally, however, the potency of natural and added vitamins and miner-als is similar. The primary purpose of processing is to increase shelf life and reduce waste. In many places around the world, simple processes like can-ning prevent large losses of fruits and vegetables.

As we learned in Chapter 5, formulated foods are mixtures of ingredi-ents. Among these ingredients are nutrients such as minerals, proteins, and vitamins. Other health-promoting compounds are also included. A careful reading of the nutritional label is necessary to understand the nutritional composition of formulated foods. Many formulated foods are primary sources of carbohydrates, proteins, and lipids with low levels of a few vitamins and minerals. Others, such as energy bars, breakfast cereals, and functional foods have high levels of many nutrients. Heavy reliance on products with high levels of nutrients and then supplementing with additional vitamins and minerals could lead to overdosing, causing metabolic imbalances.

Chilled foods include whole foods that have the nutrients typical of the food groups described above. Any preparation that requires heating can lower minerals and vitamin levels in foods. Minerals are not destroyed by the heat, but they can leach out into the cooking water. Quick cooling of cooked products helps keep them safe and slows the loss of vitamins. Unlike nutrients in processed and formulated foods, vitamins in chilled and prepared foods are perishable. Refrigeration will slow spoilage and vitamin loss, but vitamins are still not as stable in fresh foods as they are in processed and formulated foods.

12.5 Digestion and Intermediary Metabolism

As we have learned earlier, kilocalories are the unit of energy in our bodies. The dietary guidelines that provide the basis for nutritional labeling assume that the typical intake of an American is 2000 kilocalories a day. We consume approximately 1735 kilocalories to obtain all the required nutrients, allowing approximately 265 kilocalories for fun (discretionary calories). See what we can eat with 265 kilocalories in Insert 12.5. That amount, unfortunately, is much less than most of us consume.

2 medium fried wings (204)
10 breaded onion rings (230)
1, 20-ounce bottle of cola (230)
2 cups chili with beans (238)
1 glazed doughnut (242)
2 whole, large bananas (242)
3 chocolate chip cookies (243)
2 slices bakery bread (251)
1 large scoop premium ice cream (252)
30 mixed nuts (259)
1 small Wendy's hamburger (265)
1 can of cream of mushroom soup (268)
1 Dove bar chocolate ice cream (282)
3 tablespoons of peanut butter (282)
6 Oreo cookies (286)
2 slices bakery bread with 1 pat of butter (287)

INSERT 12.5
What we can do with 265 discretionary kilocalories. (Calculated from http://www.choosemy plate.gov.)

For our bodies to gain any benefit from any nutrient, it must be absorbed into the body after digestion. Digestion is a metabolic process that extracts nutrients from food products for use by our body. Digestion begins as we put the food in our mouth. The saliva we secrete moistens the food and releases amylase, an enzyme that breaks down starch. Nutritionists call this glob of food mixed with saliva the "bolus." The bolus leaves the mouth and proceeds through the esophagus on its way to the stomach. In the stomach, it is mixed with mucous, acid, and pepsin (an enzyme that starts breaking down proteins into short amino acid chains). The bolus dissolves in the stomach and is released slowly into the small intestine. In the approximately 25-feet-long journey through the small intestine, numerous enzymes break down the proteins, fats, and carbohydrates into smaller compounds like individual amino acids, fatty acids, and sugars.

The process of degrading the large molecules to smaller ones is called **catabolism. Catabolism** is necessary for absorption of nutrients across the intestinal mucosa. Digestive aids are secreted from the gallbladder, liver, and pancreas to enhance the absorption process as it releases small molecules into the bloodstream. If a nutrient is not absorbed across the intestine, it is useless to the body. Remember that dietary fiber is technically not a nutrient, but it exerts its positive effect by maintaining peristalsis and binding toxins. Any undigested parts of the bolus, including dietary fiber, proceeds to the large intestine where it is stored before propulsion out of the body. Excreted solid human waste (stool) provides the nutritionist and epidemiologist with a goldmine of information about nutrient utilization and potential causes of food-associated illness.

The small molecules absorbed into the bloodstream are either used immediately or transported to cells throughout the body. In the cells, these small molecules are reassembled into larger molecules in a process called **anabolism. Anabolism** is necessary because we need these larger molecules to maintain proper bodily functions. Proteins are needed for muscle tissue and to function as enzymes. Lipids are needed for energy storage, padding to protect organs from physical damage and as key components of cell membranes. Carbohydrates are needed for quick energy, and glycogen (animal starch) serves as a short-term energy reserve. Sugars can also be converted to other compounds our body needs. All anabolic reactions require energy to assemble these larger molecules.

Energy is derived from catabolic reactions occurring in cells as glycogen is converted to glucose, triglycerides break down into glycerol and fatty acids, and proteins are reduced to the component amino acids. Anabolism uses energy stored in the form of adenosine triphosphate (ATP) to build larger molecules. Catabolic reactions degrade larger molecules and produce ATP as a by-product. With the exception of the molecules in the lens of the eye, all other molecules are subject to turnover or replacement by other molecules. The genetic code in our DNA is what keeps us who we are despite all the modifications at the cellular and molecular level.

There are numerous things that can go wrong during digestion, and digestive disorders can reduce the quality of life. Chances for having digestive difficulties increase as we age, so here are some things we can look forward to as we get older. A low-fiber diet, low consumption of liquids, and little exercise can cause constipation. Constipation alternating with explosive diarrhea produces the symptoms of irritable bowel syndrome, which is frequently brought on by anorexia and bulimia. Swallowing air during eating can cause belching, and fermentation reactions in our intestines can cause flatulence.

Consuming large meals without sufficient liquids, lying down within 2 hours of a meal, smoking, or obesity can cause heartburn and acid reflux. Acid reflux allows the consumer to relive the dining experience over and over again, along with the stomach acid and other digestive components. Caffeine can increase the severity of acid reflux by relaxing the **epiglottis**, the structure that prevents food from reentering the mouth from the esophagus. Finally, contrary to popular opinion, ulcers are caused by a bacterium, *Helicobacter pylori*, and not by stress or fatty foods. Alcohol, aspirin, caffeine, and smoking can aggravate ulcers, but they do not cause them.

12.6 Nutritional Deficiency Diseases

Metabolic reactions through catabolism and anabolism require enzyme catalysis. For the enzyme to act, it must have its necessary cofactors, which are derived from vitamins and minerals. If we do not consume enough kilocalories, our bodies will not have sufficient energy to use for metabolism. We will not have the materials to replace the components designated for turnover of molecules within the body. Starvation, anorexia, and bulimia all prevent us from leading active lives, causing listlessness and eventually death.

Kwashiorkor is a disease affecting people who obtain adequate kilocalories but inadequate protein. Marasmus is a disease affecting people who do not obtain enough kilocalories. If we consume enough kilocalories and protein, but the proteins are incomplete sources of amino acids, the protein anabolic reactions can't continue and our body can't synthesize needed proteins. Assuming our proteins are balanced, if we do not consume enough of a vitamin or a mineral over a long period, we can develop a deficiency disease.

These deficiency diseases are unlike contagious diseases or food poisoning, which occur within a few hours or days after exposure, result in intense symptoms, and then proceed to full recovery. Nutritional deficiency diseases develop slowly over a long period. Early indications of illness may be difficult to distinguish from other disorders or diseases. Once a deficiency disease is diagnosed, it usually takes a long time to treat because the body can't absorb and assimilate large doses of nutrients over a short period.

12.7 Antioxidants, Supplements, and Antinutrients

As described in Chapter 11, vitamins A, C, and E are antioxidants that can reduce oxidation in foods and tissues. All of the so-called diseases of civilization, such as cancer, diabetes, and heart disease include a step involving oxidation of membrane lipids in cells of the body. A form of vitamin E, α-tocopherol, is a particularly effective antioxidant in membrane lipids. The tocopheroxyl free radical, formed upon oxidation, is stable and usually stops the chain reaction. This free radical cannot function as either a vitamin or an antioxidant until it is regenerated. Ascorbic acid (vitamin C) can be converted to dehydroascorbic acid, which, in turn, regenerates α-tocopherol. Dehydroascorbic acid does have some vitamin C activity, but it can be irreversibly degraded to lose all of its vitamin and regenerating capacity. Bioflavonoids found in many berries can regenerate the ascorbic acid as part of a protective cascade. As a result of this protective cascade, consumption of vitamins A, C, and E; bioflavonoids; and other compounds with antioxidant activity is increasing in an effort to avoid the diseases of civilization. Although a deficiency of these compounds may increase our chances of getting one of these diseases, clinical tests have not shown clear evidence that larger doses effectively prevent the diseases.

Consumers have become interested in supplementing the diet with higher levels of vitamins, minerals, and other compounds that appear to have health benefits but don't qualify as nutrients by classical definitions. Nutraceuticals and functional foods described in Chapter 2 fit into this category. A list of some food components with possible benefits can be found in Insert 12.6. Much information on supplements is passed from person to person and not

Potential benefit	Component	Food source
Bolster cellular antioxidant defense system	Anthocyanins	Berries, red grapes
	β-carotene	Carrots, sweet potatoes
	Sulphoraphane	Cauliflower, cabbage
May reduce risk of coronary heart disease	Beta glucan	Oat bran, rolled oats
	Omega-3 fatty acids (DHA/EPA)	Salmon, tuna
	Plant sterols and their esters	Fortified table spreads
Supports maintenance of immune system	Conjugated linoleic acid	Beef, lamb
	Dithiolthiones	Broccoli, collard greens
	Probiotic bacteria	Certain yogurts
Supports maintenance of mental function	Cyanocobalamin (Vit. B12)	Eggs, milk
	Omega-3 fatty acids (ALA)	Walnuts, flaxseeds
	Thiamin (Vit. B1)	Fortified breakfast cereals

INSERT 12.6

Potential benefits of functional components in food products. (Adapted from International Food Information Council Foundation, *Backgrounder on Functional Foods* [August 2011] at http://www.foodinsight.org/Resources/Detail.aspx?topic=Background_on_functional_Foods.)

verified by thorough scientific study. Many consumers tend to believe that if a little of a compound is good, then more of that compound is better. They do not understand that compounds can be beneficial at one level and toxic at a higher level. As more detailed scientific studies are conducted, we will be able to separate fact from fiction and design foods that are both healthy and satisfying. At present, some of these dietary supplements can interact with nutrients and drugs, leading to unintended adverse consequences.

Some naturally occurring substances in foods can lower the nutritional quality of our diets. Earlier in this chapter, we learned that excess levels of dietary fiber can bind needed nutrients, particularly minerals. Oxalates in spinach and rhubarb can bind calcium and iron as well as interfere with their absorption. We also learned in this chapter that certain minerals, when consumed in excess, can interfere with the absorption of other minerals. Antinutrients are compounds that interfere with the absorption of nutrients into the bloodstream or otherwise impede their effectiveness in the body.

Although soy is highly recommended as a protein source, it contains protease inhibitors. Proteases are the catabolic enzymes that convert proteins to individual amino acids. Protease inhibitors can help slow cancer development but can interfere with absorption of proteins. Rice contains iron-binding compounds, which can interfere with the absorption of iron if the iron is consumed at the same time as the rice. Small amounts of any antinutrient will have little effect on people consuming adequate diets. Antinutrients can have an effect on consumers who are on the borderline of getting an adequate supply of a specific nutrient. As emphasized throughout this book, it is important to consume a balanced diet.

12.8 Obesity

The obesity epidemic is becoming a major problem around the world, particularly in the United States and other western countries. Obesity is the result of accumulation of excess fat in the body such that it threatens human health. As described in Chapter 2, body mass index (BMI) is frequently used as a way to classify people according to weight, with a BMI lower than 18.5 considered to be underweight; 18.5–24.9, normal; 25.0–29.9, overweight; 30.0–39.9, obese; and higher than 40.0, morbidly obese. See Insert 12.7 for differences in body shape. The media has placed most of the blame on consumption of fast foods and processed foods, even going as far as accusing the food industry of deliberately addicting Americans through ingredients high in fat, sugar, and salt. Scientific studies suggest that the causes of obesity are more complex than what we see in the media.

Weight is primarily dependent on our energy balance. If we consistently consume more kilocalories than we burn through metabolism, we gain

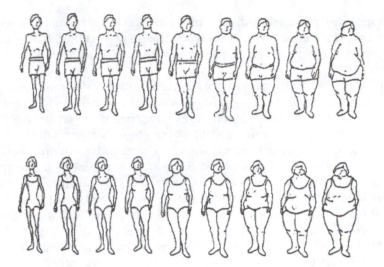

INSERT 12.7
Body shapes for male and female adults from underweight on the left to morbidly obese on the right. (© Dr. A.J. Stunkard, with permission as cited in Bulik, C.M. et al., *International Journal of Obesity Related Metabolic Disorders* 25: 1517, 2001.)

weight. If we consistently burn more kilocalories than we consume, we lose weight. Most of us reach a point where the energy consumed balances out the energy burned over a period of a week or month even if our food choices vary widely from day to day. When we reach this point, we tend to maintain a particular weight within a few pounds. Nutrient partitioning, or the amount of excess carbohydrates that are converted into protein or fat in the body, also affects how much fat is accumulated. Nutrient partitioning can be affected by genetics and by the level of physical activity.

Dramatic occurrences in our lives such as a prolonged illness, death in the family, moving out of home to go to school, trying out for an athletic team, rush, marriage, pregnancy, a new job, or a host of other circumstances can lead to a change in this balance. If these events lead to significant increases in food consumption or decreases in physical activity, we will gain weight until a new **energy-balance point** is reached. Likewise, major increases in physical activity or decreases in food consumption will lead to weight loss until a new point is reached. When we have adapted to the new situation, we may revert to the old balance point and return to the previous weight, continue with the new balance and weight, or fall somewhere in between these two endpoints.

All bodies are not created equal, however, when it comes to maintaining weight. Some people are much less affected by changes in diet and exercise than others. Obesity researchers attribute these differences to functional types based on variation in genetic, behavioral, and metabolic factors to help understand responses for individual consumers. They use many studies, which include controlled feeding of different species of animals, differences in identical or fraternal twins raised separately or together, biological and adoptive children raised in the same environment, and analysis of gene patterns.

Many factors affect the prevalence of obesity in a given population in addition to the amount of food consumed, its caloric density, and the level of physical activity. When both parents are obese, their children are more likely to be obese than if one or both parents are not obese. Mothers who have high-fat diets during pregnancy or breastfeeding tend to have more overweight and obese children than mothers who consume a low-fat diet. Dietary patterns developed in the first few years of life are difficult to break and can lead to lifetime habits and balance points established during adulthood. Genetic effects have been attributed to differences in hormonal balance as it affects metabolism. Despite the numerous pills and special diets, it is not easy to change our metabolic rate other than by increasing physical activity, and some individuals are more likely to lose weight than others.

Weight-loss diets can be successful, but most dieters regain weight unless they can incorporate a major change in lifestyle once they achieve their weight-loss goal. It appears that a tendency to obesity is programmed into many of us from the time we were conceived. Early intervention to prevent obesity before it develops is more likely to be successful than weight reduction after its onset.

12.9 Remember This!

- Many factors affect the prevalence of obesity in a given population in addition to the amount of food consumed, its caloric density, and the level of physical activity.
- Nutritional deficiency diseases develop slowly over a long period.
- Digestion is a metabolic process that extracts nutrients from food products for use by our body.
- By careful mixing of amino acids in plant sources such as grains and legumes, vegans can balance their proteins.
- Like vegetables, fruits contribute vitamins, minerals, and fiber to our diets.
- Responsible consumption of alcohol can be enjoyable and even health promoting, but too often it is misused and abused.
- The usefulness of a vitamin or a mineral in a food depends on its bioavailability.
- Carbohydrates include sugars, starches, and nondigestible cell-wall materials.

- We need to consume lipids for the essential fatty acids they provide and because lipid-soluble vitamins cannot be absorbed unless there is sufficient lipid in the intestinal tract to permit absorption.

- Antioxidants and dietary supplements are thought to contribute to health, but their role is not as clearly defined.

12.10 Looking Ahead

The book will conclude with chapters on food microbiology, food engineering, and sensory evaluation.

Testing Comprehension

1. Describe the difference between a dietician and a nutritionist. Identify three probable interactions between a food scientist and a dietician and between a food scientist and a nutritionist.

2. Compare and contrast the structures of the essential amino acids shown in Insert 12.1. What part of each structure is the same for each amino acid? What part is unique for each structure? Why are these similarities and differences important?

3. Identify five fruits that are different in color from each other and five vegetables that are different in color from each other. How do these fruits and vegetables differ in vitamins and minerals? On the basis of this information, how valid is the recommendation to vary the color of our fruits and vegetables?

4. Compare and contrast typical dietary patterns of a vegan and someone who eats meat at least twice a day. What are the primary benefits of each of these diets? What are the potential difficulties of each of these diets? What can the vegan and the meat eater do to gain the benefits of their choice without suffering from its consequences?

5. Construct the basic principles one needs to use to design a balanced diet. Compare this diet to a fad diet described on the Internet. Why do so many health professionals urge us to balance our diets rather than adopt a fad diet?

6. List five processed foods and five formulated foods that could be a regular part of a nutritious diet. List five processed foods and five formulated foods that should be consumed only occasionally. What is the rationale for placing these foods in these categories?

7. List all the food consumed in a 24-hour period. Calculate the percentage of calories consumed from carbohydrate, lipid, protein, and any other source using a website such as ChooseMyPlate.com. Is this balance typical of what is normally consumed? Is the balance relatively healthy or unhealthy? What single change in this diet would have the greatest effect on improving its nutritional quality?

8. Analyze the nutritional benefits and detriments of each of the following beverages: beer, black coffee, cappuccino, chocolate milk, energy drinks, fruit juices, low-calorie soft drinks, low-fat milk, milk shakes, mixed drinks, smoothies, sugared soft drinks, sports beverages, vitamin water, water, whole milk, and wine.

9. List all of the possible reasons why two boys of approximately the same age and height living in the same family environment can grow up and have very different weights. How can the parents identify a potential problem in the one on his way to becoming obese and prevent a lifetime of the dangers associated with obesity?

10. Appraise the statement in the chapter that obesity is much more complex than eating too many fast and processed foods. Provide evidence to either support or refute the authors' claim.

References

Bulik, C. M., T. D. Wade, A. C. Heath, N. G. Martin, A. J. Stunkard and L. J. Eaves, 2001. Relating body mass index to figural stimuli: Population-based normative data for Caucasians. *Int. J. Obes. Rel. Metab. Disord.*, 25:1517.

International Food Information Council Foundation, 2011. *Backgrounder on Functional Foods*, August. Available at http://www.foodinsight.org/Resources/Detail .aspx?topic=Background_on_functional_Foods.

Tuszynski, J. A. and M. Kurzynski, 2003. *Introduction to Molecular Biophysics*, Boca Raton, FL: CRC Press, Taylor & Francis Group.

Willett, W. C., 2005. *Eat, Drink and be Healthy: The Harvard Guide to Healthy Eating*, New York: Free Press.

Further Reading

Bock, G. and J. Goode, Eds., 2007. *Dietary Supplements and Health*, Chichester, UK: John Wiley & Sons, Ltd.

Dhingra, D., M. Michael, H. Rajput and R. T. Patil, 2012. Dietary fibre in foods: A review. *J. Food Sci. Technol.—Mysore*, 49:255.

Moss, M., 2013. *Salt Sugar Fat: How the Food Giants Hooked Us*. New York: Random House.

Webb, G. P., 2011. *Dietary Supplements & Functional Foods*, 2nd ed., Ames, IA: Wiley-Blackwell.

Whitney, E. N. and S. R. Rolfes, 2013. *Understanding Nutrition*, 13th ed., Belmont, CA: West/Wadsworth.

Wolinsky, I. and J. A. Driskell, 2008. *Sports Nutrition: Energy Metabolism and Exercise*, Boca Raton, FL: CRC Press, Taylor & Francis Group.

13

Food Microbiology

Selina majored in Food Science and graduated with a good record. She decided to stay on for her master's degree and chose to specialize in food microbiology. As part of her degree, she is conducting original research under a member of the faculty in the Food Science Department. She became interested in how *Salmonella* can get stressed under certain conditions (often when nutrients are unavailable). *Salmonella* cells can be injured and difficult to detect. Thus, the food being tested for *Salmonella* may show no signs of its presence but can still be quite dangerous. Thus, to detect the presence of *Salmonella*, an enrichment medium must be used to culture an extract of the food sample to help recover any injured cells. Selina's work is to determine at what level a specific nutrient is required to improve recovery.

Garrett's passion is molecular genetics. It was a field unheard of back in the 1960s. For his science fair project in high school, he had extracted DNA from *Arabidopsis*, a common weed. He received his bachelor's degree in Genetics with a minor in Microbiology, but he became disinterested in learning all the theoretical scientific principles. He wondered how all of this knowledge applied to real life. That's when he discovered Food Science and learned how important genetics was in working with food materials and also in the organisms that contaminate the materials. Like Selina, Garrett went on to pursue a master's degree in Food Science. He was particularly interested in the genetics of the microbes that are used to ferment milk into yogurt. His research looked specifically at the resistance of these bacteria to the bacteriophages (viruses that attack bacteria) that interfere with the conversion of milk to yogurt. He is now ready to start his PhD research and he will be looking at the genetics of the yeasts that are used in the production of beer and bread.

13.1 Looking Back

Previous chapters have focused on food topics we find in our daily lives, with the types of food products we encounter in the marketplace, and the activities that food scientists perform. In Chapter 11, we studied the importance of chemistry in understanding foods. Another basic science we need to know in order to work effectively with foods is biology, particularly microbiology. Some key points covered in previous chapters that prepare us for a basic understanding of food microbiology and other biological aspects of foods are the following:

- The Hazard Analysis and Critical Control Point system is a means of ensuring microbial safety in a product.
- The main function of a package is to preserve the physical and chemical integrity of a product including preventing microbial or chemical contamination.
- Food is preserved to make it safer by reducing or eliminating harmful microbes and to extend its shelf life by reducing or eliminating spoilage microorganisms.
- Fermentation is the only method of food preservation that encourages multiplication of microbes.
- Processing techniques for a specific food are designed with an understanding of the potential microbes present and the properties of the food.
- Preservatives are food ingredients that slow spoilage and help prevent food-associated illnesses.
- The last meal consumed is not usually the meal responsible for an outbreak of food poisoning.
- An expiration date represents the food scientist's best guess of how long a food will last before it spoils.
- Spoilage is not a good indicator of a safety risk.
- Fresh foods are more likely to contain harmful microbes than processed foods.

13.2 Food Microbiology

Microbiology is the study of the physiology, genetics, growth characteristics, survival, and behavior of microorganisms. Microorganisms generally are life forms that cannot be seen by the naked eye; however, they represent the dominant life form on earth: they are in the air we breathe, the beverages we drink, the food we eat, and everything we touch. They are also an integral part of our bodies; in fact, life would be impossible for humans without microorganisms. Microbiology is a rapidly growing field of study. The more we learn about microorganisms, the more we learn how little we really know. It is estimated that 99% of bacterial species remain undiscovered. Much of microbiology focuses on microorganisms of medical or commercial significance. Food microbiologists focus on those that can grow and survive in foods.

Some microorganisms can cause disease or death when transmitted through the food chain. These pathogens are responsible for a majority of food-associated illness, also called food-borne diseases. Spoilage microorganisms may not make people sick but can cause economic losses because of wasted food. However, not all microorganisms are bad! Without the help of some yeasts, bacteria, and molds, we could not produce bread, wine, yogurt, or many other healthy and delicious products. Food microbiologists also study how the environment may affect each microorganism's growth and behavior, how their presence will affect the food and the humans who consume it, as well as the conditions in the food itself.

With this knowledge, the food microbiologist understands how to control and manipulate microorganisms—whether to suppress pathogens from the food chain or to promote the growth of beneficial ones in fermented foods—and will be able to produce better, safer, and healthier foods. Studying food microbiology will give us a better understanding of the behavior of microorganisms and their effect on the safety, spoilage, and preservation of foods.

13.3 Types of Microorganisms in Our Foods

Among the most commonly studied microorganisms are bacteria, molds, and yeasts. Viruses and parasitic protozoa are gaining interest. Microorganisms are classified in many ways: by genus and species, size and shape (morphology), chemical reactions, nutrient requirements, metabolic products, and nucleic acid composition.

Bacteria are single-celled organisms enclosed by a cell wall. They reproduce asexually by cell division. Bacteria are classified as **prokaryotes** because they do not have defined nuclei. Under the microscope, bacteria usually are round (cocci) or oblong or rodlike (bacilli). A broad classification of bacteria is done by using the Gram stain technique, which is based on the cell wall composition. Gram-positive bacteria have a thick peptoglycan layer and stain purple while Gram-negative cells have a thin peptoglycan layer and a lipopolysaccharide layer and stain reddish-pink (see Insert 13.1 for a photomicrograph of a Gram-negative bacterium). When exposed to adverse environmental conditions, some Gram-positive bacteria can form dormant, tough, resistant structures called spores. These spores are widely found in nature (soil, water, air, even intestinal tracts of humans and animals) and allow bacteria to survive environmental stress. When favorable conditions are restored, the bacteria revert to their vegetative (nondormant) form. Certain bacteria, called starter cultures, are active agents in food fermentations and, thus, essential for the production of certain food products, whereas others may cause spoilage and food-associated illnesses.

Molds, yeasts, and mushrooms are known as fungi. Fungi are classified as **eukaryotes** because they have clearly defined nuclei. Fungi reproduce

INSERT 13.1
Gram-stained smear from a *Campylobacter jejuni* culture incubated for 48 hours at 42°C. (Photo available at http://www.asm.org/division/c/gramneg.htm and reprinted with permission by Dr. Michael J. Miller, CDC, Atlanta.)

both sexually and asexually, by budding or fission. Molds are multicellular and form long filaments called **hyphae**. A group or mass of hyphae is called **mycelium**. Yeasts are mostly single-celled organisms, but, under the right conditions, they may also form filaments. Although the individual cells of fungi cannot be seen by the naked eye, most of us have seen colonies of mold that have contaminated a food and rendered it unappetizing.

Molds and yeasts are capable of growing at temperature, pH, and water conditions that may not be favorable for bacteria. For the most part, they are considered spoilage microorganisms, but some may produce harmful myco-toxins. On the other hand, both yeasts and molds are the agents of fermentation in many common food and beverage products.

Protozoa are single-celled organisms that do not have cell walls. As they are eukaryotes, they are more organized at the cellular level than bacteria. They are also bigger in size. Some protozoa can be involved and have beneficial effects in water processing systems but those of concern to food microbiologists are parasites, which can be transmitted through food, water, and feces resulting in food-borne illnesses. The most common pathogenic protozoa are *Cryptosporidium*, *Cyclospora*, *Toxoplasma*, *Giardia*, and *Entamoeba*. While infection by protozoa will most likely result in mild to moderate gastrointestinal symptoms, sensitive populations like the infants, elderly, and those with immunodeficiencies may suffer from more severe complications. Additionally, some species may be able to affect other areas in the body.

Viruses are single or double strands of RNA or DNA, and they must infect a cell in order to be able to replicate. Although viruses can spread through the food chain and cause food-borne illnesses (hepatitis, gastroenteritis), another negative effect on the food industry is viruses that attack bacteria, also called bacteriophages or just **phages**. Phages can infect starter cultures and, therefore, delay or even completely inhibit industrial fermentation processes resulting in major economic losses. However, not all is bad when it comes to viruses! A relatively new approach uses phages to target and destroy specific harmful bacteria. This so-called phage therapy is currently used in veterinary, medicine, and agriculture applications.

13.4 Microbial Genetics

The genetic program of a cell is located in its DNA. For eukaryotes, the DNA is called the chromosome and located in its nucleus. For prokaryotes, the DNA is distributed throughout the cell. DNA is composed of two complementary chains of nucleotides and organized into units called genes, with each gene coding for a specific protein. Each nucleotide contains a five-carbon sugar, a phosphate group, and a nitrogenous base. The two chains form a double helix. DNA is replicated by separating the two strands and making a new complementary strand from each original strand resulting in a total of four strands and two identical helices.

Protein molecules that affect the cell's growth and survival are synthesized in a two-step process: **transcription** (synthesizing RNA from DNA) and **translation** (linking amino acids to synthesize proteins from RNA). Each amino acid is coded by a three-base sequence on the RNA. Not all genes are expressed (transcribed and translated) in the cell at all times as expression may be induced by environmental conditions. Indeed, the ability to withstand environmental conditions and respond to specific stresses is embedded in the genes.

Everything that a cell is or does is coded in its genes. The color, size, and shape of a cell are inherent in the code. A genotype is the basic genetic makeup of a specific organism that differentiates it from all other organisms. A mutation modifies the base-pair sequence of the DNA and thus the genotype. Manipulation of the genes within an organism to achieve a change in that organism is called genetic engineering. These changes can both promote the expression of genes that encode desirable characteristics and block the expression of genes that encode undesirable ones.

13.5 Cell Physiology and Reproduction

In contrast to the genotype, the phenotype represents the physiological response of the organism to a given environment. Frequently, microorganisms in foods are responding to environmentally stressful conditions. The reason one species can survive when another cannot is because of its ability to adapt to the environment, including the chemical composition and physical conditions of the food. Cell physiology includes all of the biochemical reactions that go on during cell replication, transcription, and translation. It includes all metabolic processes within the cell including

- The assimilation and synthesis of nutrients and their conversion to useful compounds
- The transport of these compounds to the location in which they are needed
- The breakdown of nutrients and other compounds

The eukaryotic cell contains organelles, such as mitochondria, chloroplasts, and the endoplasmic reticulum, that have specific functions in the metabolic process. The proteins that have the most immediate effect on cell metabolism are enzymes. The cell is not the static entity we see in Insert 13.2; rather, it is always under reconstruction. Cells undergo the process of turnover, constantly replacing molecules within cell structures while continuing to maintain the same outward appearance because the cell's genetic material encodes these traits. When the organism is placed under stress, a complex signaling mechanism is triggered where some genes are expressed to increase synthesis of a specific enzyme to help the cell adapt to the new conditions. Other genes may be "turned off" (not expressed) to decrease the level and activity of other enzymes.

Microorganisms reproduce themselves in many ways, but the most common way is by cell division. Basically, a cell grows to the point where it divides into two identical cells. Given the optimal conditions, bacterial

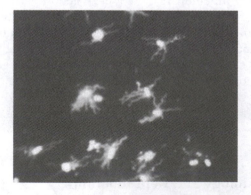

INSERT 13.2
Photomicrograph of *Salmonella typhi* cells. (Photo available at http://www.asm.org/division/c /gramneg.htm and reprinted with permission of Dr. Michael J. Miller, CDC, Atlanta.)

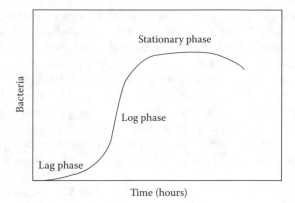

INSERT 13.3
Exponential growth curve for microorganisms.

cells can multiply rapidly, doubling in as little as 30 minutes. Such rapid multiplication can produce a million cells from one cell in a period of less than 10 hours!

When a cell is transferred into a new environment, it must adjust to the new conditions and will not multiply at an optimal rate until it has time to synthesize necessary proteins. This period of delay is called the "lag phase" (see Insert 13.3). Once the microorganism adapts to its new environment, it begins to multiply rapidly in the "log or exponential phase." At a certain point, however, the level of available nutrients is not sufficient to sustain further division and the organism enters the "stationary phase." In the stationary phase, the number of cells dividing is balanced by the numbers that are dying. Maintenance cannot be sustained forever unless the cells are transferred to a new environment. Thus, the last phase is known as the "death phase."

As mentioned earlier in this chapter, some microorganisms, mostly Gram-positive, are able to form resistant spores when the environment becomes inhospitable. If the spores are provided with rich sources of nutrients and optimal growth conditions, they will germinate into vegetative cells.

13.6 Sources of Microbial Contamination

As indicated in the first chapter, the primary sources of harmful microorganisms are soil, feces, animals, and people. When food microbiologists need to isolate a particular pathogen, the two places at which they are most likely to look are soil and feces. Most contamination of fresh fruits, vegetables, and meats is on the surface because the internal tissues of plants and animals are usually free of microorganisms. Animal intestines are colonized by both harmful and beneficial microorganisms, and feces are a rich source of these microorganisms. Our intestinal walls and immune system prevent these harmful microorganisms from getting into our bloodstream where they can do damage. Some pathogens, like *Staphylococcus*, can reside in our noses, skin, scabs, and boils. Moreover, some people may be carriers of a pathogen even if they do not show symptoms of the disease. Thus, failure to wash our hands after defecation or after touching our nose or skin can spread them to our food and mouth and, eventually, into our stomachs where they can make us very ill.

Likewise, plant tissues can become contaminated from the soil and water, from improperly manufactured organic fertilizers, and from people and animals. Animal tissues can become contaminated from hair, feathers, feces, and intestinal tracts during harvesting, collection, or milking. Adequate pasteurization of milk and juices kills harmful microorganisms and, as we learned in Chapter 10, proper sanitation is necessary to prevent the spread of microorganisms.

In the farm environment, plants come in contact with soil and animals come in contact with feces. Contaminated irrigation water can also increase the level of contamination. Thus, every step in the handling or processing of food products represents an opportunity for microorganisms to contaminate the food and for food scientists to control them. The goal of proper sanitation is to minimize the contamination in the first place. The goal of proper handling is to minimize the growth and spread of microorganisms. The goal of processing is to kill harmful microorganisms or prevent their growth. The goal of packaging is to prevent the recontamination of a safe finished product.

To reduce cross-contamination, fresh fruits and vegetables should not be shipped in trailers that have transported live animals on the previous haul. Once at a warehouse or processing plant, food storage temperatures are kept low to slow microbial growth. Equipment must be kept clean to prevent the transfer of microorganisms from contaminated equipment to food products, and food handlers must observe proper hygiene. It is particularly critical that products that will receive no heat treatment are not contaminated.

Although it is not a pleasant thought, fresh foods and raw materials are likely to contain filth. Filth in foods includes such disgusting things as fly eggs, insect parts, maggots, rodent hair and feces, and weevils. Most of these contaminants cannot be seen with the naked eye and are just as likely to be in fresh vegetables picked from a backyard garden as those bought at a farmer's market or supermarket. A systems approach to minimizing contaminants in our foods starts with the use of pesticides in the field to reduce insect and pest populations and carries through to adequate sanitation during harvesting, handling, and processing.

13.7 Environmental Conditions Affecting Microbial Growth

Contrary to popular belief, very few foods are sterile. The microflora (the microorganisms that are characteristic of or associated with a particular product) present in a food are affected by the composition of the food (intrinsic factors) as well as its environment (extrinsic factors). As we learned in Chapter 4, canned foods are sterile, but most other foods are not. Most foods contain mixed populations of microorganisms: some could be pathogens, others could cause spoilage, but many have little or no effect on the food or on the consumer.

Environmental conditions can increase, decrease, or change the types of microorganisms present. Eventually, however, one species tends to dominate. Which species predominates depends on which one is the quickest at adapting to the composition of the food and the environmental conditions. If the predominant species is pathogenic, then consumption of the food could cause serious health problems. If the predominant species causes spoilage, then the food is likely to spoil before it becomes a health hazard. The metabolites of the predominating species may result in self-inhibition (the microorganism may kill itself off) or in conditions that favor other species growth.

The temperature, relative humidity (RH), and gaseous composition of the environment affect microbial growth. The most effective way to slow microbial growth is to control the temperature. Most microorganisms grow best between the temperatures of 50°F and 95°F (between 10°C and 35°C). That is why we need to keep hot foods hot (higher than 50°C) and cold foods cold (less than 7°C). Bacteria that can survive and grow at high temperatures are called **thermophiles**; those that can grow at low temperatures are called **psychrophiles**. Bacteria grow at high RH and can outcompete other microbes. As the RH is lowered, however, bacteria lose their competitive advantage and yeast or molds are more likely to predominate. All molds require oxygen to grow and survive, but some bacteria and yeasts can grow and survive without oxygen. Organisms that can only grow in the absence of oxygen are called **anaerobes**; organisms that can grow with very small amounts of oxygen are called **microaerophiles**.

13.8 Food Compositional Factors Affecting Microbial Growth

Microbial growth in foods is affected by the chemical composition of the food. Water activity, pH, oxidation–reduction potential, nutrients, growth factors, and inhibitors affect microbial growth in foods. Every microorganism must have a carbon source and a nitrogen source for basic microbial nutrition although different species may have different growth requirements.

There are a wide variety of growth factors that help some species of micro-organisms grow at the expense of others. Most of these growth factors are vitamins.

Inhibitors are chemical compounds that slow the growth of microorganisms, with some species being more susceptible to specific compounds than others. Inhibitors added directly to foods to prevent microbial growth are called **preservatives** but many plant tissues contain inherent inhibiting substances. Water activity (A_W) is the amount of water available to the microorganism and is related to the RH within the food itself. As the acidity increases (pH decreases), bacteria are less able to grow or survive. Foods with a pH of 4.5 or higher are low-acid foods; those with a pH lower than 4.5 are high-acid foods. As a general rule, bacteria require higher water activity and pH levels than yeast and molds.

The level of oxygen (related to the oxidation–reduction potential) is another factor that affects the competitive advantages of different species as discussed in Section 13.7. Bacteria can be both aerobic and anaerobic, while most yeasts and molds are strictly aerobic, except for few species involved in anaerobic fermentations. The observant student will recognize that the conditions affecting microorganisms are very similar to those affecting enzymes. The reason is that microorganisms grow and produce chemical products through chemical reactions that are catalyzed by enzymes; thus, conditions that inhibit enzymes are likely to inhibit microbial growth.

Competition among microorganisms determines the relative populations found in food products. Some species of microorganisms require amino acids or other complex sources of nitrogen, but others can use a chemical like caffeine as both a carbon and nitrogen source. Sugars and salts bind water and thus reduce water activity. Microorganisms that can tolerate higher levels of salts than other species are called **halophiles**; those that can tolerate higher levels of sugars are called **osmophiles**. Changing the amount of sugar or salt in a product or the gases in its package can affect the competitive advantages of organisms within a food product.

One of the most popular ways of isolating and culturing microorganisms is on agar, usually in a Petri dish (see Insert 13.4 to see an example). Standard plate count agar can theoretically be used to grow all the different species (microflora) present in a food. Colonies on the agar represent billions of microbial cells but are assumed to come from a single cell. Thus, by counting the number of colonies, we can gain a rough approximation of how many microorganisms inhabit a particular food (usually expressed as colony-forming units or CFU per gram of a solid food or per milliliter of a liquid). Since some species can outcompete others in the food and on the plate, we must be careful in the conclusions we draw.

If we wish to find a certain genus, species, or related groups of microorganisms, a special agar that has growth factors, carbon sources, nitrogen sources, and inhibitors that select for specific genera or species is used. More traditional methods rely on a color change in the agar, which

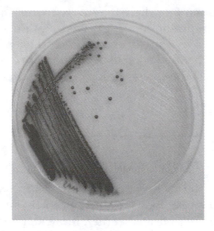

INSERT 13.4
Streak plate of *Staphylococcus aureus* on Baird Parker agar. (Photo courtesy of Samantha VanWees and Alicia Orta-Ramirez.)

provides proof of the presence of a specific organism based on a biochemical reaction characteristic of the organism. Other physical signs include the size, shape, or color of the colonies; clear rings around the colony; or production of slime. Chemical factors include the production of gas or converting specific chemicals to reaction products, usually inducing a physical change in the growth medium. Immunological tests, based on molecules called antibodies, are more specific for proteins on the outer surfaces of some microorganisms. More modern tests based on the DNA content of the microorganism can be more rapid and specific than traditional methods but also more expensive.

Certain species can become injured during the manufacturing and processing of a product. In the injured state, they might be present but not be capable of growing under ordinary circumstances. The food microbiologist might believe that there are no organisms present and may be surprised when the food causes an outbreak later. Such an event might occur because the microorganism in question was present at a sufficient level (although not a detectable level) to cause an outbreak or the conditions in the food or environment became more favorable for growth. Genera like *Salmonella* can be injured in food. The bacterium may not be detectable in this state and may cause a false-negative result. To decrease the chances of false negatives happening, the cells can be nurtured in special recovery broth to determine if any are present.

Alternatively, food microbiologists may use the detection of **indicator microorganisms** in a product as a way of ascertaining the risk of pathogens present in a product. In the broadest sense, the term **indicator organisms** can refer to any group of organisms whose presence or absence tells us something about the sample where they were found. In food microbiology, we are interested in indicator organisms whose presence in foods indicates exposure to conditions that might introduce pathogens or allow proliferation of pathogens in the food sample. Detection of coliforms is a relatively common method to test the sanitary conditions of water and food.

13.9 Fermentation Microorganisms

Although we tend to think that microorganisms in food are undesirable, some of our more popular foods are produced by beneficial microorganisms (see Insert 13.5). As indicated earlier, fermentation is the only primary method of food preservation that encourages multiplication of microorganisms. Fermentation is generally referred to as the biological process in which microorganisms induce a series of chemical reactions leading to food preservation. A stricter chemical definition of fermentation involves carbohydrate degradation in the absence of oxygen. During fermentation, the nutritional quality of foods can be improved because vitamins are synthesized. The bioavailability of vitamins and other nutrients can be enhanced during fermentation, and carbohydrates may be broken down into smaller compounds by hydrolysis.

An example of a true fermentation involves the conversion of lactose to lactic acid to produce yogurt, sour cream, and some cheeses. The smooth mouthfeel of yogurt comes from the coagulation of milk proteins. A bacterial culture (usually a mix of *Lactobacillus delbrueckii* subsp. *bulgaricus* and *Streptococcus thermophilus*) is used to start the fermentation. The distinct sour taste is caused by lactic acid, but the characteristic aroma is from acetaldehyde.

Yogurt is considered by many to be a "health food" primarily because it contains active bacterial cultures. The idea is that these active cultures can

Product	Substrate	Fermenting microorganism
Beer	Barley	*Saccharomyces cerevisae*
Bread	Wheat	*Saccharomyces cerevisae*
Pickles	Cucumber	*Lactobacillus plantarum*
Sauerkraut	Cabbage	*Leuconostoc mesenteroides*
Soy sauce	Soybeans	*Aspergillus oryae, Zygosaccharomyces rouxii*
Wine	Grapes	*Saccharomyces cerevisae*
Yogurt	Milk	*Streptococcus thermophilus, Lactobacillus delbruekii*

INSERT 13.5
Fermented products, substrates (starting material), and the responsible microorganisms.

Microorganism	*Lactobacillus bulgaricus*	*Saccharomyces cerevisiae*
Type	Gram-positive bacterium	Yeast
Food products	Yogurt	Breads and alcoholic beverages
Chemical products	Lactic acid	Carbon dioxide and ethanol
Signature	Proteolysis	Gas production
Favorable conditions	Acid/40°C–45°C	Carbohydrate-rich/30°C–35°C

INSERT 13.6
Comparison of two fermentation microorganisms.

colonize our intestines, improving our microflora and replacing or outcompeting less desirable species. Scientific research suggests that few, if any, active yogurt cultures can survive the digestion process because stomach acid can be lethal to the culture. Thus, active cultures may not significantly affect the microflora in our intestines. *Lactobacillus acidophilus*, on the other hand, is more likely to survive our stomach's environment and be beneficial. Acidophilus products, although not as popular as yogurt, are usually available in the dairy section of most supermarkets.

Many fermented products are widely available (see Insert 13.6 for responsible microorganisms). Sometimes, a single species is responsible, but at other times, it takes more than one to produce an acceptable product. In yogurt, the fermentation is started with *L. delbrueckii* subsp. *bulgaricus*, which produces lactic acid and lowers the pH to approximately 5.5, a point at which it can no longer grow effectively. Then, *S. thermophilus* starts growing and lowers the pH to the final level of 4.5. Note that the lower pH acts as a "natural" preservative because fewer species can grow in the high-acid environment that the two microorganisms have created in this synergistic effort.

Careful control of the fermentation temperature is necessary to maintain an appropriate balance between the strong acid production of the *Lactobacillus* and the greater flavor development by the *Streptococcus*. Another example is the production of kimchi, a traditional cabbage-based product in Korean cuisine, where *Lactobacillus plantarum*, *Leuconostoc*, and *Pediococcus* act sequentially to create the final product. Lactic acid bacteria are also used in the production of certain fermented sausages.

Other fermentations are produced by yeasts and molds. The production of carbon dioxide gas to help dough rise in bread baking and the production of alcohol in alcoholic beverages are remarkably attributed to the same species of yeast. *Saccharomyces cerevisiae* is responsible for most bread and alcohol products, emphasizing the importance of the specific strain and the starting substrate. Other specialized species may be used for specific applications such as *Saccharomyces carlsbergensis* for lager beers. Examples of mold-mediated fermentations are mold-ripened cheeses such as Roquefort, Gorgonzola, and Stilton, among others, and soy sauce, tempeh, and rice wine.

A successful fermentation is dependent upon the microorganisms, raw materials, type of process, and environmental conditions. The starter culture is added to begin the fermentation with the idea that a single microorganism will predominate to induce the desired chemical changes that will produce a high-quality final product. Too little of the starter may cause inadequate growth and change but too much can be expensive. An incorrect starter-culture formulation may produce a product of poor quality. Contamination of the raw material or the starter culture may promote the growth of other species and produce unwanted changes. The temperature, RH, and food compositional factors like pH should be controlled to favor the growth of the desired species. Phage infection of the starter culture will result in delay or even inhibition of the fermentation process.

13.10 Spoilage Microorganisms

By now, we should have a clear understanding that the microorganisms that cause food spoilage are not the same ones that cause food poisoning. Food spoilage produces undesirable aromas, color defects, and slime formation. Pathogens, on the other hand, do not usually alter the flavor, color, or texture of foods because the number of pathogens necessary to cause illness is fewer than the number needed to cause spoilage. Thus, aroma is not a reliable guide in determining microbial safety. Spoilage can be caused by the growth of microorganisms or by the metabolic products of microbial enzymes. Only a relatively small number of microbial genera are responsible for food spoilage. Although it is a good idea not to eat spoiled food, we are just kidding ourselves if we think we can tell when a food is safe just by using our eyes and nose.

As we learned earlier, fresh foods are more likely to contain harmful microorganisms than processed ones. Psychrotrophic bacteria are spoilage organisms that effectively outcompete other microorganisms at refrigerated temperatures. Thermophilic bacteria can survive heat treatment and can cause spoilage of pasteurized products. Bacilli bacteria can tolerate high acid levels (low pH) that normally inhibit microbial growth. Generally, symptoms of spoilage do not occur until levels above 10,000,000 microbial cells per gram. However, sometimes eliminating microorganisms from food may provide an advantage to pathogens because of lack of competition.

Cooking followed by contamination and improper storage can speed up growth of harmful microorganisms because we have killed off their competitors. That is why perishable foods should be refrigerated after they have been prepared. Objectionable odors in spoiled foods are usually breakdown products of lipids or proteins. Unsightly colors come from the synthesis of pigments. Slime can be produced by the accumulation of too many cells or the synthesis of dextran, a polysaccharide.

Some important food-spoilage bacterial genera include *Bacillus*, *Enterobacter*, *Erwinia*, *Lactobacillus*, *Pediococcus*, and *Pseudomonas*. Although considered commercially sterile, canned foods can spoil if *Bacillus stearothermophilus* spores or cells survive the heating process. *B. stearothermophilus* is more heat stable than *Clostridium botulinum*. Various species of *Bacillus* and *Lactobacillus* are responsible for the objectionable flavors encountered in spoiled, pasteurized milk. The bright fluorescent sheen on cold cuts left in the refrigerator too long is caused by *Pseudomonas fluorescens*, and the strong objectionable odor could be attributed to various *Enterobacter* or *Serratia* species.

Spoilage of fruits, vegetables, and their products is frequently caused by *Bacillus*, *Erwinia*, or *Pseudomonas* species of bacteria or *Penicillium* and *Alternaria* molds. Lactic acid bacteria and yeasts can cause the spoilage of fruit juices and salad dressings. Moldy bread is caused by *Penicillium* species and *Rhizopus stolonifer* (producing a nice black, fuzzy culture on the surface of the loaf; see Insert 13.7). Remember that the conditions in the food itself (pH, water activity, and presence of inhibitors) and the environment around the food (temperature and presence or absence of oxygen) determine which spoilage microorganism(s) will predominate.

Few things are more frustrating than to buy a food product and find that it has spoiled before we ever have a chance to eat it. One way to help avoid that problem is to look at the expiration date. Expiration dates are usually found only on perishable products like juices, milk, cold cuts, and chips, but they are becoming more common on many products. As should be obvious by now, fresh foods are more perishable than processed products. Shelf-life estimations are determined by predicting the increase of an undesirable characteristic or the decrease of a desirable characteristic. Quality losses tend to be either zero-order (linear) or first-order (semilogarithmic) reactions. Stability tests are conducted under defined conditions and mathematical models are developed. Accelerated storage tests can provide quicker but less reliable estimates of shelf life by looking at losses of product quality at temperatures higher than it would be stored normally. A prediction of shelf life is made on the basis of expected conditions, and an expiration date is placed on the product.

Despite some popular beliefs, the food does not change from perfectly good the day before the expiration date to completely spoiled the day after the expiration date. Rather, it is the cumulative result of small changes in quality. Small losses that occur each day add up to spoilage after many weeks

Microorganism	*Erwinia caratova*	*Rhizopus stolinifer*
Type	Gram-negative bacterium	Mold
Food products	Fruits and vegetables	Breads
Quality defects	Soft rots	Visible mold growth
Signature	Breakdown of cell walls	Black and fuzzy
Favorable conditions	Low oxygen/30°C	High humidity/30°C–35°C

INSERT 13.7
Comparison of two spoilage microorganisms.

or months. The estimate must be such that the product will be acceptable to most consumers at the expiration date, but it should not be such that people will toss out large amounts of perfectly good food just because the date has passed. Shelf life is primarily based on spoilage and not safety. If the product has recently expired, yet shows no indication of spoilage, it should be fine to eat. If the food is well past its expiration date, however, the prudent thing to do would be to toss it.

13.11 Pathogenic Microorganisms

The main reason food scientists are obsessed with microorganisms is that 95% of reported outbreaks in the United States are caused by microorganisms, with 4% caused by chemicals, and 1% caused by parasites. According to the Centers for Disease Control and Prevention, 1 in 6 Americans (48 million) get sick, 128,000 are hospitalized, and 3000 die per year because of food-borne illness. Based on commodities, produce is the most common source (46%) of outbreaks, followed by meat and poultry (22%), dairy and eggs (20%), and fish and shellfish (6%). A 2011 surveillance study reported that the most common pathogens associated with food-borne outbreaks resulting in the highest number of illnesses in the United States (in descending order) are Norovirus, *Salmonella* (nontyphoidal), *Clostridium perfringens*, *Campylobacter* species, and *Staphylococcus aureus*. However, the ones most associated with food-borne–related deaths (in descending order) are *Salmonella* (nontyphoidal), *Toxoplasma gondii*, *Listeria monocytogenes*, Norovirus, and *Campylobacter* species.

Food-associated outbreaks are most often caused by improper storage temperatures, poor personal hygiene, inadequate cooking temperatures, cross-contamination, and unsanitary or contaminated raw materials. Most outbreaks can be traced to a single pathogenic microorganism contaminating a single food that was either mishandled or prepared improperly.

Formulated and processed products are more susceptible to contamination by a single spoilage or pathogenic microorganism for reasons discussed earlier. Most food poisoning outbreaks are caused by one of a small number of harmful microorganisms. Food-associated pathogens affect immunocompromised individuals most severely. This group includes the very young, whose immune system has not yet fully developed, the elderly, whose immune system may be failing, pregnant women, and people suffering from chronic diseases (HIV, liver cirrhosis, etc.).

Food poisoning outbreaks are caused by either intoxications or infections. **Food intoxications** are caused by ingesting a toxin that has been produced by the contaminating microorganism. Only the toxin, not the pathogen, causes the illness. As the pathogen grows in the food, it produces the toxin. Some toxins are more heat stable than the microorganism that produces them. Although the toxin may survive a heat treatment, the bacterial cell does not. *S. aureus* and *C. botulinum* cause illness by this route. **Food infections** cause illness because ingested microorganisms that were in the food attack the human body. In some cases, the infecting microorganisms grow in the food; however, very low levels of contamination, depending on the microorganism, may be sufficient to induce illness. Typical food infections are those caused by *Salmonella, L. monocytogenes,* and *Escherichia coli* O157:H7. **Food toxicoinfections** occur when microorganisms grow to very high numbers in the food and continue to grow in the gastrointestinal tract. Toxin is then produced and released in the gut, which causes the symptoms. Examples of toxicoinfections are those by *C. perfringens* and *Bacillus cereus.*

Food poisoning outbreaks do not usually occur immediately after the consumption of the contaminated food and may not become evident until as much as 24 hours after consumption, or longer. Many symptoms of food-associated illnesses are the same, but each organism seems to have its signature symptom. These illnesses are categorized by their incubation time (time between eating the food and becoming ill), the symptoms, and the duration of the illness (see Insert 13.8). For example, botulism (an intoxication) develops within 12 to 36 hours of consumption of contaminated food. Symptoms start with constipation, fatigue, and muscle weakness, proceeding to droopy eyelids, blurred or double vision, dry mouth, slurred speech, and swallowing difficulties, ultimately leading to paralysis and respiratory failure in severe cases.

Microorganism	*Escherichia coli* O157:H7	*Listeria monocytogenes*	*Staphylococcus aureus*
Type	Gram-negative small rod	Gram-positive rod	Gram-positive coccus
Illness/symptoms	Hemorrhagic colitis; abdominal pain and vomiting; hemolytic uremic syndrome	Fever, muscle aches, and nausea or diarrhea; premature delivery or stillbirth in pregnant women	Severe nausea and vomiting; abdominal pain; possible diarrhea and fever
Incubation time	1–8 days	9–48 hours for gastrointestinal symptoms; 2–6 weeks for invasive disease	1–6 hours
Food products	Meats, sprouts, apple cider	Luncheon meats, cheese	Deli meats, salads, baked goods
Signature	Bloody stools	Grows at refrigeration temperatures	Heat-stable enterotoxins
Prevention	Pasteurization and cooking	Proper cooking	Refrigeration or heat

INSERT 13.8
Comparison of three pathogenic microorganisms.

E. coli O157:H7 can induce hemorrhagic colitis, characterized by bloody stools, hemolytic uremic syndrome, which is the leading cause of kidney failure in children, or thrombotic thrombocytopenic purpura, which combines kidney failure with brain damage. *C. perfringens*, a common source of food-associated infection, causes profuse diarrhea and acute abdominal pain within 6 to 24 hours of consumption. In most cases of bacterial toxicoinfection, the symptoms will go away without medical treatment. Use of antibiotics to treat food-associated illness is controversial because it is not clear whether they provide a cure for the illness.

13.12 Epidemiology

As mentioned in Chapter 1 the science of identifying the causes of disease outbreaks is epidemiology. The more we understand the cause of a specific outbreak, the greater the chance that future outbreaks will not occur. Most outbreaks are caused by a combination of mistakes that permit the presence or growth of one of a small number of pathogens in the contaminated food. In the investigation of a food-associated outbreak, the symptoms of those who become sick provide clues as to the responsible organism. Recent food consumption records are then collected for those who became sick and common foods are identified. The length of time between consumption of the offending foods and the beginning of the outbreak is also an important clue. Some patients may develop more severe symptoms than others. Possible explanations include variations in the amount of contaminated food consumed, the level of contamination in different locations in the food, and individual sensitivities to the pathogen.

Potential causes of the outbreak may be traced to improper handling or preparation of the food. Fecal samples from the victims are taken, as well as samples of the suspected food, which are then analyzed and compared to see if they are both contaminated with the same pathogen. Possible point(s) of contamination are identified by analyzing the distribution pattern from harvest to consumption. After the collection of all the information, a pattern usually emerges: the responsible species, the initial cause of contamination, and any human errors that allowed growth of the microorganism. Immediate efforts should then be taken to prevent further spreading of the outbreak. The case study can also be used to help set up guidelines to prevent similar occurrences from happening again.

Epidemiology is relatively simple when a large percentage of a group that attended the same social function or was part of a cruise vacation comes down with an illness 12 to 16 hours after eating the same food. It becomes more difficult when only five or six people in different locations within a large state or even different states report similar symptoms over a period of 2 weeks. Epidemiological teams from the Centers of Disease Control and Prevention in collaboration with state and local health boards have become very proficient at identifying causes of outbreaks and ways to help reduce their occurrences. Food-associated epidemiology presents a special challenge. Many victims do not seek medical treatment because they are better in a few days. As a result, cases are underreported in an outbreak.

13.13 Controlling Microorganisms in Foods

The most effective way of controlling microorganisms in foods is to kill them. Food processes are primarily designed to kill microorganisms or at least to minimize their growth. Unfortunately, the same processes that can limit microbial growth can also affect quality. Since fresh foods are more likely to be unsafe than processed ones, other techniques are needed to decrease the chances for outbreaks caused by fresh foods. "Hurdles" are barriers to microbial growth in fresh and minimally processed food products. Adequate sanitation is a key factor in preventing illness and spoilage by lowering the chances for initial contamination. Processing decreases microbial populations and packaging prevents recontamination. The hurdle concept takes advantage of the combination of several techniques to slow the growth of microorganisms, to lengthen shelf life, and to maintain safety.

Using hurdle technology, microorganisms may become injured by one technique and killed by another. For example, adding an organic acid to a product may injure the cell and then a heat treatment may kill it. A lower heat treatment can be used because the cell was already weakened by the acid. Mathematical models are developed to predict microbial growth and used to estimate the safety and stability of foods as affected by these hurdles under different storage conditions. Examples of potential hurdles include low-heat treatment, low pH, low water activity, modification of atmospheres, preservatives, and ultrahigh hydrostatic pressure.

Preservatives are food additives that prevent or retard spoilage. Sucrose (table sugar) and sodium chloride (table salt) are the two most widely used preservatives. Many foods that are advertised as having "no preservatives" are actually preserved by sucrose or sodium chloride. Both of these preservatives function mainly to reduce water activity, although sodium chloride can also directly inhibit many species of microorganisms. Organic acids like lactic and citric lower pH, inhibiting the growth of most bacteria. Benzoates and sorbates are salts of organic acids that inhibit microbial growth. Hydrogen peroxide destroys *Salmonella* in egg and dairy products. Nitrates help prevent growth of *C. botulinum* in vacuum-packaged, cured meat products. Sulfur dioxide and sulfites are added to fruit juices, dried fruit, and wines to prevent growth of unwanted species. These examples are just a few of the many applications of the preservatives that are used in the food industry.

The importance of food preparation in maintaining safety must be emphasized because improperly prepared foods can cause disease and death. Sanitation is critical with raw meats, since all raw meats should be considered contaminated with pathogenic microorganisms. Anything raw meat touches, such as a cutting board, knife, or fork can become contaminated. If these practices are then used to prepare foods that are not going to be heated (like a salad), the cross-contamination can be dangerous. Cooking kills the microorganisms on the surface of the meat, but the microorganisms in the uncooked salad will continue to multiply. In a beef steak that has not been poked with a fork or other implement, the inside of the muscle tissue is considered sterile. That is why a rare beef steak is generally considered safe to eat, but a rare hamburger (where the surface has been ground and has contaminated the rest of the meat) is not considered safe to eat. Poultry and pork need to be thoroughly cooked to be safe.

13.14 Remember This!

- "Hurdles" are barriers to microbial growth in fresh and minimally processed food products.
- Most outbreaks are caused by a combination of mistakes that permit the presence or growth of one of a small number of pathogens in the contaminated food.
- Food spoilage produces undesirable aromas, color defects, and slime formation.
- Water activity, pH, oxidation–reduction potential, nutrients, growth factors, and inhibitors affect microbial growth in foods.
- Contrary to popular belief, very few foods are sterile.
- Every step in the handling or processing of food products represents an opportunity for microorganisms to contaminate the food and for food scientists to control them.
- Everything that a cell is or does is coded in its genes.
- Among the most commonly studied microorganisms in foods are bacteria, molds, and yeasts.
- Not all microorganisms are bad! Without the help of some yeasts, bacteria, and molds, we could not produce bread, wine, or yogurt, or many other healthy and delicious products.

- Microorganisms generally are life forms that cannot be seen by the naked eye; however, they represent the dominant life form on earth: they are in the air we breathe, the beverages we drink, the food we eat, and everything we touch.

13.15 Looking Ahead

This chapter introduced the topic of food microbiology. Chapter 14 will introduce food engineering, including the design of processes to protect us from disease and foods from spoilage caused by unwanted microorganisms. Chapter 15 will describe the science associated with the use of humans to evaluate the quality of food products.

Testing Comprehension

1. Describe the three main ways microorganisms affect the food we eat. Provide examples of two beneficial microorganisms and two harmful ones. What are the main differences between beneficial and detrimental microorganisms?

2. Distinguish between a bacterium, a mold, a yeast, and a virus. Provide an example of each type of microorganism. How does each affect the quality and the safety of food?

3. Compare and contrast the properties of eukaryotes and prokaryotes. Provide three examples of each. Which type is most plentiful on earth? Why?

4. A slice of pizza is inadvertently contaminated by 100 microorganisms of the same species at 10 p.m. The slice is left out on the counter all night. Calculate the number of that species that will be present in that food the next morning at 10 a.m. if it doubles every 40 minutes. Will that slice of pizza be safe to eat for breakfast? Why or why not?

5. Compile a list of all the foods and beverages eaten in the last 24 hours. Categorize those foods as to whether they are whole, processed, formulated, fermented, prepared, or chilled. Which of these foods are most likely to spoil? Which ones are most likely to become a safety hazard? Is one category more likely to spoil or become unsafe than the others? Explain. How can the chance that they spoil or become unsafe be minimized?

6. Select a favorite food. Identify all of the extrinsic and intrinsic factors that could affect microbial growth in that food. Describe how microbial growth could be slowed in this item. Has this chapter made any foods less desirable to consume in the future? Why or why not?

7. Select a favorite fermented food. List all the ingredients needed to make that product. Diagram the probable unit operations needed to manufacture it. Can a nonfermented product be manufactured to replace it? Why or why not?

8. Garrett went to an all-you-can-eat restaurant that featured a killer salad bar. He loves cold macaroni salad, but he noticed that it had a strange odor when he started to eat it. He ate it anyway, but he did not get any more when he went back for seconds. A few hours later, he was very sick and blamed it on the macaroni salad. What really upset him was that he noticed blood in the bowl when he got up and looked down before flushing. Assuming that he indeed was a victim of food poisoning, identify the probable microorganism responsible for his illness. Explain. What should he do next?

9. Selina was one of 23 guests at a pool party. One day later, nine of them came down with a serious bout of food poisoning characterized by gastroenteritis and a fever sending four of them to the hospital. Outline the steps she would need to perform to identify the organism, food, and other factors associated with the outbreak. Why is this type of investigation needed?

Further Reading

CDC, 2014. Estimates of Foodborne Illness in the United States. Available at http://www.cdc.gov/foodborneburden/index.html.

Doyle, M. P., 2003. Foodborne Parasites: A Review of the Scientific Literature Review. FRI Briefings. Available at http://fri.wisc.edu/docs/pdf/parasites.pdf.

Doyle, M. P. and R. L. Buchanan, 2012. *Food Microbiology: Fundamentals and Frontiers*, 4th ed., Washington, DC: ASM Press.

Jay, J. M., M. J. Loessner and D. A. Golden, 2005. *Modern Food Microbiology*, 7th ed., New York: Springer Science.

Ray, B., 2013. *Fundamental Food Microbiology*, 5th ed., Boca Raton, FL: CRC Press Taylor and Francis Group.

Scallan, E., R. M. Hoekstra, F. J. Angulo, R. V. Tauxe, M. A. Widdowson, S. L. Roy, J. L. Jones and P. M. Griffin, 2011. Foodborne illness acquired in the United States—Major pathogens. *Emerg. Infect. Dis.*, 17(1):7–15.

14

Food Engineering

José I. Reyes-De-Corcuera and Robert L. Shewfelt

Nil wondered why some of his protein shakes had a better mouthfeel than others. In one of his classes, he was exposed to a science called rheology, which uses engineering principles to understand the properties of liquid and semisolid food products. He decided to do an undergraduate research project on the properties of several of the shakes he had tried to see what made some better than others. He measured the viscosity of the products and compared the values with the ingredients listed on the label. Now, he understands why it is so difficult to get those protein powders into solution. Based on what he learned in the project, he now wants to become a food engineer.

Alice just landed an internship with a new beverage processing company. She was asked to join the product and process development team. The product development leader assigned her the task of purchasing two pumps needed to process the recently formulated "Berry Outrageous" fruit punch. She contacted a salesman who asked her: "What is the available NPSH? What is the expected head at the discharge of the pump? Will they pour the ingredients into a tank or will the ingredients be mixed online?" The salesman referred her to one of the engineers who in turn asked about the flow rates expected from each pump, pipe size, and viscosity of the ingredients. Alice realized that she needed to learn more about food engineering and flow of fluids to be able to better communicate with the engineers at the processing plant as well as with equipment suppliers. She was then able to provide the right information to an engineer to help her select the best pump for her application.

Because of confidentiality concerns, Alice must not divulge the type of product she is handling, just its physical properties. When she showed the selected pumps to her supervisor, she was very excited because they turned out to be cheaper than the allocated budget. However, her supervisor told her that the pump she chose would never work in their pilot plant. Alice argued that the pump could handle the flow rates and the product, but she did not realize that although the pump was stainless steel, it was neither sanitary nor approved for handling food.

Nil and Alice are now learning that food engineers have a different mind-set than most other food scientists. They actually enjoy working with numbers and solving complex, practical problems by calculating solutions from a series of important equations that allow doing mass and energy balances, as well as to characterize the physical properties of food products, design, and specify food processing equipment and entire processing plants.

14.1 Looking Back

Chapters 11 through 13 have provided a perspective on food chemistry, nutrition, and food microbiology, respectively. To preserve foods and to understand the physical structure of foods, a food scientist must also be familiar with basic engineering principles. Concepts developed in earlier chapters that recognize the importance of food engineering include the following:

- Every step in the handling or processing of food products represents an opportunity for microorganisms to contaminate the food and for food scientists to control them.

- Supply chains involve everything used in the plant from equipment to raw materials to ingredients to packaging materials to energy and water outputs and even to its workers.

- A process developer uses a pilot plant, consisting of miniaturized pieces of equipment that mimic nonideal conditions that, unlike in the laboratory, occur in the manufacturing plant, to optimize process operations.

- In selecting the ingredients for a formulation, the food scientist must consider the quality of the food, its safety, its stability, and its cost.

- Food processors must be careful to prevent contamination, beginning with the raw materials and ingredients through every unit operation, using sanitation as the key to preventing contamination.

- Food processing and preservation increases the shelf stability of a raw material usually at the cost of nutrition and quality.

- Unit operations are distinct steps common to many food processes.

- Processing techniques for a specific food are designed with an understanding of the potential microbes present and the properties of the food.

- The higher the temperature of a heat process with the shorter time needed to kill the intended microbes, the less the loss of nutrients.

- Fresh foods are more likely to contain harmful microbes than processed products.

14.2 What Is a Food Engineer?

A food engineer uses scientific and engineering principles to better understand the properties of foods as they apply to the design of industrial food processes. By training, a food engineer uses advanced mathematics to quantify physical and chemical properties of foods and thermodynamics to calculate energy requirements to process a food. With this knowledge, the engineer can calculate mass balances to follow raw ingredients through the entire process and calculate how much of each goes into finished products, food waste, or storage for later use. These calculations are necessary for designing and optimizing efficient and economical food processes.

Therefore, mathematics is at the heart of the education of food engineers. Math gives engineers the ability to visualize properties of food materials in terms of meaningful equations. Process design, modeling, and optimization require advanced mathematics, which includes the solution of complex systems using techniques learned in algebra, calculus, and other advanced mathematical courses such as differential equations.

14.3 Engineering Fundamentals

Engineers select and apply fundamental scientific principles such as the laws of thermodynamics, Newton's laws of motion, or Fick's laws of diffusion to design processes. As we learned earlier, food processes consist of combinations of unit operations. Subdividing an entire process into smaller pieces is critical to calculating sound mass and energy balances. Furthermore, adequate selection of the part of a process around which such balances are to be made is essential. Therefore, we must first start by identifying the main types of systems as shown in Insert 14.1.

14.4 Mass Balance

The food industry uses the concept of "conservation of mass" via mass or material balance extensively. The same amount of material that comes into a processing plant in the form of raw ingredients must either leave the facility in the form of a final product, waste, or be accumulated in the warehouse as inventory for future use. Inefficiencies and losses are commonplace, especially when starting up or shutting down the processing plant and cleaning

System	Definition	Examples
Closed	No mass comes in or goes out of the system	A batch of honey mustard salad dressing once all the ingredients have been added.
Open	All continuous processes into which raw materials are continuously input, and product is continuously recovered	On-line mixing of flavors during the formulation of a soda.
Isothermal	Processes kept at the same temperature by addition or removal or heat	Fresh fruit kept in a refrigerated storage room.
Adiabatic	No heat is transferred in or out	Hot milk flowing in the thermally insulated holding section of a pasteurizer.
Isolated	Both closed and adiabatic such that no mass or energy is transferred to or from it	Hot soup kept in an insulated container such as a thermos.

INSERT 14.1
Main food systems from an engineering point of view.

up after the last shift. These losses need to be minimized to maximize profits. Thus, food scientists who become shift or plant managers need to understand and be able to calculate basic mass balances.

One of the daily tasks of a plant manager is to run a mass balance of all the plant's operations to identify bottlenecks, minimize inefficiencies, estimate profits, and adjust sales strategies. Mass balances must be done around entire processes and around individual unit operations such as drying, evaporation, concentration, peeling, cutting, canning, and so on. An example of a mass balance for orange juice is shown in Insert 14.2. Although one would think that making orange juice is a simple process, this diagram illustrates that, in reality, it involves several products (not-from-concentrate and concentrate juice) and by-products (dry peel, cold pressed oils, aroma, molasses, D-limonene). All of these products must be monitored and controlled to maximize the profitability of the processing plant, ensuring that juice yield is as high as possible and that waste and environmental impact are minimized.

Regardless of the state of matter (solid, gas, or liquid), the concept of mass balance can be applied on total mass in and out of the plant. Likewise, an understanding of how energy is distributed through the plant is necessary.

14.5 Energy Balance

Similar to the "conservation of mass," the law of "energy conservation" is also used in food engineering. The **Law of Conservation of Energy** states that energy cannot be created or destroyed; it can only be changed from one form to another. There are only two basic forms of energy: **kinetic energy**, which is associated with motion, and **potential energy**, which is associated

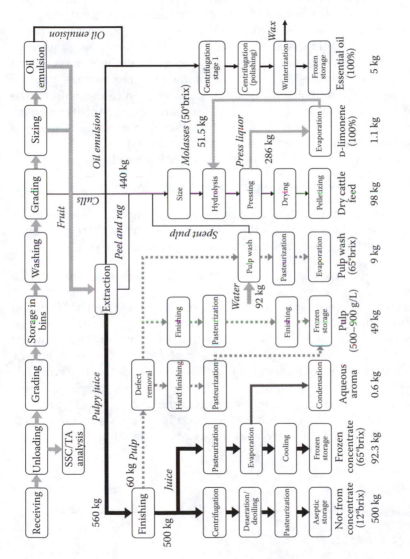

INSERT 14.2

Approximate mass balance values for orange juice and orange by-product processing. Mass balance values are approximate as they vary depending on processing conditions. (From Reyes-De-Corcuera, J.I. et al., Oranges. In *Tropical and Subtropical Fruits: Postharvest Physiology, Processing and Packaging*, Siddiq, M. et al., eds., Ames, IA: Wiley-Blackwell, 2012, Chapter 21. With permission.)

with the position/proximity to other systems. Energy use is normally computed or measured relative to some reference state. The basic measure of energy is the work required to bring the system to its designated state or condition relative to some initial reference state in an adiabatic process. The total energy of a system is the sum of its bulk kinetic and potential energies, plus all the microscopic kinetic and potential energies, or internal energy.

Thermodynamic principles involve the conversion of one form of energy into another. Food engineers are very familiar with the concept of work or the mechanical energy required in moving a given amount of mass, which is a critical factor in the design of pumping and conveying systems. Internal energy is associated with chemical bonds and useful in understanding the changes in temperature associated with **endothermic** and **exothermic** reactions. **Enthalpy**, another term of thermodynamics, is a measure of the total energy of a system. A common unit of energy is joule (J).

If a balance is made for total energy, the energy balance becomes

$$\text{Energy In} = \text{Energy Out} + \text{Accumulation} \tag{14.1}$$

From a practical point of view, food scientists and engineers are most concerned with heat, the least efficient form of energy from a thermodynamic point of view but the most important one in preserving foods.

$$\text{Heat In} + \text{Reaction Heat} = \text{Heat Out} + \text{Heat Accumulation} \tag{14.2}$$

This equation does not contradict the conservation of energy. The "Reaction Heat" term stands for heat produced or absorbed during a chemical reaction or change of phase, such as the change of ice to liquid water or liquid water to steam. Heat is sometimes produced at the expense of other types of energy such as internal energy of a chemical reaction. Some endothermic reactions or phase changes are common in the food industry. For example, a simple operation such as dissolving sugar in water requires energy leading to a temperature decrease as heat is absorbed. Therefore, heat alone is not conserved. With this knowledge, it then becomes important for us to understand how heat is transferred within food processes.

14.6 Heat Transfer

Heating and cooling are extensively used in food processing and storage. Some common examples of heat transfer processes are as follows:

- Cooling of fruits and vegetables
- Freezing of foods

- Sterilization of canned foods
- Pasteurization of milk
- Drying of foods with heat

Heat transfer is transmission of energy from a higher-temperature object to a lower-temperature object. There are three modes of heat transfer: conduction, convection, and radiation. Conduction occurs within a solid object or from one body to another in direct contact by interchange of kinetic energy between molecules being heated or cooled. Conduction can also occur in high-viscosity, motionless liquids. Convection heat transfer occurs in liquids and gases when they are placed in motion by mechanical stirring or forced convection. Also, changes in density in the fluid in some regions close to the heat source make the fluid expand. Then, the colder, denser fluid moves downward, pulled by gravity, producing mixing by natural convection.

Thermal radiation describes the electromagnetic radiation that is emitted at the surface of a body that has been thermally excited. The emitted radiation may be reflected, transmitted, or absorbed by another body. The rate at which a body reflects or absorbs radiation is termed **emissivity**. Radiative heat transfer only occurs at a surface. As the temperature of the surface of the body being heated increases, then heat is transferred to the rest of the body and its environment by conduction and convection.

Plate heat exchangers or pasteurizers are often used in dairy and beverage processing as shown in Insert 14.3. On one side of a set of parallel plates, the product flows, and in the other, heating or cooling fluids flow and heat is transferred through the plates. In this ingenious design that minimizes energy usage, the cold, unpasteurized product is pumped into a first section where it is preheated against hot pasteurized product, coming out of the **holding** section. That hot product is in turn precooled. The preheated product then flows to the heating section where it is heated against steam or hot water. Then, the product flows through a holding section where it is kept hot for a predetermined amount of time (pasteurization time) and then, as mentioned before, the product is precooled in the first section. Finally, the precooled product is cooled down against cold water.

To calculate how heat is transferred within a food, we need to determine the properties of food materials with respect to heat.

14.6.1 Thermal Properties of Materials

The ability of a material to store and conduct heat depends on the chemical composition and molecular structure of the material as well as the distribution uniformity for composite, heterogeneous materials. Any material can be characterized in terms of its thermal properties, which are intrinsic and do not depend on the mass or amount of material. The first and perhaps most easily understood thermal property is the **heat capacity** or specific heat,

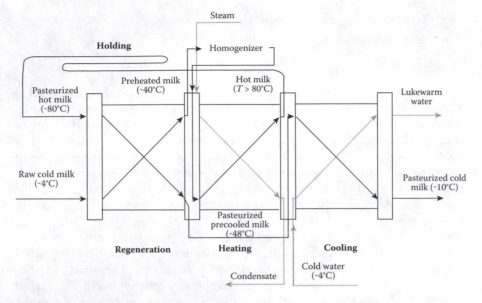

INSERT 14.3
Engineering diagram of a plate pasteurizer for pasteurization of milk (similar pasteurizers are used for fruit juices and other beverages). Note that the raw cold milk entering process is used to help cool the warm milk, which, in turn, is used to help heat up the raw milk.

denoted C_p. The heat capacity is defined as the amount of energy (in joules) required to raise the temperature of a body of a given mass in degrees Kelvin. The subscript "p" indicates that the property is determined at constant pressure. For example, the C_p of water is 4.18 J/(g·K) at 100 kPa (atmospheric pressure). In contrast, the heat capacity of stainless steel 304 L, which is the most commonly used in the food industry, is only 0.5 J/(g·K) (or 8 times smaller than water) and that of flour (13% moisture) 1.8 J/(g·K). Knowledge of the heat capacity allows us to calculate the amount of heat required to heat a material of a given mass "m" by a given change in temperature ΔT (sensible heat or Q_s):

$$Q_s = mC_p\Delta T \tag{14.3}$$

This number is extremely important because it shows the minimal amount of thermal energy required under ideal conditions, and, therefore, it is the first estimate of the energy costs of a food process. It is thermodynamically impossible for a process to cost less than what is predetermined by Q_s! In reality, the cost is much higher because of inefficiencies and heat losses that accumulate during processing. However, engineers and food scientists aim at this number when optimizing processes. This calculation only applies to foods that do not undergo phase changes. Further discussion is beyond the scope of this chapter.

The second property—the thermal conductivity "*k*"—characterizes the ability of a material to conduct heat and is used to characterize the **rate** of heat conduction. Hence, thermal conductivity is expressed in units of energy per unit of time (watts or joules per second) per distance within the material (meters) because conduction implies that heat *travels* through the material per unit of temperature (Kelvin). A greater difference in temperature will increase heat flow. In summary, an example of units for the thermal conductivity is

$$\frac{J/s}{m \cdot K} \quad \text{or} \quad \frac{W}{m \cdot K}.$$

The thermal conductivity of water, stainless steel, and glass wool insulation is 0.58, 16, and 0.04 W/(m·K), respectively. These numbers tell us that although stainless steel is not a good heat conductor for a metal, heat will conduct 30 times faster in stainless steel than in water and 10 times faster in water than in glass wool. The high thermal conductivity of metal is why it is necessary to use thermal insulation around metal pieces of equipment in processing plants where heat can be lost to the surroundings or employees can get burned when touching a hot piece of equipment.

Thermal conductivity was defined in Fourier's law as heat conduction that establishes the relationship between the heat flux ($\dot{q}_x$), the temperature difference (dT) between two points within a body, and the distance between them (dx):

$$\dot{q}_x = -k \frac{dT}{dx}. \tag{14.4}$$

This relationship is important because it allows food scientists to predict the rate of heating in solid foods and, therefore, the time required to fully cook a food in what is known as the **cold spot**. An understanding of the cold spot is crucial for food safety and food quality in meats, bakery, confections, and other types of products. The opposite of thermal conductivity is called thermal resistivity, which reflects the insulation value of a material. Many insulating materials are specified by their insulation value or *R* value.

Thermal conductivity is dependent on the characteristics of materials, moisture content, and temperature. High-moisture foods have very little air space, and their thermal conductivity is very close to that of water. Also, foods show higher thermal conductivity at higher temperatures. Finally, because many foods are nonhomogenous and nonuniform, the thermal conductivity may have a different value in a special direction than in another. A well-known example is in meat, like beef, where the value parallel to fibers is approximately 15% to 20% higher than that perpendicular to fibers.

14.6.2 Heat Transfer Coefficients

Heat transfer is even more complex when dealing with solid–liquid or solid–vapor interfaces where the fluid is in motion with respect to the solid. In these cases, it is observed that the temperature profiles appear to be discontinuous in the liquid phase as graphically illustrated in Insert 14.4a, which contrasts with Insert 14.4b that depicts conduction in two solids.

To mathematically account for the apparent discontinuity in the temperature profile at the solid–fluid interface, a **convective heat transfer coefficient** "*h*" is introduced into the equation. This coefficient relates the rate of heat transfer $\dot{Q}$ (in joules per second) to the area A (in square meters) and the temperature difference ΔT (in Kelvin):

$$\dot{Q} = \frac{dQ}{dt} = h \cdot A \Delta T. \tag{14.5}$$

In other words, the heat transfer coefficient is a proportionality factor that relates the heat flux ($\dot{q}$ = flow rate of heat per surface area) and the temperature gradient ΔT.

$$h = \frac{\dot{q}}{\Delta T} \tag{14.6}$$

Hence, the heat transfer coefficient has units of $\dfrac{J/s}{m^2 \cdot K}$, that is, joules per second, per square meter, Kelvin. This coefficient is similar to the thermal conductivity, but it accounts for the surface area through which heat is being transferred and not for the heat penetration.

Experimental determination of individual surface heat transfer coefficients is not possible because we are unable to measure accurately the surface temperature of the conducting solid. With careful experiments, however, we can obtain an approximate value. Moreover, most heat exchangers become clogged over time, and the heat transfer coefficient decreases. An understanding of heat transfer is critical in many food processes, including the manufacture of peanut butter (see Insert 14.5).

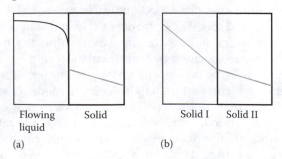

| Flowing liquid | Solid | | Solid I | Solid II |

(a)   (b)

INSERT 14.4
Temperature profiles for (a) convective heat transfer from a hot flowing liquid to a cold solid and (b) heat conduction from a hot solid (Solid I) to a cold solid (Solid II).

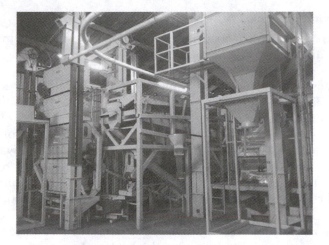

INSERT 14.5
Equipment in a peanut butter plant, R.L. Cunningham and Sons, Quitman, Georgia. (Photo provided by the Georgia Peanut Commission, taken by Jessie Turk and found at http://gapea nuttour.wordpress.com/.)

Finally, in most heating and cooling systems, there are at least two convective barriers (flowing fluids) separated by a conductive barrier (heat exchanger). For example, in the heating section of a milk pasteurizer, condensing steam or hot water is in touch with one side of a stainless steel plate or tube and on the other side is the milk that is being pasteurized. To calculate heat transfer between the steam and the milk, we must account for both surface heat transfer coefficients. In practice, this calculation is done by estimating an overall heat transfer coefficient, denoted "U." From a practical perspective, food scientists must be aware that to maximize energy efficiency, they should consult with engineers who study ways of maximizing the overall heat transfer coefficients. Air-free condensing steam is the most efficient means of heating liquids in a heat exchanger.

Heat is not the only thing that is transferred during unit operations. During mixing of ingredients and separation processes such as evaporation or centrifugation, mass is transferred from one medium or phase to another.

14.7 Mass Transfer

Mass transfer results in the transport of atoms or molecules within physical systems. Some common examples of mass transfer processes are as follows:

- **Diffusion** of salt or nutrients in food products
- **Migration** of aromatic volatiles or moisture through a package

- **Evaporation** of water during dehydration or concentration
- **Separation** of components in a distillation column or during membrane filtration

Mass transfer takes place at the interface between two phases or within a material. The driving force is a difference in concentration as the random motion of molecules causes a net transfer of mass from an area of high concentration to an area of low concentration. In the case of evaporation, heat needs to be applied to produce the phase change. For example, water evaporates from a food surface that is exposed to an unsaturated air stream that is at the same temperature as the water. In this case, the water vapor pressure at the surface is higher than that in the air and thus the evaporation of water occurs.

The required heat of evaporation is taken from the water itself. The temperature of water is lowered, causing the heat to flow from air to water at a rate proportional to the temperature difference. This action results in a dynamic equilibrium in which the water temperature does not decrease any further and the heat supplied by the air is just sufficient to balance the heat required for steady evaporation. The temperature of water under this condition is called the wet-bulb temperature, which is particularly useful in calculating drying rates and drying times.

A common unit operation during food manufacture is mixing. Mixing of components involves diffusion.

14.7.1 Fick's Law of Diffusion

Similar to conduction, diffusion of one material into another can be expressed as

$$\frac{\dot{m}_B}{A} = -D \frac{dC}{dx}, \tag{14.7}$$

where $\dot{m}_B$ is the flux of component B (in kilograms per second), A is the area through which B is diffusing, C is the concentration, x is the direction of diffusion, and D is the diffusivity in square meters per second. The units of diffusivity are intuitive and refer to the ability of a compound to diffuse. Mass transfer by diffusion occurs when the bulk of the components is stagnant; in other words, there is no convection.

14.7.2 Convective Mass Transfer

When convection occurs, whether natural or forced, a discontinuity appears in the concentration profiles between the two phases similar to what we saw with heat transfer. A mathematical treatment similar to that of heat transfer gives rise to convective mass transfer coefficients:

$$k_m = \frac{\dot{m}_B}{A(C_{B1} - C_{B2})},$$

(14.8)

where k_m is the mass transfer coefficient and C_B represents the concentration of component B at locations 1 and 2. The units of k_m are m³/(m²·s), representing a volume of component B transported per unit of time across a boundary with a given surface (m²). Further discussion is beyond the scope of this chapter. However, a food scientist must keep in mind for practical purposes that dissolving and mixing processes involving mass transfer through diffusion and convection require time.

In many processes, mass transfer can become a bottleneck. Although mass transfer time can be determined by observation or experiments, process design optimization requires knowledge of diffusivities and diffusion coefficients. The diffusivity of a component "B" into a component "A" depends to a great extent on other physical properties of component A. For example, "A" can be a gel or a liquid while chemically having the same composition. However, the diffusivity in the gel is much smaller than that in the liquid. This difference relates to the difference in rheology of the gel and the liquid. Rheology is the study of the flow behavior of fluids and is critical to understand and quantify flow of fluids, mass, and heat transfer.

14.8 Rheology

As discussed in the previous sections, the flow behavior of fluids affects heat and mass transfer dramatically. The fluids of interest in food engineering are liquid foods like beverages and semisolid foods like cream, honey, gels, pastes, puddings, purees, and sauces. It is clear that the rheological properties of a material have a direct impact in the amount of energy required to put that fluid into motion and make it flow from one place to another. For example, it takes more energy to pump honey than to pump water in the same system at the same flow rate.

A main task of food engineers is to design flowing systems for foods. Beyond the impact in equipment and process design, the rheological properties of foods have a major impact on taste and mouthfeel of a product. Viscosity is the resistance to flow of fluids. Increasing viscosity can lower flavor perception, which relies upon the ability of flavor compounds to diffuse from the food onto the tongue and reach the taste buds. An increase in temperature typically results in a decrease in viscosity and an increase in the rate of diffusion, leading to a more intense sensory experience. As we chew our food, flavor perception is enhanced by a combination of warming, dilution with saliva, and convection produced by teeth and tongue action. A typical example is melting of chocolate fat in the mouth. Thus, a food engineer in collaboration with a sensory scientist can tailor the viscosity of a product to control the diffusion of flavor or its perception over time by studying its rheological properties.

14.8.1 Rheological Properties and Types of Fluids

As for thermal and mass transfer properties, food engineers are often asked to determine rheological properties of foods that can be used to make pertinent engineering calculations or to correlate them to sensory perceptions. When a fluid is put into motion, fluid molecules slip past each other in a particular direction, which means that there is a difference in velocity between adjacent molecules. The resistance of the fluid to flow in a defined plane is called shear stress, and the velocity difference between adjacent molecules is called shear rate. The relationship between shear stress $\dot{\sigma}$ and shear rate $\dot{\gamma}$ characterizes the type of fluid.

A general equation that describes multiple types of fluids has been proposed:

$$\dot{\sigma} = \dot{\sigma}_0 + K(\dot{\gamma})^n,$$ (14.9)

where K is the consistency coefficient, which is an indication of how viscous a fluid is, and n is the flow behavior index, which is an indicator of how shear stress changes with shear rate. If $n < 1$, the fluid is called shear-thinning or **pseudoplastic** because the slope of the curve representing the apparent viscosity decreases as shear rate increases. If $n > 1$, it is called shear-thickening or **dilatant** because the slope of the curve increases with shear rate. Apple sauce and mayonnaise are pseudoplastic products as they become thinner during mastication. Some types of honey are dilatant as they become thicker when in our mouths.

Some fluids have a yield shear stress, which means that, before the fluid can start moving at all, a certain amount of shear stress $\dot{\sigma}_0$ needs to be applied. If the relationship between the shear stress and shear rate is linear ($n = 1$), and the fluid exhibits yield stress, it is a **Bingham plastic**. If a nonlinear relationship is observed with yield stress, it is called Bingham pseudoplastic ($n > 1$) or **Herschel–Bulkley plastic** ($n < 1$). Tomato paste and fat-free cream cheese are examples of a Bingham plastic product as it takes force to get them moving but then they flow uniformly. A full-fat cream cheese is an example of a Herschel–Bulkley plastic as it takes additional force to move it more rapidly out of a squeeze package. For other fluids like water, the fluid begins to move as soon as a shear stress is applied. For such fluids, Equation 14.9 reduces to

$$\dot{\sigma} = K(\dot{\gamma})^n.$$ (14.10)

This equation is called the power law, because it relates shear stress to shear rate to the nth power. Generally speaking, fluids whose behavior can be modeled with this equation are called "power law fluids." A particular case of this last equation is when $n = 1$. In that case, there is a linear relationship between shear stress and shear rate:

$$\dot{\sigma} = K(\dot{\gamma}) = \mu\dot{\gamma}. \tag{14.11}$$

Fluids that follow this simple behavior are called **Newtonian fluids** because the term was established by Sir Isaac Newton who called the proportionality constant μ "coefficient of viscosity" or simply "viscosity." Therefore, for practical purposes, viscosity is a measure of resistance to flow of a fluid, and it is determined as the slope of the curve of shear stress versus shear rate. Water, milk, and dilute sugar solutions are examples of Newtonian fluids. Viscosity of water at 20°C is 1 centiPoise (cP) and that of milk is approximately 2 cP. Viscosity is determined with capillary or rotational viscometers. Capillary viscometers are inexpensive and are based on measuring the time it takes for a given volume of a fluid to flow through a capillary of a given diameter. As viscosity decreases, so does the diameter of the capillary. The best known rotational viscometer is produced by Brookfield Engineering Laboratories (an example is shown in Insert 14.6).

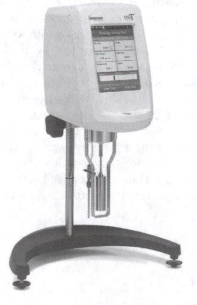

INSERT 14.6
Brookfield DV2T Touch Screen Viscometer with LV1 Spindle and Integrated Temperature Probe. Viscometers measure viscosity (resistance to flow) of liquid and semisolid products. (Image provided by Brookfield Engineering Laboratories.)

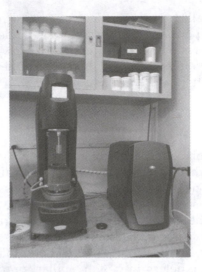

INSERT 14.7
AR 2000 Discovery Hybrid Rheometer from TA Instruments, New Castle, Delaware, installed at the University of Georgia, Food Processing Laboratory. (Photo courtesy of José I. Reyes-De-Corcuera.)

As mentioned earlier, many foods are non-Newtonian, and we can only talk about **apparent viscosity** at a particular shear rate. Rigorous characterization of such fluids requires the determination of both parameters K and n. Measurement of these parameters requires a rotational rheometer (an example is shown in Insert 14.7). That instrument is similar to a viscometer, but the geometry is such that the shear rate can be calculated. Many formulated foods require a tight control on viscosity or apparent viscosity, which can be monitored on the processing line during the manufacturing of the product. The apparent viscosity of ketchup is monitored during the blending of its ingredients: tomato paste with sugar, vinegar, and flavorings.

The effect of lipids on textural properties of cream cheese is an example of the importance of the functional properties of chemical components in a product on sensory quality. These properties become crucial in developing an understanding of how fluids flow within the processing plant.

14.9 Flow of Fluids

The handling of fluid products (fruit juices, sauce, pastes, etc.) is done by pumping them through pipes and processing equipment. Fluid motion requires energy input. Using the laws of physics, we can determine the potential energy needed if the fluid is to be pumped to a given elevation.

Since the fluid is in motion, kinetic energy must also be included in our calculations. Also, pressure must be accounted for, especially in systems that are pressurized. Finally, we need to consider that as a fluid flows through a pipe or duct, friction at the interface between the fluid and the surface of the pipe occurs. Based on the conservation of energy, mechanical energy balance can be calculated for a flowing system without accounting for friction:

$$\frac{\rho v^2}{2} + \rho g z + p = \text{constant}, \tag{14.12}$$

where ρ is the density of the fluid, v is the linear velocity, g is the acceleration of gravity, z is the elevation, and p is pressure. The first term accounts for the kinetic energy; the second, for the potential energy; and the third, for pressure. In this equation, we can see that the physical properties of the fluid also affect flow.

Both kinetic and potential energies depend on the mass of the body, which is accounted for through the use of the density. The pressure component is not directly related to any physical property of the fluid but to the conditions of the system. Finally, friction is affected by both density and viscosity. Therefore, flow of fluids depends on the viscosity, density, velocity, and the size, shape, and roughness of the pipe or duct it flows through.

Flow of fluids may be broadly characterized as laminar or turbulent. In laminar flow, the path of each molecule of fluid follows a well-defined streamline, which can be demonstrated by injecting a fine stream of dye in the flow stream when a clear fluid is pumped through a straight transparent pipe. Laminar flow happens when the flow rate or velocity of fluid is relatively low. Turbulent flow occurs when the flow velocity increases, leading to collision of fluid molecules with each other more frequently and crossing over the streamlines (see Insert 14.8). Eddy currents develop and cause certain amount of mixing in the fluid. This action can be easily demonstrated by increasing the flow rate of a colored dye during experiments for laminar flow until the mixing of dye is noticed.

The distinction between laminar and turbulent flow is made on the basis of the Reynolds number (Re), which is a dimensionless quantity. For Newtonian fluids flowing in a cylindrical pipe,

$$\text{Re} = \frac{D v \rho}{\mu}, \tag{14.13}$$

where D is the pipe diameter, v is the fluid velocity, ρ is the density, and μ is the viscosity. For Newtonian fluids, if the value of Re is below 2100, the fluid flow is laminar, and if it is higher than 4000, the flow is turbulent. However, the flow is considered transitional from laminar to turbulent for Re between 2100 and 4000. The magnitude of energy loss attributed to friction is a function of Re and is accounted for by calculating the **friction factor**. Reynolds

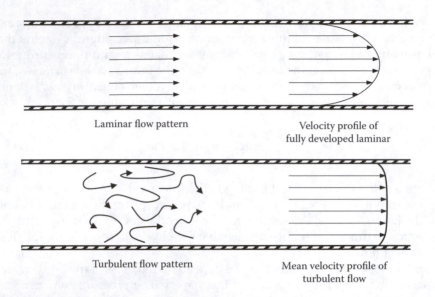

Laminar flow pattern   Velocity profile of
                                        fully developed laminar

Turbulent flow pattern   Mean velocity profile of
                                        turbulent flow

INSERT 14.8
Diagram of the differences between laminar and turbulent flow in a pipe.

number and turbulence are also important in the design of mixing operations as they are used to estimate the time required for adequate mixing, dispersing, or dissolving food components in a liquid.

The mechanical energy balance is often expressed in terms of pressure because pressure is a variable that is easy to measure. Therefore, another useful concept in understanding fluid dynamics is pressure drop. Like friction, pressure drop is a function of fluid properties like density, viscosity, and fluid velocity, as well as the dimensions and roughness of the pipe or duct in which the fluid is flowing. The pumping requirement is calculated using a mechanical energy balance on the flow system.

Flow of compressible fluids such as gases, in particular condensing steam, is extremely important in the food industry. Since this topic is beyond the scope of this chapter, interested students should pursue it in the introductory texts on food engineering provided at the end of the chapter. Food scientists must be aware, however, that compressible and incompressible fluids behave differently. Perhaps the most important fluid in any process is water.

14.10 Water Management

Water is used for food and beverage formulation, cleaning equipment, cooling containers, and may even be produced during food evaporation or drying. Water supply to food processes must be potable and free of any component that might affect the flavor of the food product such as minerals and traces of some organic matter. It may therefore be necessary to treat water before it is used. There are two types of treatments: removal of suspended solids and removal or destruction of microorganisms.

Suspended solids can be removed by allowing them to settle out in settling tanks or filtering the water through specially designed water filters. Both processes are relatively slow and large storage tanks are necessary if water is needed for washing or incorporation into the product. Additionally, water used in food preparation needs to be tasteless and have adequate mineral concentration to avoid undesired impact in the sensory properties of the end product. Water for cooling can be recirculated, which can affect overall water treatment and use.

Although some types of water filters also remove microorganisms, the easiest way of destroying them is to add chlorine solution (5–8 ppm final concentration of chlorine obtained by diluting bleach to 0.02%–0.04%). Lower chlorine levels (e.g., 0.5 ppm) are needed if the water is to be used in a product in order to prevent "off" flavors. Chlorination of water supplies can be simply arranged by allowing bleach (sodium hypochlorite) to drip, at a fixed rate, into storage tanks or pipelines. The rate of bleach addition is determined by experiment, using simple chlorine paper or more sophisticated probes to check the chlorine concentration. A common alternative that prevents off-flavors produced by chlorine or other oxidizing agents is the use of ultraviolet light or ozone treatments to sterilize (see diagram in Insert 14.9). A less suitable alternative is to boil water to sterilize it. Water should be heated to boiling and then boiled vigorously for at least 10 minutes. This operation has a high fuel requirement and will therefore increase processing costs.

Water plays many roles in food manufacturing plants. Water is frequently used as a medium for heat transfer from a heating or cooling unit to food. Boiling, steaming, and simmering are popular cooking methods that often require immersing food in water or its gaseous state, steam. To maintain adequate sanitation within a plant, frequent cleaning is necessary throughout a production shift and thorough cleaning is required at the end of each production run. Clean-in-Place uses circulation of water or other sanitizing fluids through the internal workings of equipment without the need to break the machinery down into its component parts.

Water hardness is a critical factor in food processing. Hard water has much higher levels of minerals than soft water. Water hardness is classified based on the amounts of removable calcium carbonate salt it contains per gallon. Water hardness is measured in grains; 0.064 g calcium carbonate is equivalent to 1 grain of hardness. Water is classified as soft if it contains 1 to 4 grains, medium if it contains 5 to 10 grains, and hard if it contains 11 to 20 grains.

The hardness of water also affects its pH, which plays a critical role in food processing. For example, hard water prevents successful production of clear beverages. Water hardness also affects sanitation; with increasing hardness, there is a loss of effectiveness for its use as a sanitizer. Finally, perhaps the

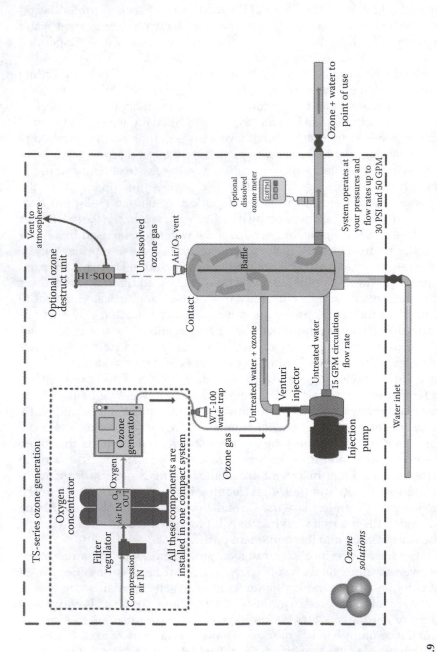

INSERT 14.9

Diagram of a system for ozone purification of water. (Image from http://www.ozonesolutions.com/info/ozone-water-treatment used with permission from Ozone Solutions Inc.)

most important issue related to hard water is the deposition of minerals in heat exchangers because these minerals foul the surface and act as thermal insulators, resulting in dramatic decreases in the heat transfer coefficients. The mineral content of water also contributes to equipment corrosion, in particular boilers. To compensate, steam, that is, energy consumption, increases. In undesirable scenarios, for example, pasteurization temperatures are no longer achieved. The hardness of water may be altered or treated by using a chemical ion-exchange system.

14.11 Remember This!

- Water is used for food and beverage formulation, cleaning equipment, cooling containers, and may even be produced during food evaporation or drying.
- Flow of fluids may be broadly characterized as laminar or turbulent.
- Increasing viscosity can lower flavor perception, which relies upon the ability of flavor compounds to diffuse from the food onto the tongue and reach the taste buds.
- Mass transfer results in the transport of atoms or molecules within physical systems.
- Thermal conductivity characterizes the ability of a material to conduct heat and is used to characterize the rate of heat conduction.
- The ability of a material to store and conduct heat depends on the chemical composition and molecular structure of the material as well as the distribution uniformity for composite, heterogeneous materials.
- Heat transfer is transmission of energy from a higher-temperature object to a lower-temperature object.
- There are only two basic forms of energy: kinetic energy, which is associated with motion, and potential energy, which is associated with the position/proximity to other systems.
- Engineers select and apply fundamental scientific principles such as the laws of thermodynamics, Newton's laws of motion, or Fick's laws of diffusion to design processes.
- The same amount of mass that comes into the processing plant in the form of raw ingredients must either leave the facility in the form of a final product or waste or be accumulated in the warehouse as inventory for future use.

14.12 Looking Ahead

Chapter 15 will describe how we evaluate quality of foods using humans instead of instruments.

Testing Comprehension

1. Describe three different situations in which a food scientist would need knowledge of engineering to be an effective employee in a food processing plant.

2. Compare and contrast the importance of heat and fluid flow in ensuring the quality and safety of formulated foods.

3. Distinguish between a batch and a continuous process. How do the two types of processes affect the determination of mass and mechanical energy balances?

4. Distinguish the effect of conduction and convection on the cold spot of a food during heating.

5. Calculate the Reynolds number of Berry Outrageous, which has a density = 1050 kg/m^3, a flow behavior index = 1, a fluid velocity = 0.276 m/s, in a circular pipe with a diameter = 0.04 m, and a viscosity = 0.006 Pa·s. What type of fluid is this (Newtonian or type of non-Newtonian)? Will the flow be laminar, turbulent, or transitional between the two? What would happen if the diameter of the pipe were increased or decreased assuming the same velocity?

6. Compare and contrast the effects of the difference in the processing operations of Berry Outrageous in its two plants—one in Maine with 0.25 g calcium carbonate and the other in Colorado with 0.75 g calcium carbonate. How will this water affect processing operations and the sensory and nutritional quality of the product?

7. Summarize the practical significance of three calculations that were described in the chapter.

8. Explain how food engineers can contribute to the manufacture of more sustainable food products.

Reference

Reyes-De-Corcuera, J. I., R. J. Braddock and R. M. Goodrich Schneider, 2012. Oranges, in *Tropical and Subtropical Fruits: Postharvest Physiology, Processing and Packaging*, Siddiq, M., Ahmed, J., Lobo, M. G. and Ozadali, F., Eds., Ames, IA: Wiley-Blackwell.

Further Reading

Fellows, P. J., 2009. *Food Processing Technology: Principles and Practices*, Cambridge, UK: Woodhead Publishing Limited.

Rao, M. A., S. S. H. Rizvi and A. K. Datta, 2005. *Engineering Properties of Foods*, 3rd ed., Boca Raton, FL: CRC Press, Taylor & Francis Group.

Singh, R. P. and D. R. Heldman, 2013. *Introduction to Food Engineering*, 5th ed., New York: Academic Press.

Tewari, G. and V. K. Juneja, 2007. *Advances in Thermal and Non-Thermal Food Preservation*, Ames, IA: Blackwell Publishing Professional.

Toledo, R. T., 2006. *Fundamentals of Food Process Engineering*, 3rd ed., New York: Springer Scientific.

Vaclavik, V. A. and E. W. Christian, 2008. *Essentials of Food Science*, 4th ed., New York: Springer Scientific.

15

Sensory and Consumer Science

Leah has read that the food industry has addicted American consumers to processed foods by adding large amounts of salt, sugar, and fat. She has learned about a new technique that scans the brain while being exposed to new foods. For her graduate project, she wants to use these scans to study the effects of foods low in salt, sugar, and fat on consumer acceptability.

Tiana remembers how great the tropical fruits were that she ate last summer on her study abroad trip to Thailand. She loved the mangoes in particular. She had not been able to find any nearly as tasty back in the States. She wants to know more about the diverse flavors she encountered in different varieties and the chemistry behind the differences.

Ignacio likes sushi more than any other food. Although he understands the importance of sushi flavor, he realizes that texture of the rice is an important aspect of its quality. He wants to combine his interest in the culinary arts and food chemistry to study the textural properties of rice in sushi products.

Leah, Tiana, and Ignacio are food scientists who need to learn sensory techniques to answer the questions they have posed. Although technology is advancing rapidly, there are still some measurements that are best made by humans rather than by instruments. These tests can involve highly trained panelists or untrained consumers. The general area of study is called sensory and consumer science.

15.1 Looking Back

Previous chapters focused on food issues we deal with in our daily lives, with the types of food products we encounter in the marketplace, activities that food scientists perform, and the basic sciences that provide the foundation for this discipline. This chapter is a continuation of Chapter 7 on Quality Assurance. Although food scientists use many instruments and other physicochemical techniques to analyze foods, some research techniques require human subjects. Sensory evaluation of food products is one of these techniques. The following key points covered in previous chapters will help prepare us for sensory studies:

- Increasing viscosity can lower flavor perception, which relies upon the ability of flavor compounds to diffuse from the food onto the tongue and reach the taste buds.

- Food spoilage produces undesirable aromas, color defects, and slime formation.
- Questions on the acceptance of new food technologies, agricultural practices, and governmental policies are being raised and studied.
- Creativity is important in designing a product or process that results in something many consumers will enjoy eating and come back for more.
- Although quality focuses on the characteristics of the product, acceptability considers the attitudes of the consumer.
- For a quality measurement to be useful, it must be accurate, precise, sensitive, and relevant.
- Quality includes sensory characteristics that can be readily detected by the five senses and hidden characteristics that are not readily detectable by consumers.
- In selecting the ingredients for a formulation, the food scientist must consider the quality of the food, its safety, its stability, and its cost.
- The conditions that affect nutritional value also affect sensory quality.
- It is not just the taste but the combination of all the sensory properties, that is, flavor, appearance, and texture, that influence our choice of food.

We perceive quality through the five senses (sight, hearing, smell, taste, and touch). Appearance is judged by sight, flavor by the senses of smell and taste, and texture by touch. When food scientists measure quality with human subjects, it is called sensory evaluation. Sensory and consumer science is important because it provides us with insight into how consumers react to the quality of a product. Sensory evaluation is performed using human panelists to make judgments on the differences in samples, describe sensory attributes, or determine consumer acceptability of food products.

15.2 Sensory Quality of Foods

Sensory quality of foods was introduced in Chapter 3 and described in greater detail in Chapter 7. There, we learned that appearance is our first indicator of whether a food is acceptable. We are also likely to inspect a product for blemishes or other visual defects, even if they are not a good indicator of a product's flavor. Flavor is the combination of taste and aroma. Flavor is what we usually associate with quality, but texture also plays a role. We reject foods if they are too hard, too mushy, or too gummy. Audible sounds when eating can also contribute to the eating experience.

15.2.1 Sensory Perception and Physiological Response

Our sensory experience usually begins by looking at the food. We see the color or colors of a particular food, shininess, bruises, and visual texture. We may then feel the texture of the food as we handle it and smell the aroma in the air. Aroma is the perception of volatile compounds by receptors in the nose both before (orthonasal) and during (retronasal) the eating process. Taste is perceived by receptors on our tongues and classified as sweet, sour, bitter, salty, and umami. Flavor perception is a complex process that integrates responses of the palate to a mixture of organic and inorganic chemicals as well as how the food feels in the mouth. These perceptions change during chewing.

To separate taste sensations from aromatic sensations, we can block our nasal passages with a nose clip or chew with our mouth closed. These two simple techniques prevent aroma perception while permitting full taste perception. Some individuals are super tasters in that they have a very low threshold for taste compounds, particularly bitter. They tend to be much more sensitive to small changes in formulations that affect taste. Regardless of how we interact with the sensory properties of the food, signals are sent from the receptor site (nerve, taste bud, etc.) through a complex biochemical pathway to the brain for interpretation (see Insert 15.1). These messages are communicated through a series of chemical impulses that can be recorded.

15.2.2 Appearance

The colors we see in a food product are the result of natural pigments in the food or the addition of natural or artificial colorants. Among the natural colorants are those produced in plants and animals or by microbes. Colors of plant pigments include red to purple anthocyanins, orange to red carotenoids, green chlorophyll, and yellow flavanols. The purple pigment in fresh meat is myoglobin. **Oxymyoglobin** provides the bright red of fresh hamburger after it has been exposed to oxygen. **Nitrosomyoglobin** is the pigment responsible for the characteristic color of luncheon meats like bologna. Oxymyoglobin turns to **metmyoglobin** as the uncooked meat turns brown. Browning of fresh fruits and vegetables is attributed to the formation of quinine polymers from the action of the enzyme polyphenoloxidase. The brown of chocolate and bread crust is attributed to melanoidins formed by Maillard browning reactions.

Plant and animal pigments tend to be unstable, frequently deteriorating more quickly than flavor, thus causing us to reject food that is otherwise safe and flavorful. Food processes, particularly those involving heat, cause colors to fade because of the degradation of the pigments. Artificial colorants are brighter and more stable than many natural pigments. They are also usually more potent and can be added in much smaller quantities to achieve the same effect on product color. Thus, they are the ingredients of choice for

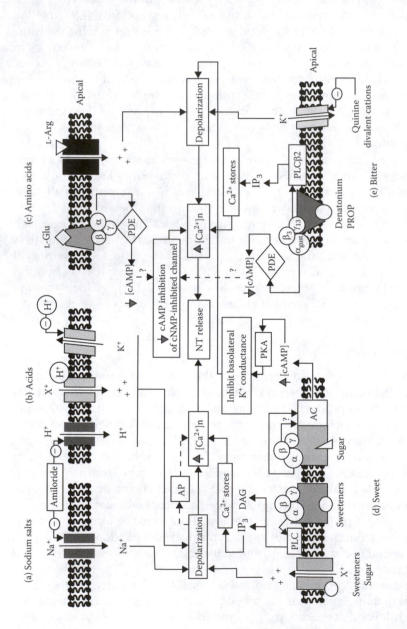

INSERT 15.1

Complex mechanism of signal transduction of the five basic tastes (a) salty, (b) sour, (c) umami, (d) sweet, and (e) bitter from the taste buds to the brain. (From Rawson, N.E. and Li, X., The cellular basis of flavour perception: Taste and aroma. In *Flavor Perception*, Taylor, A.J. and Roberts, D.D., eds., Ames, IA: Blackwell Publishing, 2004, Chapter 3. With permission.)

most formulated foods. Food labels that have ingredients such as Yellow 5, Blue 1, or Red 40 contain artificial colorants.

Color perception is affected by more than food chemistry. Individuals who are color blind have difficulty distinguishing between certain colors, such as red and green. The color of foods may not be as meaningful to consumers who are color blind as they are to those who are not. The amount and type of light can also affect our color perception. The appearance of a fresh apple under fluorescent lighting may not be as appealing as it is in bright sunlight. Certain colors clash with other colors, whereas some colors are complementary. This knowledge is important to designers of food packages who face the challenge of attracting the attention of food purchasers and motivating them to buy the product.

15.2.3 Flavor

Taste is the perception of specific compounds on the tongue. Sugars like sucrose and fructose, as well as artificial compounds, interact with receptors on the tongue to elicit a sweet taste. Organic acids, like citric acid in oranges and acetic acid in vinegar, are responsible for the taste of sourness. In some sweet fruits, the perception of sweetness is related to the ratio of sugars to acids. Sodium chloride registers as salty on the tongue, whereas chemicals like caffeine, quinine, and tannins are bitter. Monosodium glutamate is the compound most closely associated with umami, but parmesan cheese can also be used as an ingredient to impart it in food products.

Aroma is much more complex than taste. Thousands of chemical compounds interact with receptors in our nose, either orthonasally or retronasally (during mastication), to convey characteristic aromas. Some foods have character-impact compounds in which a single compound can convey the aroma of that food. Raspberries, for example, contain 4-(4-hydroxyphenyl)-butan-2-one, a character-impact compound also known as raspberry ketone. This compound has been advertised as a miracle weight-loss compound at doses much higher than we would find in nature. Benzaldehyde is the character-impact compound for cherries and almonds. Chemical structures of some character-impact compounds are shown in Insert 15.2. The characteristic odor of most foods, though, is attributed to an interaction of many compounds.

Aromatic compounds of fresh fruits develop during ripening. When these compounds accumulate at too high a level, the fruit is considered overripe. The tree-ripe mangoes Tiana likes so much are picked and consumed close to their peak flavor. Supermarket mangoes, however, are picked before they reach their peak flavor to allow for shipment to their destination. Early picking is done so that the mangoes will not be overripe by the time they reach the supermarket.

Physiological changes in fresh meats during storage can produce both desirable and undesirable aromas. Likewise, cheese aroma develops over time in a process also known as ripening, accounting, at least in part for the differences in mild and sharp cheddar. Heating during cooking and other

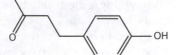

4-(4-Hydroxyphenyl)-butan-2-one

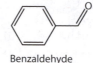

Benzaldehyde

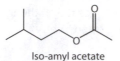

Iso-amyl acetate

Nootkatone

INSERT 15.2
Character-impact compounds of raspberries (4-(4-hydroxyphenyl)-butan-2-one), cherries (benzaldehyde), bananas (iso-amyl acetate), and grapefruit (nootkatone).

food processes transforms flavor compounds into those we associate with toasted bread, grilled chicken, pasteurized milk, hot chocolate, and vegetable casseroles.

Flavor perception involves a complex series of reactions of the food with our nose, tongue, and other parts of our mouth (see Insert 15.3). Perception starts with the peeling of an orange, brewing of coffee, or baking of fresh bread, which sends volatile aromatic compounds into the air. The volatile compounds travel to the olfactory receptors in our nose and start our saliva and digestive juices flowing. When the food enters the mouth, chewing breaks the food down into smaller components releasing nonvolatile-taste and volatile-aromatic compounds. These compounds interact to produce a unique flavor for each food item. Flavor perception changes as we continue to chew. Most consumers integrate these sensations into a single response that is generally considered pleasant, neutral, or unpleasant. Expert tasters, however, can detect specific flavor notes and evaluate the changes in perception during chewing with time-intensity techniques.

Flavor profiles can be developed by a panel of expert tasters for each food product. Flavor compounds contribute to the initial impact of the product, referred to as the top note. Other compounds may not contribute directly to a specific flavor but they may enhance or block other flavor notes by bringing out pleasant notes and suppressing unpleasant ones. Still other molecules provide a product with a background that adds richness to the flavor. In addition, some compounds contribute to an aftertaste, which can either be beneficial or detrimental to the overall eating experience.

As discussed in Chapter 7, analytical chemists use chromatographic techniques to determine the chemical components of food products that contribute to taste and aroma. High-performance liquid chromatography is used to separate individual sugars and organic acids. Gas chromatography (GC) is used to

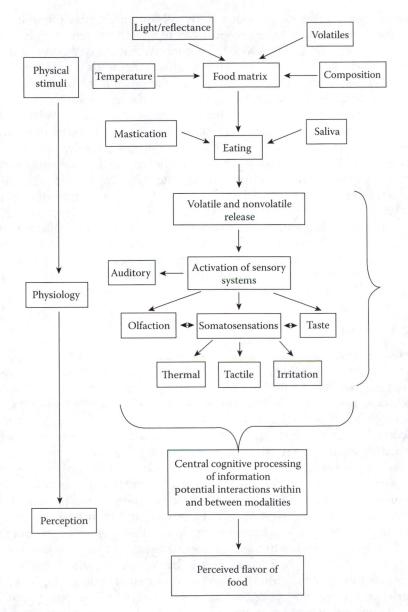

INSERT 15.3
Diagram of complex nature of flavor perception. (From Keast, R.S.J. et al., Flavor interactions at the sensory level. In *Flavor Perception*, Taylor, A.J. and Roberts, D.D., eds., Ames, IA: Blackwell Publishing, 2004, Chapter 8. With permission.)

separate volatile aromatic compounds. By splitting the signal, the individual compounds can be sent to a nose port where an analyst can sniff them and describe the specific aroma associated with that compound. When GC is coupled with mass spectrometry (MS), the volatile compounds can be identified.

Another instrumental approach to flavor evaluation is the use of electronic noses and tongues. These instruments use a series of sensors to detect different patterns of response to the chemicals present, either the volatile components in the headspace above the sample or the components in solution. Advanced statistical analysis can then be used to compare the patterns with each other and cluster similar patterns. Although earlier versions of these instruments provided no information on the chemical composition of the products, they can be useful in quality control to identify items that do not provide a close enough match to the standard. Thorough testing must be conducted to calibrate these instruments to ensure that items classified as similar to the standard are acceptable and that those classified as not similar are not acceptable as determined by sensory tests. Instruments also have a tendency to "drift," meaning that, after continued use, they may provide different responses to the same samples. Periodic recalibration is necessary.

15.2.4 Texture

The texture of a food relates to the sense of touch. Although just looking at a product can give us an idea of whether it is rough or smooth, firm, or mushy, many times we will touch the product with our hands or with a utensil to decide whether we wish to consume it. A hard peach or tomato is not likely to be eaten. Many items that cannot be cut by the side of a fork are considered unacceptable for eating. The proper texture of rice that Ignacio seeks when preparing a meal is the result of many factors in preparation.

Once we get a product into our mouth, the texture of the product becomes even more important in determining if it is acceptable. For example, most consumers like their chips and celery to be crisp, their shakes to be thick and creamy, their meat and vegetables to be tender, and their bread to be light and fluffy. Conversely, most consumers do not like their creamed potatoes to be lumpy, their okra or luncheon meats to be slimy, their peaches or cherries to be crunchy, or their fruit juices to be watery. We also have textural sensations known as chemical feeling factors that contribute to the eating experience, for example, pungency (onions), heat (peppers), cool (menthol), and astringency (green tea or red wine). All of these textures that we feel, whether with our hands or in our mouths, affect our perception of quality.

There are instruments that measure textural properties of food products. Individual instruments have been designed to measure the firmness and toughness of fruits and vegetables, the toughness of wieners and other meat products, or the consistency and viscosity of semisolid and liquid products. One instrument incorporates a set of dentures to help determine the effect of chewing on the breakdown of foods. Electromechanical measuring devices, such as the one shown in Insert 7.2b, allow an analyst to perform different types of tests on many different types of foods. The Texture Profile Technique is accomplished using an instrument to measure such characteristics as gumminess, chewiness, and adhesiveness and can be matched to sensory equivalents evaluated by a trained sensory panel.

15.3 Sensory Tests

Although there are advantages to using instruments to measure sensory characteristics, some attributes are very difficult to determine accurately with instruments. Sensory panels are often used to measure quality because the results can be more relevant to consumer acceptability than those obtained from instrumental tests. Some food scientists dislike sensory tests because they consider them to be "subjective" and not "objective." Sensory scientists argue that a sensory test that follows a given protocol closely can be as accurate and precise as an instrument. They also contend that a well-conducted sensory test that measures an attribute relevant to consumer perception of quality is better than an "objective" test that has no relevance to consumers.

All quality tests must be designed carefully to obtain meaningful information, but attention to detail is even more critical in sensory testing because of the difficulties associated with using human subjects. Human subjects are more likely to be rushed, less likely to work at nights and weekends, more likely to complain, less willing to repeat an experiment, and more likely to get sick than instruments. These reasons are why sensory testing requires careful planning and more complex logistics than most experiments. Any sensory test must have a clear-cut objective. A specific test is then chosen to match the objective of the study. In universities, any test involving human subjects, such as sensory panelists, must be approved by an Institutional Review Board to ensure that such subjects are not at risk.

Sensory samples must be prepared using proper sanitary standards and served at the appropriate temperature for consumption. Samples are presented to the panelists in random order to prevent panelist bias. The panel room is held at a comfortable temperature for the panelists and free from distractions such as noise and interfering odors (see a panel room in Insert 15.4). Panelists should be separated so that they are unable to compare responses, either verbally or nonverbally.

Sensory tests can take many forms based on the objective. For example, if a company wants to tell if there is a difference between the leading brand and its copycat version or between the current formulation and a new one with less expensive ingredients, there are difference tests that can provide the answer. If there are differences between two products, a sensory descriptive panel can determine the specific differences and help quantify those

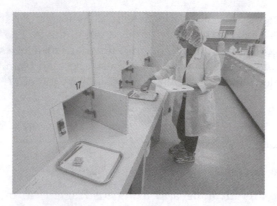

INSERT 15.4
Analytical sensory tests are conducted in controlled booths. (Photo courtesy of John Amis.)

differences. Consumer tests can help establish what consumers like and what they don't like.

15.3.1 Difference Tests

Many times, we just want to know whether two samples are different from each other. Too often, experimenters design elaborate sensory tests when a simple difference test is what is really needed. Difference tests are very useful when we want to know if a product is comparable to the competition, what effect a new ingredient has on the acceptability of a current or new product, or if the quality of a product is deteriorating during storage. Several types of tests can be used to determine differences. Traditionally, the triangle test is preferred, in which a panelist is presented three samples, of which two are similar and one different and asked to choose the different sample. Gaining in popularity is the tetrad test in which the panelist is provided four samples of two different groups of two similar samples and asked to correctly identify which samples belong in which group.

These tests are very good at identifying a sample that is different, but they have limitations. Sometimes, a test is designed to determine differences in flavor, but panelists are able to distinguish differences on the basis of color or texture. To solve this problem, colored lights can be used to screen out differences in color. Texture, however, is more difficult to hide. Also, because of the statistical tests used, negative results don't necessarily mean there is no difference. It just means that any differences are not detectable using that test. In most cases, the lack of a statistically significant difference is good enough to conclude that the samples are similar, but occasionally such conclusions can prove costly.

For example, a beverage company reformulated its product using a less expensive ingredient, performed a difference test, found no difference, and changed its formulation. Over the next 2 years, they made more changes in ingredients and performed a series of difference tests on the subsequent formulations. When a marked drop in sales of their product was reported, a sensory scientist compared their current product with the original one and found that the two were quite different. Although each change in itself was not enough to produce a noticeable difference, the sum of the changes was large enough to produce consumer dissatisfaction and decreased sales.

Another limitation of difference tests is that they don't tell us which sample is better or why. One way to get more information is to use a difference-preference test, which asks the panelist which sample they prefer and why they prefer it. The problem with such questions is that they can take a panelist's mind off the task at hand and can provide erroneous results. Also, a preference test usually requires a much larger sample size than a difference test to determine if there is a true preference. This problem can be solved by performing a difference test first. If it is determined that there is a difference, then a preference test with a larger panel can be performed to find out which sample is best. A descriptive test with a trained panel can also be conducted to help understand why one sample is different from another.

15.3.2 Thresholds

Threshold testing is performed to determine the level at which an ingredient or chemical compound can be detected or recognized. This type of testing is done when it is important to know if an ingredient or a compound is making a difference in a product. There are two types of thresholds, detection and recognition. A **detection threshold** is the concentration of a substance at which a panel can consistently detect a difference from more dilute samples. A **recognition threshold** of a substance is the level at which the panel can determine the identity of the substance. For example, if peppermint was added to a chewing gum, the detection threshold would be the amount of peppermint present that would make a difference in the aroma or flavor of the gum but not recognized as peppermint. More peppermint would need to be present to clearly identify the flavor as peppermint. The threshold for a given substance is calculated as the **geometric mean** of panelist responses.

Thresholds can be very useful, but the tests are very labor intensive and time consuming. Only one substance can be tested at a time, and it must be sampled at many dilutions. Frequently, the compound is diluted with water, which may or may not be related to its role in a food product with many other ingredients.

15.3.3 Sensory Descriptive Analysis

Many times, we need to know more about a product or sample than just the difference or about an ingredient than its threshold. Sensory descriptive analysis is performed to provide a description of the components of sensory quality that can be detected. These components are called notes. The notes can be quantified to better understand the relative contribution of each note. Differences between samples can be evaluated to help understand why they are different and what can be done to improve food quality.

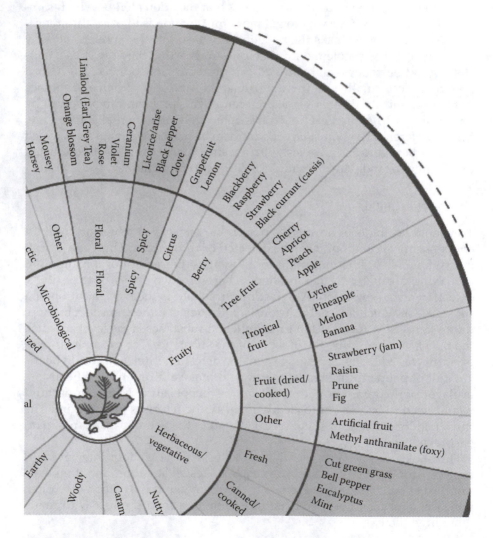

INSERT 15.5

A portion of the wine aroma wheel that illustrates the complexity of some sensory descriptive lexicons. (The Wine Aroma Wheel. Copyright 1990, 2002 A.C. Noble, http://www.winearoma wheel.com. With permission.)

Sensory descriptive tests are very complex and require extensive preparation. Panelists are screened for the ability to detect small differences. They
are then trained to ensure that the panel generates consistent results.

Descriptive panels are more sensitive to small differences in products than
the general public. Thus, it is not a good idea to include trained descriptive
panelists in other types of panels. For many products, there are published
lexicons, lists of specific descriptive notes for specific products. Extensive
lexicons have been developed for specific products such as the wine aroma
wheel shown in Insert 15.5. If there is no lexicon for a product, the panel
director works with the panel to develop a lexicon. Typical notes include
sweet, acid or sour, salty, bitter, fruity, and earthy, but the notes vary from
product to product.

There are many different types of descriptive analysis. In many of them, a
set of standards is developed for each note such as different concentrations
of sugar for the sweet note and of caffeine for the bitter note. Descriptive tests
can also be used to partition taste and aroma. As mentioned earlier, taste and
aroma are partitioned by using a swimmer's nose plug to block the nasal
passage of panelists so that taste can be detected, but aroma is not perceived.
The taste notes can then be evaluated first followed by the aromatic notes
once the nose clips have been removed.

Sensory descriptive tests provide a profile of the notes that contribute to
the flavor or texture of a sample. Differences between samples can be demonstrated by spider-web graphs as shown in Insert 15.6. Like other types of
sensory tests, descriptive analysis has limitations. Although a trained panel

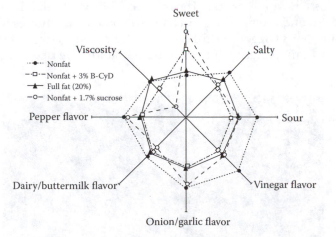

INSERT 15.6
Effect of selected food additives on the sensory quality of reduced-fat, ranch-type salad dressings. Note the differences on the treatments with cyclodextrin (3% B-CyD) added and with
sucrose (1.7%) added. (From Reineccius, T.A. et al., *Journal of Food Science* 69: FCT334, 2004. With
permission.)

may find pronounced differences in different products, an untrained panel may not be able to detect overall differences in the samples. Sensory descriptive analysis also does not determine which product is best. Preference testing is needed to determine which products are best.

15.3.4 Time Intensity

These tests evaluate the changes in intensity of a particular note during mastication. Our initial reaction to a food may be very different from what we perceive later as we chew. Tastes and aromas may increase as we burst open cells or other compartments in the food or diminish after the initial burst of flavor disappears. A pleasant flavor may be undermined by a bitter aftertaste. Mouthfeel may undergo dramatic changes. Such changes are most relevant to consumers who chew gum, but they can be important in salted snacks, sauces, squid, and numerous other products. These intensity changes over time can all be evaluated by trained panelists.

15.3.5 Functional Magnetic Resonance Imaging

A relatively new technique, functional magnetic resonance imaging (fMRI), is being used to see how certain food sensations affect the brain by scanning it to see what areas respond. Through such scans, it is possible to differentiate consumers who find very sweet sugar solutions to be pleasant from those who find them unpleasant and how monosodium glutamate functions as a flavor enhancer. These scans also have helped identify how certain tastes and aromas affect each other. Some fMRI studies have shown that certain foods trigger reward centers. Other studies suggest that certain foods show brain patterns similar to those of addictive drugs and could be

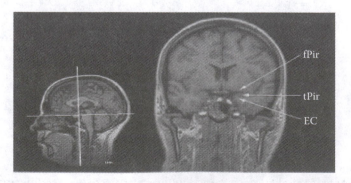

INSERT 15.7
Primary olfactory cortex in the brain–coronal section by fMRI scan. fPir, frontal piriform cortex; tPir, temporal piriform cortex; EC, entorhinal cortex. (Reprinted from Wiesmann, M. et al., Functional magnetic resonance imaging of human olfaction. In *Flavor Perception*, Taylor, A.J. and Roberts, D.D., eds., Ames, IA: Blackwell Publishing, 2004, Chapter 7.)

responsible in the development of obesity. At present, it is difficult to separate out differences in brain scans between addiction, craving, and pleasure. Further research is needed to determine how useful these techniques will be to sensory and consumer scientists and how much they will reveal about brain responses to food. The areas of the brain that are most affected are shown in Insert 15.7.

15.3.6 Integrating Sensory and Physicochemical Tests

Sensory tests are difficult to conduct. They require hours of sample preparation and the participation of motivated sensory panelists. Sensory panelists usually have other duties and responsibilities and are rarely fully compensated for their time and effort. Many food scientists would prefer to develop a physical test using an instrument or direct chemical test to make comparisons between products or to trace quality changes of that product during storage. Statistical relationships are generally used to provide a rough idea of what tests may be useful. Mathematical models are developed to establish predictive relationships.

If a single physicochemical test or combination of tests helps predict the results of the sensory panel, the food scientist can use that mathematical model as an indicator of sensory quality. The indicator can then be used for routine testing in quality control or new product development instead of gathering together sensory panels. It is generally a good idea to test the model occasionally with sensory testing to make sure that the model is still valid.

15.3.7 Consumer Testing

Sensory testing is divided into two types—**analytical** and **affective**. Difference, threshold, descriptive, and time-intensity tests are analytical. Preference or consumer tests are affective. Consumer testing is less controlled than other types of sensory testing, and consumers are less reliable as panelists than those typically used in analytical tests. The only way to find out what consumers think, however, is to ask the consumer. Three main types of consumer testing involve the use of focus groups, large consumer panels, and home-use testing. **Focus groups** are used by marketing specialists to test new product concepts on consumers before a product is developed. They may also be used later in the development process to determine if developers are on the right track. Large sensory panels are usually used late in the development process to determine if a product is acceptable or if one prototype is preferred over another one. **Home-use tests** are particularly beneficial when some preparation is required by the consumer.

Focus groups usually contain 8–12 people who have an interest in the product. They are led by a group leader who attempts to elicit a wide range of responses from the group. Focus groups present ideas that can be developed further. Through careful probing of the participants, the group leader can uncover valuable information about why certain consumers like certain food quality characteristics and why they don't like others. They can also be useful in sorting out market segments, such as mild, medium, sharp, and extra sharp cheese.

Large consumer panels are usually conducted to determine acceptability or preference. A series of samples is presented, and the consumers are asked to select the best sample, rank them in order from best to worst, or rate them on a nine-point Hedonic scale (as shown in Insert 7.8). Sometimes, large consumer panels are used to determine differences between two samples as well.

In home-use testing, the consumer is provided one or two products to be used under normal conditions in the home. Then, one person is asked to complete a questionnaire on responses by members of the household to the product, any complaints or concerns they had with it, and any difficulties in preparation or serving of the item. Home-use tests trade off less control over the product and the panelists for information on how that product performs under more realistic conditions.

In conducting a consumer test, it is critical to separate typical consumers from potential consumers and nonconsumers of the product or product type. Each group may have a very different reaction to the product being tested. It is also important to look at market segments. For example, if we are interested in genetically modified organism (GMO) rice, we must understand that most consumers who grew up in Asia are much more sensitive to subtle differences in rice flavor than most consumers who grew up in the United States. Golden rice is a GMO that was bred to improve the nutritional status of consumers whose primary staple is rice and do not obtain sufficient vitamin A in their diet. Unfortunately, the carotenoids that are responsible for the golden color and nutritional value can also contribute to the flavor. These compounds might be below the flavor thresholds of a typical American, but they could be objectionable to Asians who eat rice as a staple food.

Focus groups can be very useful in helping product developers decide which product concepts to reject and which concepts to develop further. There are not enough participants in a focus group, however, to detect differences or measure preference. Large consumer panels can tell us what consumers like and what they don't like, but they can't tell us why. If the consumer tests are conducted without an understanding of potential market segments, the results may not be clear or useful.

15.3.8 Integrating Sensory and Consumer Tests

Fundamental differences exist in traditional sensory (analytical) and consumer (affective) tests. Consumer tests tell us what consumers like and dislike. Other sensory tests help determine if products are different from each

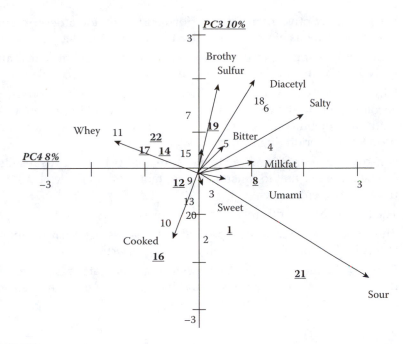

INSERT 15.8

Principal component analysis of mild cheddar cheeses where the numbers represent different cheeses presented to a sensory descriptive analysis. The bold underlined numbers represent cheeses that were then presented to a consumer panel. (From Drake, S.L. et al., *Journal of Food Science* 73: S449, 2008. With permission.)

other (difference), how they differ, and by how much (descriptive analysis). None of these tests, when done separately, give us a complete picture of a product. When they are conducted sequentially or simultaneously, however, we can get a much better understanding of what factors affect the acceptability of a food product. We can also learn what characteristics contribute to acceptability and what we can do to improve acceptability. A mathematical model integrating sensory and consumer tests is shown in Insert 15.8.

15.4 Remember This!

- Fundamental differences exist in traditional sensory (analytical) and consumer (affective) tests.
- The only way to find out what consumers think is to ask the consumer.
- fMRI is being used to see how certain food sensations affect the brain by scanning it to see what areas respond.

- Sensory descriptive analysis is performed to provide a description of the components of sensory quality that can be detected.
- Threshold testing is performed to determine the level at which an ingredient or chemical compound can be detected or recognized.
- Difference tests are very useful when we want to know if a product is comparable to the competition, what effect a new ingredient has on the acceptability of a current or new product or if the quality of a product is deteriorating during storage.
- Sensory panels are often used to measure quality because the results can be more relevant to consumer acceptability than those obtained from instrumental tests.
- The texture of a food is related to the sense of touch.
- The colors we see in a food product are the result of natural pigments in the food or the addition of natural or artificial colorants.
- Flavor perception is a complex process that integrates responses of the palate to a mixture of organic and inorganic chemicals as well as how the food feels in the mouth.

Testing Comprehension

1. List all of the quality characteristics associated with a specific food product. How many are sensory characteristics and how many are hidden characteristics? How would these characteristics be measured in a QC laboratory?
2. Differentiate the use of sensory techniques used in QA and its use in product development. Why are the two approaches different?
3. Construct a series of sensory tests to determine the best alternate ingredient for a formulated food when a critical ingredient becomes unavailable. What factors must be considered in determining which alternate ingredient is best?
4. Generate a plan for a series of sensory tests that would be needed in the development of gluten-free, refrigerated cookie dough.
5. Outline an approach to studying the acceptability of a newly developed chewing gum that serves as a delivery system for vitamins and minerals. Which vitamins and minerals should be used in this product? Which of these added nutrients might present a problem? Why?

6. Compare and contrast the strengths and weaknesses of difference tests and sensory descriptive analysis. Provide three examples of appropriate use of each test.

7. Distinguish between the definition of craving and the two definitions of addiction in the glossary. Which of the three definitions appears to be the most appropriate for our attraction to products containing fat, salt, sugar, or any combination of the three types of ingredients? Does the same definition apply for all three types of ingredients or is there a difference? What can food scientists do to decrease the levels of these ingredients in food products?

8. Calculate the average Hedonic rating obtained in a preference test Alice conducted on Berry Outrageous and what will be its closest competitor using a Hedonic scale as shown in Insert 7.8. The test was conducted over three consecutive days with 326 consumers evaluating the products. Nine participants did not follow directions, and their data must be discarded. Also calculate the percentage of participants who indicated that they liked each product versus those who were neutral or disliked it. Based on these calculations, which product was best? Should Alice recommend that a multicity marketing test be conducted or should it go back to the product developers? Here are the results for the test:

	Berry Outrageous	Competitor
9—Like extremely	0	0
8—Like very much	4	9
7—Like moderately	133	86
6—Like slightly	99	133
5—Neither like nor dislike	64	89
4—Dislike slightly	17	0
3—Dislike moderately	0	0
2—Dislike very much	0	0
1—Dislike extremely	0	0

References

Drake, S. L., P. D. Gerard and M. A. Drake, 2008. Consumer preferences for mild cheddar cheese flavors. *J. Food Sci.*, 73:S449.

Keast, R. S. J., P. H. Dalton and P. A. S. Breslin, 2004. Flavor interactions at the sensory level, in *Flavor Perception*, Taylor, A. J. and Roberts, D. D., Eds., Ames, IA: Blackwell Publishing.

Rawson, N. E. and X. Li, 2004. The cellular basis of flavour perception: Taste and aroma, in *Flavor Perception*, Taylor, A. J. and Roberts, D. D., Eds., Ames, IA: Blackwell Publishing.

Reineccius, T. A., T. L. Peppard and G. A. Reineccius, 2004. Potential for beta-cyclo-dextrin as partial fat replacer in low-fat foods. *J. Food Sci.*, 69:FCT334.

Wiesmann, M., B. Kettenmann and G. Kobal, 2004. Functional magnetic resonance imaging of human olfaction, in *Flavor Perception*, Taylor, A. J. and Roberts, D. D., Eds., Ames, IA: Blackwell Publishing.

Further Reading

Ennis, J. M., 2012. Guiding the switch from triangle testing to tetrad testing. *J. Sens. Stud.*, 27:223.

Krueger, R. A. and M. A. Casey, 2008. *Focus Groups: A Practical Guide for Applied Research*, 4th ed., Thousand Oaks, CA: Sage Publications, Inc.

Lawless, H. T. and H. Heymann, 2010. *Sensory Evaluation of Food: Principles and Practices*, 2nd ed., New York: Springer.

Meilgaard, M., G. V. Civille and B. T. Carr, 2006. *Sensory Evaluation Techniques*, 4th ed., Boca Raton, FL: CRC Press.

Moskowitz, H. R., J. H. Beckley and A. V. A. Resurreccion, 2012. *Sensory and Consumer Research in Food Product Design and Development*, 2nd ed., Ames, IA: Wiley-Blackwell.

Stone, H., R. Bleibaum and H. A. Thomas, 2012. *Sensory Evaluation Practices*, 4th ed., Waltham, MA: Elsevier Inc.

Glossary

3D printing: use of an instrument that produces a product one layer at a time using a template from an inventory of available ingredients.

Accuracy: the property of a measurement with respect to how close the estimate comes to the real value.

Acid reflux: stomach acid traveling back up the esophagus and entering the mouth leading to a bad taste and potential damage to tooth enamel.

Acidification: lowering the pH of a food to inhibit microbial growth by the addition of a food-grade acid.

Acidity: the capacity of the acids present in a food to resist being neutralized by addition of a base.

Acidulant: an ingredient that lowers the pH of a product to slow spoilage and impart a sour or tart taste.

Aciduric: bacteria that are tolerant of a high-acid environment (low pH).

Addiction: dependence on a specific chemical compound to the point of an inability to stop using it OR a pattern of behavior that continues by a person despite the knowledge that it is harmful.

Adiabiatic system: one in which no heat is transferred in or out.

Affective sensory test: determines preference for a food using a large number of naïve consumer panelists.

Aftertaste: the residual flavor after an item has been swallowed.

Agricultural Marketing Service (AMS): component of the United States Department of Agriculture (USDA) that offers its services to provide quality grades for animal and plant products.

Allergen: a compound that elicits an abnormal immune response in a susceptible individual.

Amino acid: the fundamental unit of a protein characterized by an amino group and a carboxylic group.

Amygdalin: toxic molecule found naturally in peach and apricot pits that releases cyanide and was once sold as a cure for cancer.

Amylase: enzyme that breaks down starch into sugars.

Anabolism: the part of intermediary metabolism that builds large molecules like lipids, proteins, and glycogen from small molecules like fatty acids and glycerol, amino acids, and simple sugars.

Anaerobe: bacteria that can live in an environment free of oxygen.

Analytical sensory evaluation: use of trained or experienced panelists to determine specific aspects of a food.

Anaphylactic shock: extreme allergenic reaction that can result in an inability to breathe normally and even death if left untreated.

Anorexia: eating disorder resulting from not consuming enough food and which leads to malnutrition.

Anthocyanin: water-soluble pigment found in plants characterized by a red, blue, or purple color.

Antibiotic: molecule that halts or inhibits microbial growth and is used to fight disease in humans and animals.

Anticaking agent: food additive that prevents hygroscopic (water-loving) materials from absorbing water and clumping up.

Antimicrobial agent: food additive that inhibits microbial growth.

Antinutrient: a compound that binds or otherwise impedes a nutrient such as a mineral or vitamin from being absorbed into the bloodstream and thus rendering it ineffective in the body.

Antioxidant: a natural component or food additive that inhibits oxidation of lipids.

Antioxidant vitamin: vitamins A, C, and E, which can either act directly as an antioxidant or otherwise contribute to retarding or stopping lipid oxidation.

Apparent viscosity: ratio of shear stress to shear rate of a non-Newtonian fluid at a given shear rate.

Appetite suppressant: ingredient or supplement that inhibits the hunger response.

Applied research: science that focuses on developing solutions for practical problems.

Aquatic: of or pertaining to water; in food science, resources associated with fresh- and saltwater fish.

Aromatic: of or pertaining to the generation of an odor.

Artificial colorant: a food additive derived from an inorganic source that imparts color to a food product.

Artificial ingredient: one not normally found in nature and prepared by chemical synthesis.

Artificial sweetener: a food additive that can replace the sweetness of sugar, generally leading to reduced calories and less volume or weight in a product for the same level of sweetness.

Aseptic processing: preservation of a food, usually by heat, to kill all micro-organisms present before packaging and where the package is filled in a microbial-free environment.

Aspartame: artificial sweetener composed of the bonding of the amino acids aspartic acid and phenylalanine.

Astringency: chemical feeling factor that causes the mouth to pucker.

Atherosclerosis: heart disease resulting from the accumulation of plaque in the arteries leading to restricted blood flow.

Atopic reaction: adverse reaction to a compound in food without producing an antibody.

Azodicarbonamide (ADA): food additive that is used in bread-making to condition the dough by making it more rubbery in texture. It is also found in yoga mats.

Backhauling: a truck returning to near the original shipment point with a load of goods such that the wasting of fuel to transport an empty truck can be minimized.

Bacilli: bacteria that have an oblong or rodlike shape.

Bacteriophage: virus that infects bacteria.

Balanced diet: one that provides all the necessary nutrients without contributing to excess calories.

Basic research: science that contributes to a fundamental understanding of the world with no immediate or direct application to practical problems.

Batch process: as opposed to a continuous process, a batch process takes place typically in a container where mixing (ingredient addition), reaction, and heat exchange occur with no product exiting the container until the process is completed.

Beverage: a liquid food.

Binge-and-starve diet: eating disorder that alternates between excessive consumption of food followed by long periods of little or no food.

Bingham plastic: a fluid that shows yield stress and acts as a solid at low shear stress but as a Newtonian fluid at high shear stress.

Bingham pseudoplastic: a fluid that shows yield stress, acts as a solid at low shear stress, but flows as a pseudoplastic (shear-thinning) fluid as additional stress is applied.

Bioactive compound: a molecule that induces a physiological response inside the body.

Bioavailability: the amount of a bioactive compound that can be absorbed into the body and induce a physiological response.

Biochemical pathway: a series of steps in a living system catalyzed by enzymes.

Biodegradable: materials that will break down into components that can be used for composting or other applications instead of accumulating in a landfill.

Bioenergy crops: plants grown specifically to be converted into ethanol or other compounds for use as fuel.

Bioflavonoid: class of compounds found primarily in plants that produces a reducing environment in a cell, thus contributing to regeneration of antioxidants.

Bioinformatics: study of the biological properties of natural products using advanced computer techniques.

Biological hazard: a microorganism or its toxins that could lead to food poisoning.

Bitter: a sharp and unpleasant taste associated with beer, dark chocolate, and other foods and is frequently confused with sour.

Blanching: short heat treatment during preparation of a food, generally before canning or freezing, conducted primarily to inactivate enzymes.

Body mass index (BMI): a method of measuring healthy relationships between weight and height equal to weight in kilograms divided by the square of the height in meters.

Bolus: the mass of food as it leaves the mouth and travels down the esophagus and through the small intestine into the large intestine.

Bottleneck: a point in an overall process at which a unit operation cannot keep up with the amount of incoming material, resulting in slowing down production and decreasing efficiency.

Botulinum toxin: molecule produced by *Clostridium botulinum* that causes food poisoning.

Botulism: disease condition frequently resulting in numbness, blindness, and death due to inadequate processing of foods contaminated by *Clostridium botulinum*.

Bulimia: eating disorder that results from purging a meal by vomiting, use of laxatives, or other means between the time it is consumed and the time it is digested.

Bulking agent: food additive that increases mass and volume of a product particularly when fat or sugar are reduced during formulation of such product.

Bulking up: gaining weight, particularly muscle mass, generally done to enhance athletic performance.

Butylated hydroxyanisole (BHA): synthetic antioxidant added to foods to prevent development of rancidity.

Butylated hydroxytoluene (BHT): synthetic antioxidant added to foods to prevent development of rancidity.

By-product: a secondary product that can be formed from what is left over in the manufacturing of a primary product.

Calibration: the process of testing an instrument with a known standard to ensure that the measurements are consistent from one use to another.

Caloric density: the amount of calories present in a food relative to its size.

Calorie: common name used for a kilocalorie of energy.

Can seam: the part of the can that is sealed to the lid and which could permit contamination if improperly sealed.

Cancer: a category of related diseases characterized by abnormal cell growth in a particular part of the body resulting in malignancy and which can spread to the rest of the body.

Capsaicin: compound in hot peppers responsible for the sensation of heat.

Carbohydrate: a compound in food that contains carbon, oxygen, and hydrogen typically composed of one or more simple sugars which contributes to 4 kilocalories per gram.

Carbon footprint: the contribution to the production of greenhouse gas production and thus to global warming.

Carotenoid: lipid-soluble pigment found in plants and animals characterized by a red, yellow, or orange color.

Case-ready meats: meat that has been packaged into consumer trays at a manufacturing plant and then sent to a supermarket or other retail outlet.

Casual-dining restaurant: usually part of a chain that serves a standard set of entrées, sides, beverages, and desserts that have been processed off-site and are sold at a moderate price.

Catabolism: the part of intermediary metabolism that breaks down large molecules like lipids, proteins, and glycogen to small molecules like fatty acids and glycerol, amino acids, and simple sugars.

Catering: transport of meals from a central location to the place of consumption.

Celiac disease: an autoimmune response to the gluten found in wheat, barley, rye, and perhaps oats.

Cell membrane: a semipermeable structure surrounding every cell (plasma membrane) and many organelles within each cell that is composed primarily of phospholipids and proteins. It contains the components of the cell or organelle and helps regulate flow from one side to the other.

Cellular compartmentation: separation of organelles in animal, microbial, and plant cells to permit physiological specialization.

Cellulose: a complex carbohydrate, made up of long chains of glucose, and which is not able to be digested by humans but can be digested by ruminants such as cattle.

Centers for Disease Control and Prevention (CDC): governmental agency that monitors disease outbreaks around the country and the world to identify causes and strategies and prevent similar outbreaks.

Character-impact compound: single molecule that conveys the primary flavor note of a food.

Chelating agent: a molecule that binds minerals.

Chemical: any substance composed of atoms held together by bonds that cannot be broken to its components by physical means without breaking these bonds.

Chemical feeling factor: sensation on the tongue or elsewhere in the mouth, such as heat, coolness, pungency, or astringency, which is neither a taste nor an aroma.

Chemical hazard: a compound either as a component or a contaminant in a food that could lead to food poisoning.

Chemical preservation: addition of food additives to delay spoilage or decrease the chances of a safety hazard.

Chemometrics: in-depth use of statistics to detect patterns in large data sets of chemical analyses.

Chilled foods: ones that have been refrigerated from the farm or processing plant through a cold distribution chain until purchase by the consumer.

Chinese Restaurant Syndrome: disease characterized by headaches and dizziness experienced by susceptible individuals who consume large amounts of monosodium glutamate or similar substances.

Chlorophyll: lipid-soluble pigment found in plants characterized by a green color.

Chloroplast: organelle in bacterial or green-plant cells that conducts photosynthesis.

Chocolate liquor: liquid chocolate composed of cocoa butter and cocoa powder.

Cholesterol: an important lipid component of the body that serves as a precursor for certain hormones and a stabilizer of cell membranes, but it can also contribute to formation of plaque in arteries and contribute to heart disease.

cis **fatty acid:** unsaturated lipid component that is found naturally in plant and animal products and is characterized by hydrogen atoms located adjacent to each other across a double bond.

Clarification: removing pulp and cloudiness and any impurities to make a clear juice.

Clean label: an ingredient statement on a food package that contains only easy-to-pronounce ingredients without any chemical-sounding names.

Clean-in-Place: automatic circulation of a sequence of rinses, caustic soap, and acidic sanitizing solutions through equipment, valves, pipes, and fittings to sanitize it without requiring a breakdown into its components.

Climacteric: property of some fruits to ripen up after harvest by self-generation or external application of ethylene.

Closed system: one in which no mass goes in or out.

Cluster analysis: statistical technique that helps separate or group together different samples or treatments.

Coagulation: precipitation of proteins in a food product, usually induced by heat or acid, that results in a gel or solid structure.

Coalesce: clumping together of small particles or bubbles in a product to form a bigger particle or bubble.

Cocci: bacteria that have a round shape.

Cocoa butter: the lipid portion of chocolate liquor that is yellowish-white in color used to make white chocolate.

Cocoa powder: the nonlipid portion of chocolate liquor used to make hot chocolate.

Codex Alimentarius: collection of internationally recognized standards, codes of practice, guidelines, and other recommendations relating to foods, food production, and food safety.

Coenzyme: an organic compound that enables an enzyme to change a metabolic substrate to a metabolic product.

Cofactor: an inorganic compound that enables an enzyme to change a meta-bolic substrate to a metabolic product.

Cold plasma: partially charged material that is neither gas, liquid, nor solid and exhibits unique properties that can be used in food packaging.

Cold shortening: excessive toughening in fresh meat resulting from too rapid chilling of the muscle after harvest such that glycogen cannot be converted to lactic acid.

Cold spot: the location within a product being heated that is the last to receive heat.

Colloidal suspension: a discontinuous phase made of very fine, insoluble particles dispersed in a continuous phase.

Colony-forming unit (CFU): group of microorganisms grown from a single cell.

Color: a general term to indicate all aspects of the appearance of a food.

Colorant: a natural or synthetic food additive that changes the color of a product.

Colorimeter: an instrument used to measure the color of a food in terms of hue (color name like red, yellow, green, and blue), lightness (light to dark or white to black), and chroma (degree of brightness).

Commercial sterilization: inactivation of all microorganisms that could affect the quality of a food including those that ferment or spoil the product or lead to a safety hazard.

Commercially sterile: a product that has no viable spoilage microorganisms or pathogens but could have some microorganisms that have no effect on the quality or safety of that product.

Composting: use of biodegradable materials to break down components into organic fertilizer usually through self-generated heat.

Concentration: removal of water from a beverage to increase the level of solids.

Conching: a slow-mixing operation in chocolate manufacturing that reduces particle size and results in a smoother texture.

Conduction: transfer of heat in solids from one molecule to another imme-diately adjacent proceeding from the heat source to the cold spot.

Confection: a sweet food product including all candies and some baked goods like cakes, cookies, and donuts.

Constipation: a stoppage of flow through the digestive tract resulting in an inability to excrete solid waste and an accumulation of that waste in the intestines.

Consumer acceptability: the probability that an individual consumer within a population will like a food.

Consumer test: affective sensory technique to determine acceptability of a food.

Continuous phase: the portion of a dispersion that is present at the greatest concentration.

Continuous process: one in which new materials are being added at one end and finished products are being collected at the other end.

Controlled atmosphere storage: process of maintaining a specific gas composition in a storage facility to slow the natural spoilage processes.

Convection: transfer of heat in fluids through patterns of currents.

Craving: a desire to consume a specific food.

Critical Control Point (CCP): specific unit operation within a process where, if something goes wrong, the food product will be unsafe.

Cross-contamination: the transfer of microorganisms from a contaminated food or utensil to another food, usually one that will not be further heated or processed, potentially leading to food poisoning.

Cross-docking: breaking down a large load of product from a supplier into smaller mixed loads for distribution to a retailer without the need to store items in a wholesale warehouse.

Cryogenic freezing: use of super-cold fluids such as liquid nitrogen or propylene glycol to rapidly freeze a food product.

Culinary: pertaining to food preparation in a kitchen with particular emphasis on chefs who have been trained to enhance the appeal of a meal.

Curing: preservation of meats by adding one or more preservatives such as nitrates, nitrites, salt, or sugar.

Customer: the direct purchaser of a food or ingredient such as a manufacturer for an ingredient supplier and a restaurant chain or supermarket for a finished product.

Customization: manufacturing of a product that meets the needs of an individual consumer.

Dairy product: a food that contains milk as a primary ingredient.

Death phase: the portion of the microbial growth curve in which cell death exceeds cell division.

Deficiency disease: a serious ailment caused by the lack of the sufficient intake of a specific nutrient such as protein, a vitamin, or a mineral.

Degumming: removal of phospholipids and other materials in the purification of vegetable oils.

Dehydration: drying process of a food product or the loss of water in the body resulting in reduced metabolism.

Denaturation: unfolding of a protein chain, without disruption of the primary structure, brought on by heat, solvent, or the physiochemical event leading to loss of normal function.

Dental caries: specific unit operation within a process where, if something goes wrong, the food product will be unsafe.

Deoxyribonucleic acid (DNA): compound found in the nucleus of a cell that contains the genetic code for the organism.

Descriptive note: a sensation (aromatic, color, taste, or textural) that can be defined, identified, and quantified by a sensory descriptive panel.

Detection threshold: the minimal concentration of a compound that changes the perception of aroma or taste without recognition of the character of the sensation.

Diabetes: a disease resulting from the inability of the body to adequately metabolize sugar because of an insufficient production of insulin by the pancreas or inadequate response to the insulin produced and which results in an inability to control blood sugar levels.

Dietary fiber: complex carbohydrates that provide little or no calories because they are indigestible but can help prevent constipation and provide additional health benefits.

Dietary supplement: any compound added to food or medicine to provide a health benefit, regulated under the guidelines outlined in Dietary Supplement Health and Education Act (DSHEA) and not subject to the restrictions of the Food Additives Amendment of the Pure Food and Drug Act.

Dietary Supplement Health and Education Act (DSHEA): law governing Food and Drug Administration (FDA) regulation of use and marketing of dietary supplements.

Dietician: a scientist with a background in nutrition who designs meals and meal plans for individuals with specific dietary needs and for institutions like hospitals, the military, school lunch programs, and prison systems.

Difference-preference test: one which determines whether a difference can be detected between two treatments and which treatment is preferred. Generally, these tests are not considered appropriate as the requirements for an effective preference test clash with those for an effective difference test.

Difference test: one which determines whether there is a significant difference between two samples.

Differentiation: a clear distinction between one product and another, usually referring to two brands within a similar product category.

Diffusion: random distribution of particles within a fluid as they transfer from a higher to a lower concentration.

Digestion: the process of breaking down of nutrients in the bolus to permit absorption across the intestinal mucosa and delivering them into the bloodstream.

Dilatant: shear-thickening fluid such that the viscosity increases as the shear stress increases.

Disaccharide: carbohydrate consisting of two simple sugars linked together by a glycosidic bond.

Discontinuous phase: the portion of a dispersion that is present at the lowest concentration.

Dispersion: a suspension of two normally incompatible substances with a smaller discontinuous dispersed in a larger continuous phase.

Distribution: everything that happens to a food product from the manufacturing plant to the consumer.

Downcycling: recycling packaging materials to another use other than a primary package.

Drift: the tendency of instrumental measurements to change over time, necessitating recalibration of the instrument.

Drum drying: removal of water in a liquid product by forming a thin film on a heated, rotating drum and then recovering the dry material by scraping the surface of the drum with a knife edge.

Early adopter: adventurous consumer who likes to try new products and is willing to share likes and dislikes with friends and relatives.

Eating disorders: behavioral problem in consumption of foods that leads to nutritional imbalances.

Ecotoxicity: pollution of the environment through natural or synthetic stress from biological, chemical, or physical means.

Efficacy: ability to perform its function, that is, the degree to which an ingredient functions in a product with respect to its intended purpose.

Electrochemical sensor: analytical tool that sends signals to a receiver and reduces the need to perform more cumbersome chemical testing.

Electrolyte: charged ions of an ionic compound when dissolved in water or other polar solvent.

Electron-beam radiation: use of ionizing radiation to surface sterilize foods or kill living insects on fresh fruits and vegetables.

Electronic nose: instrument that can differentiate aromas of foods using an array of sensors.

Electrospinning: layer-by-layer accumulation of material at the micro or nano levels using an electric charge.

Electrospraying: layer-by-layer application of a fine mist at the micro or nano level using an electric charge.

Emissivity: rate at which a body reflects or absorbs radiation.

Emulsifier: a compound that helps form and maintain an emulsion as it is partially soluble in both water and lipid.

Emulsion: a dispersion of water and lipid components that does not separate out into phases.

Endoplasmic reticulum: organelle within a cell that consists of an invaginating membrane and participates in protein synthesis and lipid metabolism.

Endothermic: type of chemical reaction that requires the absorption of heat.

Energy: in nutrition, the stored capacity in the body to maintain metabolic processes, generate heat, or perform physical activity measured in the form of kilocalories; in engineering, the ability to do work.

Energy balance: distribution of energy within a system.

Energy-balance point: weight at which an individual is likely to maintain by matching the energy consumed in foods with the energy burned in physical activities over a period.

Energy bar: a product generally shaped in the form of a candy bar that usually contains protein, vitamins, and minerals and is frequently used as a quick snack or meal replacement.

Energy drink: a beverage that provides a quick source of energy in the form of sugars generally containing caffeine. Note that a sugar-free energy drink provides no energy in the form of calories but stimulates the body to burn energy.

Enrichment broth: liquid media used to recover injured microorganisms that may not be detected otherwise.

Enrobing: unit operation in chocolate manufacture in which a formed center passes under a chocolate waterfall to evenly coat it.

Enthalpy: measure of the total energy within a system.

Environmental Protection Agency (EPA): governmental agency responsible for protecting the environment and with a particular interest in the safety of pesticides in food.

Enzyme: a protein that will catalyze an organic reaction in biological organisms or in processing vessels.

Epidemiologist: scientist who uses a wide range of data to help identify the cause of a disease outbreak and the possible course for prevention of repeat episodes.

Epidemiology: science of identifying the cause of a disease outbreak and the possible course for prevention of repeat episodes by analyzing a wide range of data.

Epiglottis: the valve at the top of the esophagus that prevents flow of gastric juices from entering the mouth.

Essence: volatile aromatic compounds that evaporate during concentration of a juice are captured by condensation and returned to the concentrated beverage.

Ethanol: a simple alcohol that is produced during fermentation of fruits, grains, and starches to make beer, wine, and other alcoholic beverages. It contributes 7 kilocalories per gram.

Ethnic foods: items specifically identified with a specific culture or nationality.

Ethylene: a gas that functions as a plant hormone that can be generated by a plant to promote fruit ripening, as a wound response or artificially from ethanol. Some plant tissues such as lettuce leaves are very sensitive to ethylene.

Eukaryote: organism consisting of one or more cells with a well-defined nucleus surrounded by a membrane.

Eutrophication: accumulation of nutrients such as acids, nitrogen, phosphorus, and potassium to the point that they decrease the oxygen in water or plant fertility in soil.

Exhausting: unit operation in canning to remove all the air in the can or jar after filling and before sealing.

Exothermic: type of chemical reaction that releases heat.

Expiration date: the end of the estimated shelf life of a food product as marked on the product label.

Extraction: chemical process that removes a component from a substance such as aromatic compounds from a spice or water-soluble compounds from tea leaves or ground coffee.

Extrinsic factors: conditions outside a food that affect the growth of the microflora in that food.

Extrusion: complex food process that involves mixing and kneading to force the formulated food through an orifice under pressure to a desired size and shape.

Fad diet: popular trend primarily to reduce weight that is nutritionally inadequate.

Fair-trade: a marketing term used to designate products that have been sustainably produced in developing countries and adequate wages have been paid to the growers and workers.

Fast-food restaurant: one that minimizes the time between ordering a food and serving it: alternatively known as Quick Service Restaurants.

Fasting: voluntary reduction in or elimination of food consumption over a designated period generally motivated by political, religious, or spiritual reasons.

Fat: a lipid that is solid at room temperature or lipid stored in the body.

Fat replacer: a food additive that possesses some of the functional properties of fat without the calories and is added to reduce fat in a product.

Fatty acid: a portion of a lipid composed of a carbon chain, a carboxyl group at one end of the molecule, and hydrogen atoms attached to the carbon atoms.

Fecal sample: one taken from the solid waste of a human or other animal to determine if it is a carrier or victim of a specific food-borne pathogen.

Feces: solid waste from a human or other animal usually rich in pathogenic microorganisms and a potent contaminant of foods.

Federal Food Drug and Cosmetic Act (FFDCA): the law that authorizes the regulations promulgated by FDA to ensure safety in the food supply and prevent fraud by manufacturers and distributors.

Fermentation: conversion of a raw food into a processed product by adding microorganisms that will change the chemical composition of the food and decrease the chances of it spoiling.

Fiberboard: strong, reinforced packaging material made from paper and wood fibers and used in shipment of food packages.

Fick's laws of diffusion: provide the basic mathematical relationship for the flux of one chemical species into another. Diffusion is a function of concentration gradient and distance and allows the calculations of diffusivity.

Fieldprint: calculation of the contribution of a specific field to greenhouse gas production, water use, and other environmental impacts.

FIFO: First-In, First-Out inventory management scheme to ensure rapid turnover of stock.

Filth: contaminants in food such as fly eggs, insect parts, maggots, rodent hair and feces, and weevils.

Fine-dining restaurant: one that specializes in high-quality food with a longer time between ordering and service than other establishments and in which the meal can be prepared under the direction of a chef, generally with an emphasis on presentation and at a premium price.

Finished product: a formulated food product that is ready for distribution and sale.

First-order reaction: semilogarithmic degradation of a component or attribute over time.

Flatulence: intestinal buildup and expression of gas resulting in socially unacceptable sounds and odors.

Flavanol: water-soluble pigment characterized by a yellow color found in plants.

Flavor: sensory sensation of a food combining the perception of taste and aroma.

Flavor enhancer: a compound or combination of compounds that has little direct effect on flavor but increases the intensity of other flavor compounds in the food.

Flavor profile: a description of the impact of the aromatic and taste notes of a food.

Flavorant: a natural or synthetic food additive that contributes to the flavor of a product.

Flow behavior: the effect on the shear rate of a fluid when it is exposed to increasing levels of shear stress.

Fluid: gases, liquids, and semisolid objects that are put into motion upon application of shear stress.

fMRI: or functional magnetic resonance imaging, a method used to determine brain activity in response to a stimulus.

Focus group: a small panel of consumers who are asked to describe their opinions about a specific food or product category to provide qualitative information useful in developing and marketing products.

Folate and folic acid: B vitamin critical in proper development of the fetus during pregnancy.

Food additive: an ingredient placed in a food product to achieve a specific function.

Food and Drug Administration (FDA): the primary US government agency responsible for safety of ingredients and food products.

Food-associated illness: one that is caused in whole or part by consumption of a contaminated food.

Food-borne illness: one that is caused in whole or part by consumption of a contaminated food.

Food gel: a semisolid structure in a food product or menu item that provides unique textural properties.

Food infection: a type of food poisoning caused by consumption of a food contaminated by a microorganism that grows inside the person.

Food intoxication: a type of food poisoning caused by consumption of a food that contains a toxin usually produced by microorganism.

Food pathogen: a microorganism that causes illness by an infection or intoxication of contaminated food.

Food poisoning: an illness caused by a food infection or intoxication.

Food preservation: any method that extends the shelf life of a product by slowing or halting decay or quality loss of a whole food by killing or inhibiting microorganisms or inhibiting chemical reactions in the food.

Food processing: modification of raw food ingredients to improve safety, extend shelf life, or enhance quality.

Food Safety and Inspection Service (FSIS): branch of USDA responsible for enforcing regulations on meat and poultry products shipped in interstate commerce.

Food Safety Modernization Act (FSMA): law that updates the powers of FDA to shift the focus from responding to food contamination to preventing it.

Food scientist: a professional who has received technical training in the safety, chemistry, preservation, quality and analysis of food materials, ingredients, and resultant products.

Food sensitivity: an adverse reaction to a specific food or ingredient that is not detected by production of antibodies.

Food service: preparing and serving of meals for consumers by a business or institution for consumption on site, pick up, or delivery.

Food toxicoinfection: a type of food poisoning caused by consumption of a food contaminated by a microorganism that produces a toxin in the gastrointestinal tract.

Food trends: changes in the purchase and consumption patterns of a significant portion of the population.

Formulated food: a product resulting from the mixture of ingredients.

Fourier's law: provides the basic mathematical relationship for the flux of heat from one point in space to another. It is a function of temperature gradient and distance and allows the calculations of thermal diffusivity.

Free radical: highly reactive molecule that has an unpaired electron that leads to initiation, propagation, and termination of oxidation reactions particularly with lipids and proteins.

Freezer burn: visual defect in improperly packaged frozen foods resulting from the sublimation of ice to water vapor leading to surface dehydration.

Fresh-cut produce: a whole fruit or vegetable that has been washed, cut to bite-sized pieces, and packaged to provide convenience for the consumer.

Freshman fifteen: the typical weight gain in pounds of a first-year student in college.

Friction factor: term in rheological calculations that accounts for the effects of friction on the energy required to produce the flow of a fluid.

Fruit: an edible, ripened ovary of a plant's reproductive system.

Functional food: a raw food or formulated product that provides health benefits not included in basic nutritional properties.

Functional property or functionality: the ability of an ingredient to perform a specific function in a food product owing to the physical and chemical properties of the component compounds in the ingredient.

Fundamental scientist: one who pursues basic science without any immediate or direct application in mind.

Gas chromatography: an analytical technique that separates individual compounds after volatilization and is used in many applications including the composition of flavors in fresh and processed foods.

Gas permeability: the degree to which gases such as oxygen, carbon dioxide, and ethylene can pass in or out of a package with glass and metal being impermeable and all others, including hard plastics, permitting some passage.

Gastroenteritis: illness of the bowels characterized by vomiting, cramps, and diarrhea.

Gelatinization: degradation of the starch molecule in the presence of water and heat to increase its solubility and improve its consumer acceptability.

Gelato: an Italian version of ice cream that tends to have less fat, less overrun, and more sugar than American ice cream.

Gene expression: signaling process from the nucleus to synthesize a specific compound in the cell.

Generally Recognized as Safe (GRAS): food additives that have been shown to be acceptable for use in the food supply based on general use over a long period, scientific research, and thorough review by scientific panels.

Genetic engineering: manipulation of a genome to modify the behavior of an organism.

Genotype: the genetic makeup of an organism that differentiates it from all others.

Geometric mean: the weighted average of values using within a base 10 logarithmic scale.

Glass-transition temperature: point during freezing at which all the molecules within a food become immobile.

Gliadin: one of the protein components of gluten and the portion that is generally considered responsible for the development of celiac disease and other sensitivities to gluten.

Glucagon: a hormone that helps regulate sugar concentration in the bloodstream by raising blood glucose levels when they become too low.

Gluten: a protein complex of glutenin and gliadin formed during hydration and mixing of flour from grains such as wheat and barley.

Gluten-free product: one made from grains or other materials that do not possess the gluten protein complex and are acceptable to eat by consumers with celiac disease.

Glycogen: long chain of glucose molecules stored in the liver and skeletal muscle that serves as a ready reserve of energy for the body.

GMO: genetically modified organism by manipulation of the DNA.

Golden rice: genetically modified to prevent interference with iron absorption and provide β-carotene, which is yellow in color.

Good Agricultural Practices (GAP): guidelines developed to reduce the chances of contamination of raw materials on the farm.

Good Handling Practices (GHP): guidelines developed to reduce the chances of contamination of harvested crops after they leave the farm and before they reach the market or manufacturing plant.

Good Manufacturing Practices (GMP): guidelines developed to provide for systems that assure proper design, monitoring, and control of manufacturing processes and facilities.

Governmental regulation: rules made by federal, state, and local agencies that govern the growing, handling, manufacturing, and distribution of foods.

Grade standards: guidelines developed and used by USDA to classify plant and animal products on the basis of quality.

Grain: a plant and the food it produces that is grown primarily for its seeds to be used for human food or animal feed.

Greenhouse gas emissions: production of carbon dioxide, methane, and other gases that contribute to global warming.

Gum: a food additive developed from natural sources that functions as a thickener, gelling agent, or other form of stabilizer in a formulated food.

Halal: foods permitted by Islamic tradition or law.

Halophile: microorganism that can tolerate higher levels of salt than most species.

Handling system: a series of steps or unit operations, from the growing location for a plant or animal to the market to be sold as fresh items or to the manufacturing plant for further processing.

Haram: foods not permitted by Islamic tradition or law.

Harvest: separation of an edible part from the plant or sacrifice of an animal for food.

Hazard Analysis and Critical Control Point (HACCP): a systematic approach to identifying dangers in a segment of the supply chain, manufacturing or distribution chain, and monitoring operations where the dangers are most likely to be controlled.

Hazard Analysis and Risk-based Preventive Controls (HARPC): a "preventive control plan" with similarities to HACCP in that it covers hazard analysis, monitoring, records, corrective actions, and verification of food products and processes that do not have a requirement for a critical limit as in HACCP plans.

Heart disease: restricted flow of blood into the heart that eventually leads to the organ's inability to function and to death.

Heat capacity: the amount of energy required in raising the temperature of a body of a given mass.

Heat exchanging: the transfer of heat from one substance to another such as from a hot coil to a liquid or a warm food to a freezing surface.

Heat flux: rate of heat transfer per unit area.

Heat of evaporation: the heat required to convert a liquid at the boiling temperature to a gas.

Heat transfer: transmission of energy from a higher-temperature object to a lower-temperature object.

Hemicellulose: complex carbohydrate that is found in plants, indigestible and a component of dietary fiber.

Herb: in culinary or food formulation applications, a spice that is derived from leafy green plants such as parsley, sage, rosemary, and thyme.

Hidden quality characteristics: those attributes of a food that cannot be directly determined by the consumer, such as nutritional value and safety.

High-density lipoprotein (HDL): a molecule composed of cholesterol bound to a protein, also known as the "good" cholesterol.

High-performance liquid chromatography (HPLC): an analytical technique that separates individual compounds in a food extract without requiring volatilization of the compounds.

High-pressure processing: nonthermal technique that uses pressure to inactivate microorganisms.

Home-use test: one where the consumer is provided with a product to be evaluated in a realistic environment and which is followed up by survey questions.

Homogenization: the process of breaking fat globules to very small particles in a beverage such as milk to prevent separation of the fat from the water phase.

Hotspot: point in a life cycle of a product that can be modified to improve sustainability of that product.

Human subjects: participants in an experiment and requiring approval by an Institutional Review Board.

Hurdle: barrier to microbial growth.

Hydrocarbon: an organic molecule containing only carbon and hydrogen atoms.

Hydrocolloid: a food additive that is able to bind water through a large number of hydrogen bonds that can act as a gelling agent, thickener, or other form of stabilizer in formulated foods.

Hydrogen bond: an attraction between a hydrogen atom in a molecule and an atom in an adjacent molecule such as oxygen.

Hydrogenation: the addition of hydrogen across a double bond in an unsaturated fatty acid to achieve better melting properties and mouthfeel of a product at the expense of forming *trans* fatty acids.

Hydrolysis: chemical reaction that results in the release of water from an organic molecule.

Hydrophile/Lipophile Balance (HLB): ratio of the hydrophilic character of a stabilizer to its hydrophobic character.

Hydrophilic: the degree to which a molecule is compatible with water.

Hydrophobic: the degree to which a molecule is not compatible with water.

Hydroxyl group: portion of an organic molecule consisting of an oxygen atom and a hydrogen atom and is important in cohesion of substances through hydrogen bonding.

Hypercalcemia: a high level of calcium in the bloodstream, which could be an indication of metabolic problems.

Hyphae: long filaments formed by molds.

Hypoglycemia: low blood sugar that, left untreated, can lead to fainting, seizures, brain damage, and even death.

Image quality characteristics: those attributes of a food that are established in the mind of the consumer by marketing, the media, and recommendations by friends.

Immiscible: inability of one fluid to mix with another fluid.

Immunocompromised: a condition that renders a person more susceptible to an illness than the general population.

Immunodeficiency: inability of an individual's immune system to adequately defend itself from threats that most others can.

Immunological test: diagnostic procedure used to identify specific microorganisms involving an immune reaction.

Incubation time: the time in hours or days between the consumption of a contaminated food and the evidence of symptoms of food poisoning.

Indicator microorganism: one whose presence or absence tells us something about the sample where they were found.

Individual quick freezing (IQF): technique involving direct contact of each piece of food with the freezing medium.

Industrial food system: market-driven and intensive production, processing, and distribution of foods for company profit.

Ingredient: a raw material or food additive that performs one or more specific functions in a food product.

Ingredient statement: a required item on a food label that lists all ingredients from the greatest to the smallest amount by either their common or chemical names.

Inhibitor: compound that slows or blocks enzyme reactions or microbial growth.

Institutional Review Board: committee that evaluates studies with human subjects to ensure that ethical procedures will be used.

Insulin: a hormone that helps regulate sugar concentration in the bloodstream by lowering blood glucose levels when they become too high.

Integrated cropping systems: intensively produced foods that combine efforts to improve sustainability and profitability by using waste from one operation to provide nutrients for other operations.

Integrated Pest Management (IPM): technique used by growers of plant crops to determine when and how often to apply pesticides in contrast to the use of a preplanned schedule of application whether the crop needs it or not.

Interesterification: rearrangement of fatty acids in a lipid molecule to affect its melting temperature and thus its desirability as a food ingredient.

Intermediary metabolism: the combination of digestion, catabolism, and anabolism that allows the body to regenerate itself.

Intermediate-moisture food: one with a water activity that is low enough to inhibit microbial growth without being considered dry, many of which are shelf stable at room temperature.

International Organization for Standardization (ISO): association that establishes guidelines for business practices in many areas of product manufacturing including quality assurance and food safety to facilitate global trade.

Intestinal mucosa: a membrane that lines the intestines and selectively absorbs small molecules across into the bloodstream for transport to the cells as a critical part of digestion.

Intrinsic factors: conditions within a food that affect the growth of the microflora in that food.

Inulin: a carbohydrate polymer consisting of a long chain of fructose molecules.

Ion exchange: a separation system in which ions (charged atoms or molecules) in a fluid are switched with those bound to a solid matrix (a resin) as the fluid passes through a container packed with the solid.

Irradiation: use of ionizing radiation to preserve foods.

Irritable bowel syndrome: a disease state that inhibits digestion and frequently leads to constipation followed by explosive diarrhea.

Isolated system: process where no mass or heat is transferred in or out, that is, both closed and adiabatic.

Isothermal system: process kept at the same temperature by adding or removing heat or by the use of thermal insulation.

Junk food: a food product with little or no nutritional or health benefit that is consumed primarily for pleasure.

Ketone body: a molecule that is formed during metabolism when a protein is used to supply energy.

Ketosis or ketoacidosis: a disease state that results from the production of ketone bodies when protein becomes the primary source of energy for the body.

Key Quality Attributes (KQAs): quality characteristics of a specific product that relate directly to wants and needs of consumers of that product.

Kilocalorie: the more appropriate term for what we normally consider as calories equivalent to the energy required to raise the temperature of a kilogram of water by 1°C.

Kinetic energy: energy in motion.

Kosher: foods permitted for consumption by Jewish law.

Kwashiorkor: a deficiency disease associated with the lack of enough protein and calories in the diet.

Laboratory bench: assigned space of a product developer where initial formulations are produced for testing.

Lactic acid fermentation: conversion of a raw food by a microorganism into a product that has a sour taste attributed to the formation of lactic acid.

Lacto-ovo vegetarian: a person who consumes a plant-based diet but is permitted to consume dairy and egg products.

Lactose: a disaccharide composed of a molecule of glucose bound to a molecule of galactose and is the primary sugar found in milk.

Lactose intolerance: inability to digest normal levels of lactose leading to discomfort caused by production of gas by anaerobic, intestinal bacteria.

Lag phase: the beginning of the microbial growth curve in which cell division is steady but slow.

Laminar flow: pattern in which the path of each molecule of fluid follows a well-defined streamline.

Law: an act passed by a legislative body that is signed by the executive authority and becomes binding to the population.

Law of Conservation of Energy: energy cannot be created or destroyed; it can only be changed from one form to another.

Lean Finely Textured Beef (LFTB): by-product of beef processing that recovers meat that is 95% lean and treated with ammonium hydroxide to improve safety; popularly known as pink slime.

Leavening agent: a food additive that causes breads or other bakery products to rise owing to the production of CO_2 either biologically by yeast or chemically from baking soda.

Lecithin: an emulsifier found naturally in egg yolks or soybeans and which is composed predominantly of phosphatidylcholine.

Life cycle: everything that happens to a food product during growth of raw materials and ingredients, manufacture, distribution, and consumer use.

Life-cycle analysis: identification of all inputs and outcomes into a product and its packaging during its life cycle to help determine how it can be produced more sustainably and profitably.

Life expectancy: the length of time in years a person with a specific demographic category is likely to live.

Lignin: a polymer found in cell walls of plant tissue that functions as dietary fiber.

Line extension: changes in a product feature, such as flavor, content, size, name, or packaging.

Lipid: the technical term for a fat or oil characterized by its insolubility in water and which contributes 9 kilocalories per gram.

Lipid hydrolysis: breaking of a bond in a triacylglycerol or phospholipid to release water and a free fatty acid.

Lipid oxidation: degradation of fats and oils in a food leading to rancid odors.

Lipopolysaccharide: complex molecule characterized by a combination of a lipid and a complex carbohydrate.

Lipoprotein: a molecule that contains both a lipid, usually cholesterol, and a protein.

Log phase: the portion of the microbial growth curve in which cell division greatly exceeds cell death leading to exponential growth.

Low-density lipoprotein (LDL): a molecule composed of cholesterol bound to a protein, which also known as the "bad" cholesterol.

Lycopene: a bright red carotenoid that functions as a potent antioxidant and is found primarily in watermelon, tomatoes, and their products.

Macrobiotic diet: one which avoids meat and processed foods consisting mainly of grains and vegetables.

Macronutrient: a component of foods that contributes kilocalories.

Maillard browning: complex series of nonenzymic reactions that produces a golden-brown color from the combination of a reducing sugar and a free amine.

Malnutrition: inadequate consumption of essential nutrients.

Marasmus: a deficiency disease associated with the lack of enough calories in the diet.

Market test: presentation or distribution of an advanced prototype to a large group of consumers to determine whether the item can be launched or needs more research.

Marketing: the group within a company that connects the company to the consumer with an ultimate aim of increasing market share of all of its products.

Mask: a compound or combination of compounds that may have little direct effect on flavor but decreases the intensity of other flavor compounds in food.

Mass balance: mathematical relationship accounting for the mass of matter that comes into a process or unit operation in the form of raw ingredients and for the mass of matter that leaves the process or unit operation in the form of an intermediate product, final product, by-product, waste, or that is accumulated at any stage of the process within a practical time frame.

Mass spectrometer: analytical instrument that systematically breaks larger molecules into fragments to help identify the chemical structure of the original molecule by comparing the pattern of fragments to a library of compounds.

Mastication: the process of chewing a solid food to form it into the bolus and making it easier to swallow.

Materials handling: movement of raw materials, ingredients, partially processed foods, and finished products from one location to another usually within a food manufacturing facility.

Meat analog: a formulated food that contains no meat and sometimes no animal-produced ingredients designed to have the appearance, flavor, and texture of a meat product.

Mechanical energy balance: mathematical relationship accounting for the distribution of mechanical energy within a system required to pump, convey, or otherwise transport products within a processing plant.

Megadose: excessive consumption of a compound such as a vitamin or mineral that has adverse consequences on health.

Meta-analysis: statistical procedure that accumulates data from a large number of studies in a specific area of research to draw concrete conclusions from seemingly conflicting information.

Metabolism: a series of enzyme-catalyzed processes in the body that allow it to function properly; with respect to food and nutrition, the primary processes are anabolism and catabolism.

Metmyoglobin: brown pigment that is produced from the degradation of oxymyoglobin in meat as it ages in the presence of oxygen.

Microaerophile: microorganism able to survive and grow at very low oxygen concentrations.

Microbial contamination: deliberate or incidental incorporation of undesirable microorganisms to a food.

Microfiltration: purification of a fluid through a porous solid membrane with pores typically smaller than 10 µm to remove fine particles.

Microflora: the sum of all microorganisms in a finite environment such as a specific food.

Micronutrient: a component of foods, such as a vitamin or mineral, that does not provide kilocalories but is essential to health and well-being.

Microstructure: the architecture of compounds at the molecular level or organisms at the cellular level.

Microtechniques: laboratory methods that use very small levels of solvents and reagents to reduce accumulation of toxic waste materials.

Microtechnology: processes that use very small particles (less than a micrometer) to form customized materials.

Migration: movement of compounds in a package, particularly plastic, into the food it contains.

Milling: grinding of larger food particles into smaller ones such as grains into flour.

Mineral: an inorganic element present in a food that can be essential or toxic depending on human needs and the amount present.

Minimally processed: food that has undergone some unit operations such as cutting or packaging with little or no major preservation step such as heating, freezing, or drying.

Mitochondria: organelle within a living cell that functions to synthesize ATP as a means of storing energy.

Modified atmosphere packaging (MAP): container in which initial conditions of gas composition have been set in the package to slow spoilage of a food.

Modified starch: a complex carbohydrate that has been chemically treated to improve its functional properties in a formulated food.

Moisture sorption isotherm: the mathematical relationship between water content and water activity in a food, usually expressed in graphical form.

Molecular gastronomy: the merging of food science and culinary arts to better understand the chemical and physical changes that occur during cooking and other forms of food preparation.

Molecular mechanism: the series of chemical steps required to produce a specific outcome in a biological system.

Molecular mobility: ability of a compound in a food or tissue to move from one location to another.

Monosaccharide: a single sugar molecule, such as glucose or fructose, which cannot be broken down by hydrolysis without losing its status as a sugar.

Monosodium glutamate (MSG): the sodium salt of the amino acid, glutamic acid, known for its ability to enhance the flavor of foods by contributing to umami and also associated with Chinese Restaurant Syndrome.

Monounsaturated fatty acid: one which contains one double bond and thus is not susceptible to lipid oxidation.

Mouthfeel: the perception of the physical properties of a food in the mouth.

Muscle contraction: a shortening of the muscle during exercise that involves binding of actin and myosin.

Muscle foods: those derived from the muscular tissue of animals and which go through rigor to become meat.

Muscle relaxation: a lengthening of the muscle during exercise that involves release of actin from myosin.

Mutation: a modification of the genetic material in an organism.

Mycelium: group or mass of hyphae.

Mycotoxin: toxic substance produced by a mold.

Myoglobin: meat protein that is purple when the muscle is first cut, turns into oxymyoglobin (red) when exposed to air and to metmyoglobin (brown) upon longer storage.

MyPlate: guidelines for a healthy diet as recommended by USDA and found at www.choosemyplate.gov.

Nanoparticle: substance that is extremely small in structure on the order of billionths of a meter.

Nanotechnology: processes that use extremely small particles (atomic or molecular levels) to form unique products.

Natural food: theoretically one that has not been modified or preserved by humans but frequently described by food processors, restaurants, and supplement suppliers as one that contains no artificial ingredients.

Natural ingredient: a food item that has been derived from animal, microbial, or plant substances without chemical modification.

Natural resources: air, soil, water, crops, and livestock in the environment.

Natural toxin: one that occurs in a raw or whole food without any modification or preservation by humans.

Net weight: the amount of food in a primary package minus the weight of the package.

Newton's laws of motion: describe the relationship between a solid object and the external forces that put it into motion or change its trajectory.

Newtonian fluids: liquids, gases, and semisolid substances that have a linear relationship between shear stress and shear rate with respect to flow.

Nitrites: salts that are used to preserve meats by maintaining color in the form of nitrosomyoglobin (frankfurter pinkish red) and preventing growth of *Clostridium botulinum*.

Nitrosamine: potentially carcinogenic molecule that forms during curing of meats or in the stomach when nitrites react with free amines in proteins.

Nitrosomyoglobin: the pigment fixed in red meats during curing with nitrates and nitrites in combination with other ingredients.

Nonclimacteric: property of many fruits and vegetables that fail to ripen after harvest.

Nondestructive measurement: quality evaluation by an instrument that does not result in loss of the item measured.

Nonenzymic: chemical reaction or physical change in living tissue or a food item that does not involve catalysis by an enzyme.

Non-Newtonian fluids: liquids, gases and semisolid substances that have a nonlinear relationship between shear stress and shear rate with respect to flow.

Nonthermal processing: food manufacturing operations that use means other than heat to preserve foods and result in little or no increase in ambient temperatures during manufacture.

Nucleic acid: compound that carries the genetic code of an organism.

Nutraceutical: a formulated medicinal product made from health-promoting ingredients.

Nutrient: an essential compound that contributes to energy (carbohydrate, lipid, protein) or metabolic processes (vitamin, mineral).

Nutrient partitioning: with respect to obesity, the percentage of excess carbohydrate in the body that goes into fat accumulation relative to the amount that goes into producing protein to increase muscle mass.

Nutrigenomics: scientific discipline that combines a knowledge in chemistry with that of molecular biology to better understand how ingredients in foods contribute to human health.

Nutrition: sustenance of living organisms by essential molecules in food or related materials and the study of this process.

Nutrition Labeling and Education Act (NLEA): law that enables FDA to set regulations for Nutrition Facts statements on packaged food products.

Nutritional label: information on the product that provides the ingredient statement as well as the amount and the Percent Daily Value of selected nutrients.

Nutritional quality: the ability of ingredients or foods to contribute to health and well-being.

Nutritionist: a scientist who studies how nutrients affect the health and well-being and provides advice on healthy eating.

Obesity: accumulation of too much body fat such that it jeopardizes health equivalent to 25% or more fat of total body weight in a male and 35% or more fat of total body weight in a female but frequently classified as having a BMI equal to or greater than 30.

Ohmic heating: use of electricity to generate thermal energy to preserve foods.

Oil: a lipid that is liquid at room temperature.

Oilseed: a grain or legume that is a significant source of edible lipid.

Oleogel: a lipid-soluble molecule made by combining an oil with a carbohydrate polymer that aids in gelation of lipid-based food systems.

Oligofructose: a chain of nine or less fructose molecules linked together by glycosidic bonds, usually a hydrolysis product of inulin.

Oligosaccharide: a chain of three to nine sugar molecules linked together by glycosidic bonds.

Omega-3 fatty acid: a polyunsaturated lipid that is essential for good health.

Organic fertilizer: one derived from plant, animal, or food waste that is used to return the unused nutrients into the soil as opposed to those produced synthetically from petroleum.

Organic food: one produced with no synthetic fertilizers, pesticides, hormones, or other agricultural chemicals.

Orthonasal: perception of aroma of a food through the nose without eating it.

Orthorexia: eating disorder that limits the diet to "healthy" foods to the extent that it becomes so extreme that it cannot provide sufficient nutrients to maintain health.

Osmophile: microorganism that can tolerate higher levels of sugar than most species.

Osmotic pressure: the amount of water pressure inside of and outside of a cell as determined by the resistance of the cell membrane to being permeated.

Osteoporosis: disease state resulting from inadequate consumption of available calcium and results in fragile bones.

Outbreak: development of food poisoning to a group of people attributed to consumption of food from a single source.

Overhydration: excess consumption of water leading to intoxication and possible death.

Overrun: incorporation of air into a product to improve its texture.

Overweight: according to the CDC and World Health Organization (WHO), a person whose BMI is 25 or above.

Oxidation: a chemical process in living organisms associated with reactive oxygen species that degrades lipids, proteins, and nucleic acids.

Oxidation–reduction potential: the degree to which a molecule can add electrons; in a food, it is related to the amount of oxygen present and the likelihood its components will become oxidized.

Oxymyoglobin: the red pigment in red meats produced when myoglobin is exposed to oxygen.

Pale Soft Exudative (PSE): a defect in meat, particularly pork but also noted in poultry, characterized by objectionable light color, soft texture, and excessive juice release.

Palletized: individual containers stacked on a standard pallet for shipment to and storage in a warehouse.

Parasite: an organism that derives some or all of its needs from another organism.

Partially hydrogenated vegetable oil: lipid ingredient that has been modified by increasing the degree of saturation of its component fatty acids to improve its functional properties at the cost of producing *trans* fatty acids.

Particulate: small solid piece of food such as a corn kernel or an individual pea that is suspended in a liquid.

Pasteurization: a partial heat treatment that kills some but not all microorganisms to extend shelf life with minimal loss of flavor or nutritional quality.

Pathogenic microorganisms or pathogens: those that can cause illness by an infection or intoxication.

Pectic enzyme: protein that catalyzes the breakdown of pectin, a key component of plant cell walls, which results in softening of the tissue.

Pectin: a carbohydrate component of plant cell walls that functions as dietary fiber.

Peptoglycan: complex molecule characterized by a combination of protein and carbohydrate.

Peristalsis: the process of moving the bolus through the digestive system and into the large intestine.

Pesticide: a molecule applied to crops to prevent damage caused by insects, microbial decay, weeds, or other factors that affect crop yield.

pH: the negative base 10 logarithm of the hydrogen ion chemical potential (in practice concentration) on a scale from 0 to 14 where a value below 7 is acidic, a value of 7 is neutral, and a value above 7 is alkaline or basic.

Phase: the physical state of all or part of a food such as solid, liquid, or gas; a distinct component of a dispersion either continuous or discontinuous; or the portion of a growth curve that refers to predominant behavior of cells within an organism such as lag, log, stationary, or death.

Phase change: transformation of a compound from one state to another, generally related to solids, liquids, and gases.

Phenotype: the observable set of characteristics in an organism that are a result of its genotype and the adaptation to the environment.

Phospholipid: a polar lipid that is soluble in both aqueous and nonaqueous solutions and is a component of cell membranes.

Photochemical ozone: a pollutant generated by incomplete combustion of fossil foods.

Physical hazard: a danger in a food attributed to the presence of a solid object such as shards of glass, metal, or small pebbles.

Physical properties: fundamental physical attributes of a substance or product that can be directly measured such mass, volume, density, or viscosity, or complex attributes such as color or texture, which is a complex measurement of a single or a combination of multiple physical properties that correlate to human perception.

Physicochemical test: a method to determine the physical or chemical properties of an ingredient or food.

Phytosterol: lipid with a basic sterol structure derived from plants.

Pilot plant: laboratory that includes small-scale manufacturing equipment and is used to identify potential problems in processing a new product and produce enough material for a market test.

Pink slime: popular term for lean finely textured beef.

Plant sterol: a lipid present in fruits, vegetables, and grains that inhibits cholesterol absorption during digestion.

Plasma: highly charged state of matter that is the major component of the universe, found in stars including our sun.

Plasma membrane: a semipermeable barrier around every living cell composed primarily of phospholipids and proteins.

Polycyclic hydrocarbon (PAH): one of a class of toxic compounds found in foods that have been heated above 120°C.

Polygalacturonase: enzyme that breaks down pectin leading to tissue softening.

Polyphenoloxidase: enzyme that breaks down phenolic compounds in plants leading to browning.

Polysaccharide: a long chain of simple sugars linked together by glycosidic bonds.

Polyunsaturated fatty acid: one that contains more than one double bond, increases the fluidity of cell membranes and is susceptible to lipid oxidation.

Postmortem physiology: chemical reactions that occur in muscle foods after harvest.

Potable water: that which is safe and acceptable for drinking.

Potential energy: stored energy.

Prebiotic: nondigestible substance that stimulates the growth of beneficial microorganisms in our intestines.

Precision: the property of a measurement with respect to how close the estimate comes to repeated measures on the same sample.

Precursor: a compound in a living system that can be converted into a more functional one through biological, chemical, or physical processes.

Preference test: affective sensory technique to determine the acceptability of different treatments.

Prepared entrée: the main course of a meal that is ready to eat or heat and eat.

Prepared foods: ones that are ready to eat or heat and eat with the exception of whole fruits and vegetables.

Prerequisite Program (PRP): a set of programs such as Good Management Practices that must be in place before a HACCP plan can be established.

Preservative: a compound added to food to inhibit microbial growth or halt other spoilage processes helping to extend shelf life and ensure a safe product.

Preventive Control Program: risk-based system put into a processing operation to anticipate food safety problems before they happen.

Primary package: the package directly in touch with a food product.

Primary structure: chain of amino acids in a protein linked together by peptide bonds.

Prion: a protein that infects cells, causing neurodegenerative conditions.

Probiotic: microorganism that, when digested, has beneficial aspects in the body.

Process control: means of ensuring that unit operations in food manufacturing are operating correctly.

Process optimization: maximization of profitability by maximization of process efficiency (e.g., minimizing bottlenecks and inefficiencies in unit operations needed to produce a product) within economic constraints that include capital and operating costs as well as market demand.

Processed food: a product that has been modified to improve its safety, extend the shelf life, enhance its quality, and improve its convenience.

Product development: all aspects involved in design of new commercial items including initial formulation, package design, process development, sensory testing, scale-up from bench to pilot plant to manufacture, and producing a marketing plan.

Product launch: introduction of a new product to the market.

Prokaryote: organism without a clearly defined nucleus.

Protein: a molecule composed of a long string of amino acids that can function as an enzyme, cellular transporter, structural component, or nutrient, which contributes 4 kilocalories per gram.

Protein peptide: a short chain of amino acids usually a fragment from a protein molecule.

Protozoa: group of single-celled eukaryotes that are capable of movement.

Pro-vitamin: a precursor molecule that does not have vitamin activity until it is broken down into one that can act as a vitamin.

Pseudoplastic: shear-thinning fluid such that the apparent viscosity decreases as the shear stress increases.

Psychrophile: microorganism that can survive and outcompete others at low temperatures above freezing.

Pulsed electric field: a series of short bursts of electricity used in the preservation of foods.

Pungency: a chemical feeling factor in the mouth such as the sharp reaction to fresh-cut onions.

Pureé: finely chopped and cooked item, particularly fruits and vegetables.

Quality: properties of a food that distinguish it from similar foods and affect its preference by consumers.

Quality Assurance (QA): a means of ensuring quality and safety of a food by focusing on keeping the process in control.

Quality Control (QC): a means of ensuring quality and safety of a food by testing the finished product.

Quality Management (QM): a means of ensuring quality by means of modifying the process to more closely fit the wants and needs of the consumer.

Quaternary structure: linkage of two or more peptide chains within a protein to form the functional molecule.

Quorn: a protein produced by a mold used as source for meat analogs suitable for consumption by vegans.

Radiation: transport of electromagnetic waves including heat in a vacuum or gases.

Radurization: a partial treatment with ionizing irradiation to kill some (primarily pathogens) but not all microorganisms to extend shelf life with minimal loss of flavor or nutritional quality. Comparable to pasteurization.

Rancidity: an off-flavor attributed to the oxidation of lipids.

Raw materials: whole foods such as fruits, grains, meats, and vegetables.

Reaction heat: heat produced or absorbed during a chemical reaction.

Recall: action taken by a company or government agency to send out a notice to consumers and distributors regarding a product manufactured and introduced into the market that may be contaminated or mislabeled and should not be consumed.

Recognition threshold: the minimum concentration of a compound that permits positive identification of the character of the sensation.

Recontamination: unintentional introduction of undesirable chemicals or microorganisms into a processed food.

Recyclable: a package of a product made of materials that can be recovered for further use.

Refining: unit operation that separates out complex mixtures of components into distinct fractions such as sugar from molasses and white flour from ground wheat.

Relative humidity (RH): partial pressure of vapor relative to the complete saturation at a given temperature and atmospheric pressure.

Relevance: the property of a measurement with respect to how it matches the needs and desires of the ultimate consumer.

Reliability: the property of an instrument to produce measures that are accurate and precise.

Replication: in microorganisms, the division of a cell into two identical cells.

Research Chef: one certified by the Research Chefs Association on the basis of demonstrated knowledge of food science and the culinary arts.

Resources: anything needed to produce a product including its package.

Restructured meats: ground meat that has been reformed into a muscle-like texture.

Retort: a jacketed steam kettle used to can foods by heating under pressure.

Retrogradation: the process of expelling water by a starch leading to staling.

Retronasal: perception of aroma of a food through the nose while chewing it.

Reynolds number: dimensionless quantity that engineers use to calculate whether the flow of a specific fluid will be laminar or turbulent.

Rheological properties: attributes of a fluid that affect its flow behavior.

Rheology: study of the deformation of solids and fluids. It helps characterize the flow behavior of fluids.

Rheometer: instrument that measures flow behavior of fluids.

Ribonucleic acid (RNA): compound carrying genetic information of an organism and that can be synthesized from DNA during transcription.

Rigor mortis: muscle shortening after harvest owing to the irreversible binding of the proteins actin and myosin and which results in tough meat.

Ripening: a complex set of reactions in a fruit that generally results in a color change, sweetening, and softening, or the changes in a fermented cheese from raw milk to the final product.

Sales: the group within a company that is directly in touch with the customers to meet their needs (note that the customer is not usually the ultimate consumer).

Salty: a usually pleasant taste associated primarily with the presence of sodium chloride.

Sanitation: the process of keeping an area clean and relatively free of contaminating chemicals and microorganisms.

Sanitation Standard Operating Procedure (SSOP): mandatory guidelines for keeping areas clean.

Sashimi: literally Japanese for raw fish.

Satiety: the feeling of fullness.

Saturated fats: those in which the component fatty acids contain no double bonds.

Saturated fatty acid: one that contains no double bonds, is not susceptible to lipid oxidation, and is associated with increased risk of heart disease.

Scale-up: producing larger amounts of a product prototype from bench to pilot plant or pilot plant to manufacturing, generally resulting in new challenges and problems.

Scalping: movement of chemical compounds, particularly vitamins or odorants, in a food into the packaging material.

Scurvy: deficiency disease resulting from inadequate consumption of vitamin C.

Secondary package: one that contains one or more primary packages.

Secondary structure: folding of the primary structure of a protein caused by interactions between amino acids in proximity to form α-helix or β-sheet shapes.

Segment: a part of the consuming population that prefers a specific variation of a food or food product such as tart or sweet apples, mild or sharp cheese, or medium or hot chili sauce.

Semisolid food: a product that acts like a solid when there is no shear stress but acts like a fluid when shear stress is applied.

Sensitivity: the level of detection of an instrument.

Sensor: a device inserted into a processing line that can detect small differences in an attribute such as color, pH, sugar concentration, or viscosity.

Sensory descriptive analysis: the technique of identifying and quantifying the intensity of specific quality characteristics by a panel of human subjects.

Sensory evaluation: a series of techniques using human subjects to identify, describe, or analyze those characteristics that can be perceived in an ingredient, raw material, or finished food product using one or more of the five senses.

Sensory panel: a group of human subjects that participate in an analytical or affective sensory test.

Sensory perception: human response to a stimulus by one or more senses.

Sensory quality: characteristics of a raw material, ingredient, or food product that can be perceived by the five senses and usually confined to appearance, flavor, and textural properties.

Sequestrant: molecule or ingredient that binds metal ions to prevent them from oxidizing fats that would cause flavor problems.

Shear rate: velocity at which shear stress is applied to a fluid.

Shear stress: stress (force per unit area) that results from the shear applied to a fluid.

Shelf life: the length of time a food can maintain its acceptability to the consumer.

Shelf stable: the property of a food that permits a long shelf life at room temperature.

Shewhart Control Chart: a plot of a specific property of a food product to determine if the process is under control, is beginning to drift out of control, or has gone out of control.

Shrink: the amount of a food item that is lost in a supermarket generally calculated in terms of dollars and cents.

Solanine: a natural toxin found in potatoes that have been exposed to sunlight after harvest.

Solubility: the degree to which a molecule, usually a solid, will dissolve in another compound, usually a liquid such as water or oil, to form a homogeneous solution.

Solvent: a compound, usually a liquid, which dissolves other molecules, usually solids.

Sour: a usually unpleasant taste associated primarily with the presence of organic acids and frequently confused with bitter.

Source reduction: reducing the amount of packaging material in a food product.

Sourcing: identifying suppliers for raw materials, ingredients, packaging materials, or anything else needed for a food product.

Spice: a plant part such as bark, root, seed, or other vegetative tissue that has been dried and used to add flavor or color to a food.

Spider-web plot: circular graphic display of the differences in treatments used in sensory and environmental studies.

Spoilage: degradation of quality of a product to the point that it becomes unacceptable because of a change in flavor, appearance, texture, or other characteristics.

Sports nutrition: field of study that addresses specific needs of athletes.

Spray drying: dehydration process that involves forcing a liquid through an atomizer to produce a fine mist that leads to the evaporation of the water and collection of a fine powder.

Spreadability: the ease of a butter, margarine, or similar product to be evenly distributed on a solid food, particularly a bakery product.

Stabilizer: an ingredient that inhibits the breakdown of a formulated food with particular reference to preventing loss of texture.

Staling: the insolubility of starch in a baked product owing to retrogradation, resulting in an unacceptable product.

Staple food: comprises a major part of diet of a particular group or culture.

Starch: a complex carbohydrate made up of long chains of simple sugars that is able to be digested by humans.

Starter culture: a single strain or combination of microorganisms added to a raw material to produce a controlled fermentation.

Stationary phase: the essentially dormant portion of the microbial growth curve in which cell death is roughly equivalent to cell division.

Statistical Process Control (SPC): a method used to determine if a process is in control using standard mathematical methods.

Stereospecificity: mechanism of a reaction that results in molecules that are nonsuperimposable mirror images of each other.

Sterile: absent of any living microorganisms.

Sterol: multiringed lipid derived from plant or animal sources that serves as an important component of the body and is a precursor for certain hormones and a stabilizer of cell membranes.

Substrate: a compound that is transformed by an enzyme to form a chemical product.

Sucralose: an artificial sweetener that has a taste and a molecular structure similar to sucrose.

Sucrose ester: a compound in which fatty acids are covalently attached to a sucrose molecule that is not absorbed in the intestine and can be added to a food as a low-calorie fat replacer.

Sugar: a simple carbohydrate that is rapidly metabolized to provide quick energy.

Supercritical fluid: gas under pressure that exhibits properties of both a gas and a liquid.

Supplier: an individual or company that provides resources for a food product.

Supply chain: the collection of all individuals or companies who provide resources for a food product.

Surfactant: a compound that disrupts surface tension of a liquid.

Sushi: literally Japanese for "with rice" but generally used for any refrigerated product of raw fish with rice in American English.

Suspension: dispersion of discontinuous particles in a continuous phase.

Sustainability: "meeting the needs of the present without compromising the ability of future generations to meet their needs" (http://lct.jrc .ec.europa.eu/glossary).

Sustainability Consortium: collection of corporations, government agencies, and social-service organizations that have banded together to decrease the environmental impact of consumer-based products.

Sustainability index: a designation that will communicate directly to a consumer the sustainability of a specific food product.

Sustainable food: "designed, manufactured, and sourced under process guidelines, based on the efficient use of natural resources, the minimization of all kinds of waste, and the reduction of negative impact in surrounding communities along their life cycle" (http://www .sustainabilityconsortium.org/glossary/).

Sweet: a pleasant taste associated primarily with the presence of sugars, particularly fructose and sucrose, and artificial compounds that mimic this taste.

Syneresis: the difference between moisture sorption isotherms of a food during dehydration and rehydration.

Systems approach: evaluation of a set of operations as a whole and not merely the sum of its parts.

Tannin: complex polyphenolic molecule that is brown in color and can function as an antioxidant.

Taste: the perception of bitter, salty, sour, sweet, and umami by a chemical reaction with an ingredient or food on the tongue.

Temperature gradient: difference in temperature in adjacent points in space.

Tempering: the process of heating chocolate above the melting temperature and then slowly cooling to solidify it in the proper crystal structure.

Tertiary structure: folding of the primary structure of a protein caused by interactions between amino acids that are not in proximity.

Tetrad test: difference test in which four samples are presented consisting of two pairs of two samples with those in a pair the same as each other, and the panelist is asked to identify the samples belonging to each pair.

Texture: the property of food as perceived by the sense of touch by hand, mouth (mouthfeel), or utensil.

Texture Profile Technique: analytical method that measures specific textural characteristics either by instruments or sensory panel.

Textured vegetable protein: a derivative of plant proteins processed to convey the texture of familiar food products such as its use in meat analogs.

Thermal conductivity: physical property that quantifies the ability of a material to conduct heat.

Thermal properties: attributes of a substance that allow it to store or conduct heat.

Thermodynamics: study of transfer of energy and its conversion from one form to another form.

Thermogenesis: the metabolic processes that generate heat in the body.

Thermophile: microorganism that can tolerate higher temperatures than most species.

Third-party audit: an organization not affiliated with either the supplier or the manufacturer that inspects the facilities of the supplier to ensure that it is operating within proper guidelines.

Threshold test: one that evaluates a series of dilutions of a compound to determine the minimal levels at which it can be detected or recognized.

Thrombosis: restriction of blood flow in the arteries attributed to clotting of platelets and that can result in a heart attack.

Time intensity test: one that evaluates the changes of sensory characteristics during mastication and swallowing.

Time–temperature indicator: device that integrates the exposure of a food product to various temperatures over the duration of storage to estimate the product's remaining shelf life.

Top note: the predominant flavor sensation elicited by a specific food or ingredient.

Total Quality Management (TQM): a means of ensuring quality and safety of a food by encompassing the entire process from the supply chain through distribution.

Toxicology: the study of toxic substances and the risk they pose to living organisms.

Traceability: the degree of ease in determining the source of a food or ingredient.

trans **fats:** those in which the component fatty acids contain at least one double bond where the orientation of the hydrogen atoms are on opposite sides of the bond. *Trans* fats are produced during hydrogenation of unsaturated fats and are undesirable in a food product.

Transcription: synthesis of RNA from DNA.

Transformation: genetic modification of DNA in the nucleus of a cell to change the traits of an organism.

Translation: synthesis of proteins by sequentially linking amino acids together as coded by RNA.

Triacylglycerol: a lipid that contains three fatty acids linked by an ester bond to a glycerol backbone.

Triangle test: the most common difference test in which three samples are presented, two of which are the same and the other is different, and the panelist is asked to identify the different sample.

Turbulent flow: pattern that, as the velocity of a fluid increases, collisions of fluid molecules with each other occur more frequently and cross over the streamlines leading to disruption.

Ulcer: disturbance in the lining of an organ such as the stomach that leads to irritation and bleeding.

Ultrahigh pressure: nonthermal preservation technique that kills microorganisms by implosion when exposed to very high levels of pressure.

Umami: a pleasant taste perceived as brothy or meaty and associated primarily with salts of specific amino acids, particularly monosodium glutamate but found in many ingredients such as soy sauce and parmesan cheese.

Unit operation: step in a manufacturing process that affects the final quality and safety of a product.

United States Department of Agriculture (USDA): the agency in the American government responsible for developing and enforcing grade standards of fresh items as well as conducting continuous inspection of all meats sold in the country.

Unsaturated fats: those in which the component fatty acids contain at least one double bond.

Unsaturated fatty acid: one that contains at least one double bond and may be susceptible to lipid oxidation.

Value: the acceptability of a product at a given price.

Value chain: a supply chain that emphasizes the values of sustainability.

van der Waals forces: noncovalent attractions between molecules or portions of molecules such as between amino acids within a protein.

Vegan: a person who avoids the use of any animal-derived products.

Vegetable: any edible plant part that is not a seed or other part of the plant's reproductive system.

Vegetarian: a person who avoids meat but may consume some other animal-based products.

Vegetative cells: those in a phase and environment that promotes growth.

Vertical farm: a futuristic idea of using a series of high-rise buildings to recycle wastes as nutrients for inner-city farms that can produce foods and make the city environment more sustainable.

Virus: an entity that infects cells.

Viscometer: instrument that measures viscosity of fluids.

Viscosity: resistance to flow.

Vitamin: an organic compound essential to human health that can be obtained by eating a balanced diet.

Volatile: the property of a molecule to leave the surface of a food and enter the atmosphere as a gaseous substance; many volatile components of foods contribute to that food's aroma.

Water activity (A_w): the vapor pressure in a food relative to that of distilled water. Water activity relates to the availability of water to participate in chemical reactions or support growth of microorganisms.

Water footprint: the amount of water that is used in a field to grow a crop or in the production of a food product.

Water hardness: degree of minerals present in water with the higher concentration of minerals relating to greater hardness.

Water holding capacity (WHC): the ability of a food to retain water, which relates to its juiciness and texture.

Water intoxication: disease state owing to excess consumption of water.

Water vapor transmission rate: the speed at which water in the gaseous state passes through a specific packaging material.

Wet bulb temperature: temperature of a small volume of liquid (water) when surrounded by a steady flow of a gas (air). In combination with dry bulb temperature (i.e., the temperature of the stream of air), it is used to determine the humidity of air.

Whole food: a raw material that is recognizable with respect to its original form and has had little or no processing.

Wholesale: a market that sells products primarily to retail outlets but may sell them to the ultimate consumer, usually in large quantities.

Xanthophyll: yellow pigment found in fruits and vegetables.

Zero-order reaction: linear degradation over time that is independent of the concentration of the reactant.

Index